Really Essential Medical Immunology

PROFESSOR IVAN ROITT

Department of Immunology,
Royal Free and University College Medical School,
London,
UK

AND

PROFESSOR ARTHUR RABSON

Department of Pathology,
Tufts University School of Medicine,
Boston,
USA

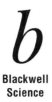

Blackwell Science

© 2000
Blackwell Science Ltd
Editorial Offices:
Osney Mead, Oxford OX2 0EL
25 John Street, London WC1N 2BL
23 Ainslie Place, Edinburgh EH3 6AJ
350 Main Street, Malden
  MA 02148-5018, USA
54 University Street, Carlton
  Victoria 3053, Australia
10, rue Casimir Delavigne
  75006 Paris, France

Other Editorial Offices:
Blackwell Wissenschafts-Verlag GmbH
Kurfürstendamm 57
10707 Berlin, Germany

Blackwell Science KK
MG Kodenmacho Building
7–10 Kodenmacho Nihombashi
Chuo-ku, Tokyo 104, Japan

The right of the Authors to be
identified as the Authors of this Work
has been asserted in accordance
with the Copyright, Designs and
Patents Act 1988.

First published 2000

Set by Excel Typesetters Co., Hong Kong
Printed and bound in Italy
by G. Canale & C. SpA, Turin

The Blackwell Science logo is a
trade mark of Blackwell Science Ltd,
registered at the United Kingdom
Trade Marks Registry

DISTRIBUTORS

Marston Book Services Ltd
PO Box 269
Abingdon, Oxon OX14 4YN
(*Orders*: Tel: 01235 465500
         Fax: 01235 465555)

USA
Blackwell Science, Inc.
Commerce Place
350 Main Street
Malden, MA 02148-5018
(*Orders*: Tel: 800 759 6102
          781 388 8250
    Fax: 781 388 8255)

Canada
Login Brothers Book Company
324 Saulteaux Crescent
Winnipeg, Manitoba R3J 3T2
(*Orders*: Tel: 204 837 2987)

Australia
Blackwell Science Pty Ltd
54 University Street
Carlton, Victoria 3053
(*Orders*: Tel: 3 9347 0300
        Fax: 3 9347 5001)

A catalogue record for this title
is available from the British Library

ISBN 0-632-05506-5

Library of Congress
Cataloging-in-publication Data

Roitt, Ivan M. (Ivan Maurice)
    Really essential medical immunology/
    Ivan Roitt, Arthur Rabson.
        p.   cm.
    Includes bibliographical references.
    ISBN 0-632-05506-5
    1. Clinical immunology.
    I. Rabson, Arthur.
    II. Title.
    [DNLM: 1. Immunity.
    2. Allergy and Immunology.
    QW 540 R741r 2000]
    RC582 .R65 2000
    616.07′9—dc21

                        00-023045

For further information on
Blackwell Science, visit our website:
www.blackwell-science.com

Contents

CHAPTER 1

Innate immunity

We live in a potentially hostile world filled with a bewildering array of infectious agents against which we have developed a series of defense mechanisms at least their equal in effectiveness and ingenuity. It is these defense mechanisms which can establish a state of immunity against infection (Latin *immunitas*, freedom from) and whose operation provides the basis for the delightful subject called 'Immunology'.

A number of nonspecific antimicrobial systems (e.g. phagocytosis) have been recognized which are **innate** in the sense that they are not intrinsically affected by prior contact with the infectious agent. We shall discuss these systems and examine how, in the state of **specific acquired immunity**, their effectiveness can be greatly increased.

EXTERNAL BARRIERS AGAINST INFECTION

The simplest way to avoid infection is to prevent the microorganisms from gaining access to the body. The major line of defense is of course the skin which, when intact, is impermeable to most infectious agents; when there is skin loss, as for example in burns, infection becomes a major problem. Additionally, most bacteria fail to survive for long on the skin because of the direct inhibitory effects of lactic acid and fatty acids in sweat and sebaceous secretions and the low pH which they generate. An exception is *Staphylococcus aureus*, which often infects the relatively vulnerable hair follicles and glands.

Mucus, secreted by the membranes lining the inner surfaces of the body, acts as a protective barrier to block the adherence of bacteria to epithelial cells. Microbial and other foreign particles trapped within the adhesive mucus are removed by mechanical stratagems such as ciliary movement, coughing and sneezing. Among other mechanical factors which help protect the epithelial surfaces, one should also include the washing action of tears, saliva and urine. Many of the secreted body fluids contain bactericidal components, such as acid in gastric juice, spermine and zinc in semen, lactoperoxidase in milk, and lysozyme in tears, nasal secretions and saliva.

A totally different mechanism is that of microbial antagonism associated with the normal bacterial flora of the body. This suppresses the growth of many potentially pathogenic bacteria and fungi at superficial sites by competition for essential nutrients or by production of microbicidal substances. To give one example, pathogen invasion is limited by lactic acid produced by particular species of commensal bacteria which metabolize glycogen secreted by the vaginal epithelium. When protective commensals are disturbed by antibiotics, susceptibility to opportunistic infections by *Candida albicans* and *Clostridium difficile* is increased.

If microorganisms do penetrate the body, two main defensive operations come into play, the destructive effect of soluble chemical factors such as bactericidal enzymes and the mechanism of **phagocytosis**—literally 'eating' by the cell (Milestone 1.1).

PHAGOCYTIC CELLS KILL MICROORGANISMS

The polymorphonuclear neutrophil

This cell shares a common hematopoietic stem cell precursor with the other formed elements of the blood and is the dominant white cell in the bloodstream. It is a nondividing, short-lived cell with a multilobed nucleus (figures 1.1 & 1.2a,b) and an array of granules which are of two main types: (i) the **primary azurophil granule**, which develops early and contains myeloperoxidase together with most of the nonoxidative antimicrobial effectors, including defensins, bactericidal/permeability increasing (BPI) factor and cathepsin G (figure 1.1), and (ii) the peroxidase-negative **secondary specific granules**, containing lactoferrin and

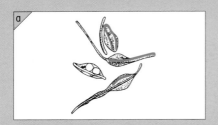
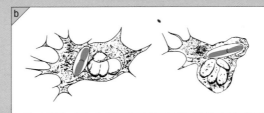
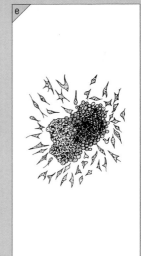
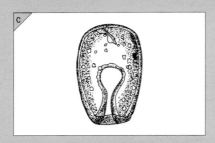
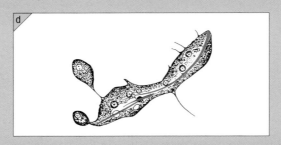

Figure M1.1.1 Reproductions of some of the illustrations in Metchnikoff's book, *Comparative Pathology of Inflammation* (1893). (a) Four leukocytes from the frog, enclosing anthrax bacilli. Some are alive and unstained, others which have been killed have taken up the vesuvine dye and have been coloured. (b) Drawing of an anthrax bacillus, stained by vesuvine, in a leukocyte of the frog. The two figures represent two phases of movement of the same frog leukocyte which contains stained anthrax bacilli within its phagocytic vacuole. (c and d) A foreign body (colored) in a starfish larva surrounded by phagocytes which have fused to form a multinucleate plasmodium, shown at higher power in (d). (e) This gives a feel for the dynamic attraction of the mobile mesenchymal phagocytes to a foreign intruder within a starfish larva.

The perceptive Russian zoologist, Elie Metchnikoff (1845–1916), recognized that certain specialized cells mediate defense against microbial infections, so fathering the whole concept of cellular immunity. He was intrigued by the motile cells of transparent starfish larvae and made the critical observation that a few hours after the introduction of a rose thorn into these larvae, it became surrounded by these motile cells. A year later, in 1883, he observed that fungal spores can be attacked by the blood cells of *Daphnia*, a tiny metozoan which, also being transparent, can be studied directly under the microscope. He went on to extend his investigations to mammalian leukocytes, showing their ability to engulf microorganisms, a process which he termed **phagocytosis**.

Because he found this process to be even more effective in animals recovering from infection, he came to a somewhat polarized view that phagocytosis provided the main, if not the only, defense against infection. He went on to define the existence of two types of circulating phagocytes: the poly-morphonuclear leukocyte, which he termed a 'microphage', and the larger 'macrophage'.

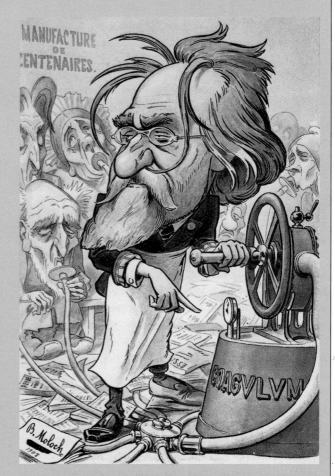

Figure M1.1.2 Caricature of Professor Metchnikoff from *Chante-clair*, 1908, No. 4, p. 7. (Reproduction kindly provided by The Well-come Institute Library, London.)

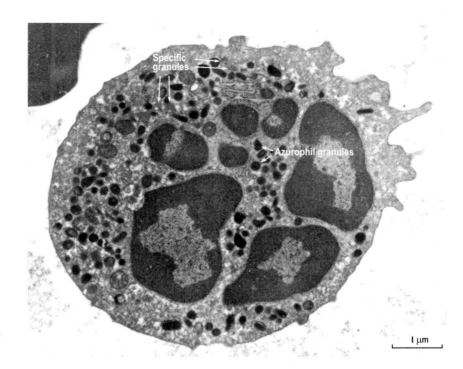

Figure 1.1 Ultrastructure of neutrophil. The multilobed nucleus and two main types of cytoplasmic granules are well displayed. (Courtesy of Dr D. McLaren.)

much of the lysozyme, alkaline phosphatase (figure 1.2c) and membrane-bound cytochrome b558 (figure 1.1).

The macrophage

These cells derive from bone marrow promonocytes which, after differentiation to blood monocytes (figure 1.2a), finally settle in the tissues as mature macrophages where they constitute the **mononuclear phagocyte system** (figure 1.2d). They are present throughout the connective tissue and around the basement membrane of small blood vessels, and are particularly concentrated in the lung (figure 1.2f, alveolar macrophages), liver (Kupffer cells), and lining of spleen sinusoids and lymph node medullary sinuses, where they are strategically placed to filter off foreign material. Other examples are mesangial cells in the kidney glomerulus, brain microglia and osteoclasts in bone. Unlike the polymorphs, they are long-lived cells with significant rough-surfaced endoplasmic reticulum and mitochondria, and whereas the polymorphs provide the major defense against pyogenic (pus-forming) bacteria, as a rough generalization it may be said that macrophages are at their best in combating those bacteria (figure 1.2e), viruses and protozoa which are capable of living within the cells of the host.

Microbes are engulfed by phagocytosis

Before phagocytosis can occur, the microbe must first adhere to the surface of the polymorph or macrophage. Depending on its nature, a particle attached to the surface membrane may initiate the ingestion phase by activating an actin–myosin contractile system which extends pseudopods around the particle (figures 1.3 & 1.4a); as adjacent receptors sequentially attach to the surface of the microbe, the plasma membrane is pulled around the particle just like a 'zipper' until it is completely enclosed in a vacuole (phagosome; figures 1.3 & 1.4b). Within 1 minute the cytoplasmic granules fuse with the phagosome and discharge their contents around the imprisoned microorganism (figure 1.4c), which is subject to a formidable battery of microbicidal mechanisms.

There is an array of killing mechanisms

Killing by reactive oxygen intermediates

Trouble starts for the invader from the moment phagocytosis is initiated. There is a dramatic increase in activity of the hexose monophosphate shunt generating reduced nicotinamide-adenine-dinucleotide phosphate (NADPH).

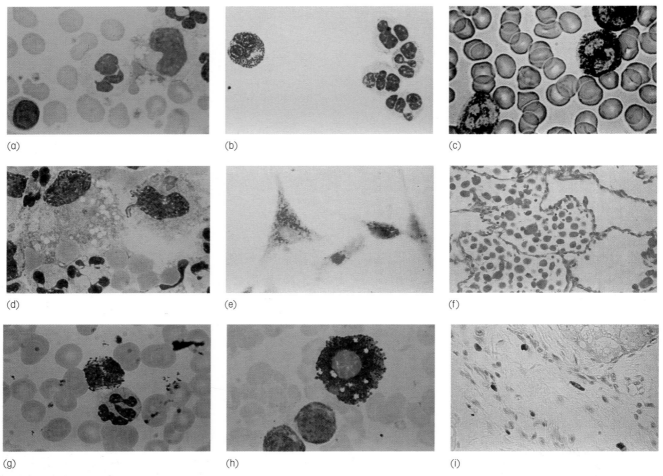

Figure 1.2 Cells involved in innate immunity. (a) Monocyte, showing 'horseshoe-shaped' nucleus and moderately abundant pale cytoplasm. Note the three multilobed polymorphonuclear neutrophils and the small lymphocyte (bottom left). Romanowsky stain. (b) Four polymorphonuclear leukocytes (neutrophils) and one eosinophil. The multilobed nuclei and the cytoplasmic granules are clearly shown, those of the eosinophil being heavily stained. (c) Polymorphonuclear neutrophil showing cytoplasmic granules stained for alkaline phosphatase. (d) Inflammatory cells from the site of a brain hemorrhage showing the large active macrophage in the center with phagocytosed red cells and prominent vacuoles. To the right is a monocyte with horseshoe-shaped nucleus and cytoplasmic bilirubin crystals (hematoidin). Several multilobed neutrophils are clearly delineated. Giemsa. (e) Macrophages in monolayer cultures after phagocytosis of mycobacteria (stained red). Carbol-Fuchsin counterstained with Malachite Green. (f) Numerous plump alveolar macrophages within air spaces in the lung. (g) Basophil with heavily staining granules compared with a neutrophil (below). (h) Mast cell from bone marrow. Round central nucleus surrounded by large darkly staining granules. Two small red cell precursors are shown at the bottom. Romanowsky stain. (i) Tissue mast cells in skin stained with Toluidine Blue. The intracellular granules are metachromatic and stain reddish purple. (The slides from which illustrations (a), (c), (d), (g) and (h) were reproduced were very kindly provided by Mr M. Watts of the Department of Haematology, Middlesex Hospital Medical School; (b) was kindly supplied by Professor J.J. Owen; (e) by Drs P. Lydyard and G. Rook; (f) by Dr Meryl Griffiths and (i) by Professor N. Woolf.)

Electrons pass from the NADPH to a unique plasma membrane **cytochrome (cyt b558)**, which reduces molecular oxygen directly to superoxide anion (figure 1.5). Thus the key reaction catalysed by this NADPH oxidase, which initiates the formation of reactive oxygen intermediates (ROI), is:

$$NADPH + O_2 \xrightarrow{\text{oxidase}} NADP^+ + \cdot O_2^- \qquad \text{(superoxide anion)}$$

The superoxide anion undergoes conversion to hydrogen peroxide under the influence of superoxide dismutase, and subsequently to hydroxyl radicals $\cdot OH$. Each of these products has remarkable chemical reactivity with a wide range of molecular targets making them formidable microbicidal agents; $\cdot OH$ in particular is one of the most reactive free radicals known. Furthermore, the combination of peroxide, myeloperoxidase and halide ions constitutes a potent halo-

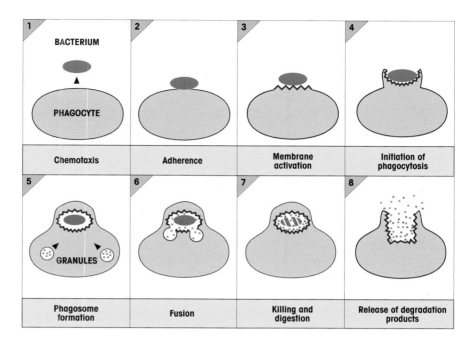

Figure 1.3 Phagocytosis and killing of a bacterium.

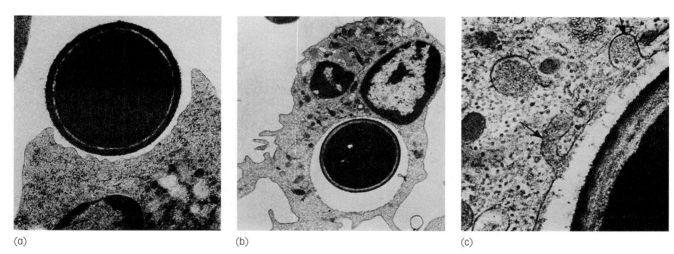

(a)   (b)   (c)

Figure 1.4 Adherence and phagocytosis. (a) Phagocytosis of *Candida albicans* by a polymorphonuclear leukocyte (neutrophil). Adherence to the surface initiates enclosure of the fungal particle within arms of cytoplasm (× 15 000). (b) **Phagolysosome formation** by a neutrophil 30 minutes after ingestion of *C. albicans*. The cytoplasm is already partly degranulated and two lysosomal granules (arrowed) are fusing with the phagocytic vacuole. Two lobes of the nucleus are evident (× 5000). (c) Higher magnification of (b) showing fusing granules discharging their contents into the phagocytic vacuole (arrowed) (× 33 000). (Courtesy of Dr H. Valdimarsson.)

genating system capable of killing both bacteria and viruses (figure 1.5).

Other killing mechanisms

Nitric oxide can be formed by an inducible NO synthase (iNOS) within many cells of the body but particularly in macrophages and human neutrophils where it generates a powerful antimicrobial system. Whereas the NADPH oxidase is dedicated to the killing of extracellular organisms taken up by phagocytosis and cornered within the phagocytic vacuole, the NO mechanism can operate against microbes which invade the cytosol; so, it is not surprising that the majority of nonphagocytic cells which may be infected by viruses and other parasites are endowed with an iNOS capability.

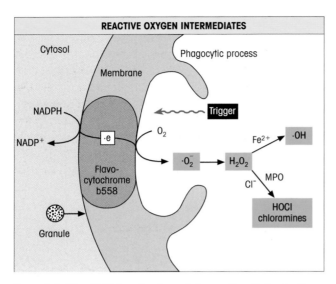

Figure 1.5 Microbicidal mechanisms of phagocytic cells. Production of reactive oxygen intermediates. Electrons from NADPH are transferred by the flavocytochrome oxidase enzyme to molecular oxygen to form the microbicidal molecular species shown in the boxes.

If this were not enough, further damage is inflicted on the bacterial membranes by neutral proteinase (cathepsin G) action and by the bactericidal or bacteriostatic factors, lysozyme and lactoferrin and a group of proteins called defensins. Finally, the killed organisms are digested by hydrolytic enzymes and the degradation products released to the exterior (figure 1.3).

COMPLEMENT FACILITATES PHAGOCYTOSIS

Complement and its activation

Complement is the name given to a complex series of some 20 proteins which, along with blood clotting, fibrinolysis and kinin formation, forms one of the triggered enzyme systems found in plasma. These systems characteristically produce a rapid, highly amplified response to a trigger stimulus mediated by a cascade phenomenon where the product of one reaction is the enzymic catalyst of the next. The activated or the split products of the cascade have a variety of defensive functions and the complement proteins can therefore be regarded as a crucial part of the innate immune system.

Some of the complement components are designated by the letter 'C' followed by a number which is related more to the chronology of its discovery than to its position in the

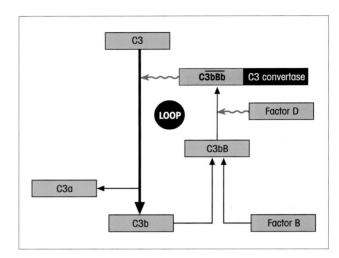

Figure 1.6 The C3 convertase feedback loop. Represents an activation process. The horizontal bar above a component designates its activation.

reaction sequence. The most abundant and the most pivotal component is C3.

C3 undergoes slow spontaneous cleavage

Under normal circumstances, small amounts of C3 are continuously broken down into the split product C3b, or a functionally similar molecule designated C3i or $C3(H_2O)$. In the presence of Mg^{2+} this can complex with another complement component, factor B, which then undergoes cleavage by a normal plasma enzyme (factor D) to generate $C\overline{3bBb}$. Note that conventionally a bar over a complex denotes enzymic activity, and that on cleavage of a complement component the larger product is generally given the suffix 'b' and the smaller 'a'.

$C\overline{3bBb}$ has an important new enzymic activity: it is a **C3 convertase** which can split large amounts of C3 to give C3a and C3b. We will shortly discuss the important biological consequences of C3 cleavage in relation to microbial defenses, but under normal conditions there must be some mechanism to restrain this process to a 'tick-over' level since it can also give rise to even more $C\overline{3bBb}$. That is, we are dealing with a potentially runaway **positive-feedback** or **amplification loop** (figure 1.6). As with all potentially explosive triggered cascades, there are powerful regulatory proteins in the form of factor H and factor I which control this feedback loop.

C3 convertase is stabilized on microbial surfaces

A number of microorganisms can activate the $C\overline{3bBb}$ convertase to generate large amounts of C3 cleavage products by stabilizing the enzyme on their (carbohydrate) surfaces, thereby protecting the C3b from factor H. Another protein, properdin, acts subsequently on this bound convertase to stabilize it even further. This series of reactions provoked directly by microbes leads to the clustering of large numbers of C3b molecules on the microorganism and has been called the **alternative pathway** of complement activation (figure 1.7).

The post-C3 pathway generates a membrane attack complex

Recruitment of a further C3b molecule into the C$\overline{3bBb}$ enzymic complex generates a C5 convertase, which activates C5 by proteolytic cleavage releasing a small polypeptide, C5a, and leaving the large C5b fragment loosely bound to C3b. Sequential attachment of C6 and C7 to C5b forms a complex with a transient membrane binding site and an affinity for C8. The C8 sits in the membrane and directs the conformational changes in C9 which transform it into an amphipathic molecule capable of insertion into the lipid bilayer and polymerization to an annular **membrane attack complex** (MAC; figures 1.8 & 2.3). This forms a transmembrane channel fully permeable to electrolytes and water, and due to the high internal colloid osmotic pressure of cells, there is a net influx of Na$^+$ and water, frequently leading to lysis.

Complement has a range of defensive biological functions

These can be grouped conveniently under three headings:

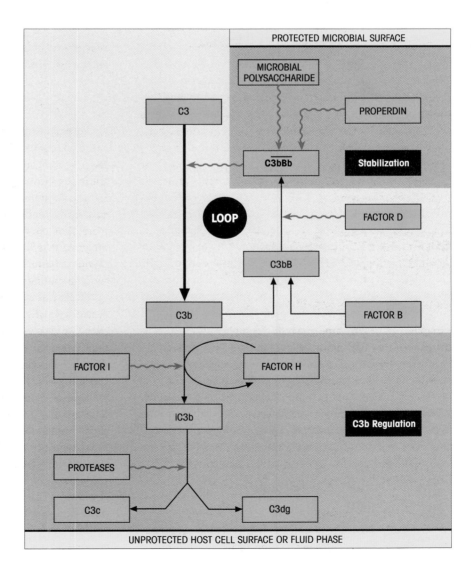

Figure 1.7 Microbial activation of the alternative complement pathway by stabilization of the C3 convertase (C$\overline{3bBb}$), and its control by factors H and I. When bound to the surface of a host cell or in the fluid phase, the C3b in the convertase is said to be 'unprotected' in that its affinity for factor H is much greater than for factor B and is therefore susceptible to breakdown by factors H and I. On a microbial surface, C3b binds factor B more strongly than factor H and is therefore 'protected' from or 'stabilized' against cleavage — even more so when subsequently bound by properdin. Although in phylogenetic terms this is the oldest complement pathway, it was discovered after a separate pathway to be discussed in the next chapter, and so has the confusing designation 'alternative'.

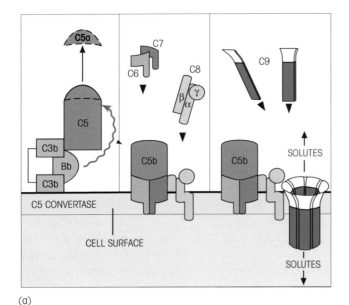

(a)

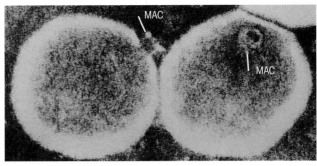

(b)

Figure 1.8 Post-C3 pathway generating C5a and the C5b–9 membrane attack complex (MAC). (a) Cartoon of molecular assembly. (b) Electron micrograph of a membrane C5b–9 complex incorporated into liposomal membranes clearly showing the annular structure. The cylindrical complex is seen from the side inserted into the membrane of the liposome on the left, and end-on in that on the right. (Courtesy of Professor J. Tranum-Jensen and Dr S. Bhakdi.)

1 C3b adheres to complement receptors

Phagocytic cells have receptors for C3b (CR1) which facilitate the adherence of C3b-coated microorganisms to the cell surface. This process, called opsonization, is more fully discussed on p. 97 but is perhaps the most important function resulting from complement activation.

2 Biologically active fragments are released

C3a and C5a, the small peptides split from the parent molecules during complement activation, have several important actions. Both act directly on phagocytes, especially neutrophils, to stimulate the respiratory burst associated with production of reactive oxygen intermediates and to enhance the expression of surface receptors for C3b. Also, both are **anaphylatoxins** in that they are capable of triggering mediator release from mast cells (figures 1.2i, 1.9 & 1.10) and their circulating counterparts the basophils. As you will read later these mediators have a variety of actions important in host defence. Both C3a and C5a are also potent neutrophil chemotactic agents which have a striking ability to act directly on the capillary endothelium to produce vasodilatation and increased permeability, an effect which seems to be prolonged by leukotriene B_4 released from activated mast cells, neutrophils and macrophages.

3 The terminal complex can induce membrane lesions

As described above, the insertion of the membrane attack complex into a membrane may bring about cell lysis.

COMPLEMENT CAN MEDIATE AN ACUTE INFLAMMATORY REACTION

We can now put together an effectively orchestrated defensive scenario initiated by activation of the alternative complement pathway (see figure 1.10).

In the first act, C$\overline{\text{3bBb}}$ is stabilized on the surface of the microbe and cleaves large amounts of C3. The C3a fragment is released but C3b molecules bind copiously to the microbe. These activate the next step in the sequence to generate C5a and the membrane attack complex.

The next act sees C3a and C5a (anaphylatoxins), together with the mediators they trigger from the mast cell, acting to recruit polymorphonuclear neutrophils and further plasma complement components to the site of microbial invasion. Under the influence of the chemotaxins, neutrophils slow down and the surface adhesion molecules they are stimulated to express cause them to marginate to the walls of the capillaries where they pass through gaps between the endothelial cells (diapedesis) and move up the concentration gradient of chemotactic factors until they come face to face with the C3b-coated microbe. Adherence to the neutrophil C3b-receptors then takes place, C3a and C5a at relatively high concentrations in the chemotactic gradient activate the respiratory burst and, hey presto, the slaughter of the last act can begin!

The processes of capillary dilatation (redness), exudation of plasma proteins and also of fluid (edema) due to hydrostatic and osmotic pressure changes, and accumulation of neutrophils are collectively termed the **acute inflammatory response**.

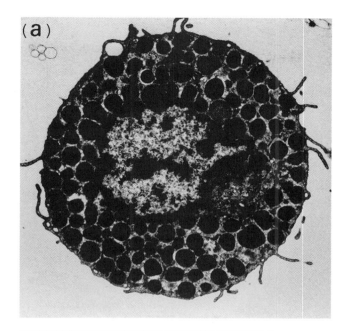

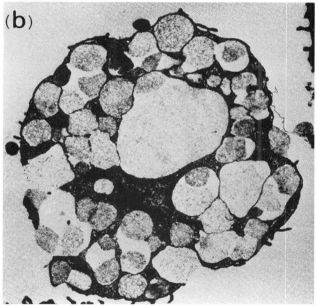

Figure 1.9 The mast cell. (a) A resting cell with many membrane-bound granules containing preformed mediators. (b) A triggered mast cell. Note that the granules have released their contents and are morphologically altered, being larger and less electron dense. Although most of the altered granules remain within the circumference of the cell, they are open to the extracellular space. (Electron micrographs × 5400.) (Courtesy of Drs D. Lawson, C. Fewtrell, B. Gomperts and M.C. Raff from (1975) *Journal of Experimental Medicine* **142**, 391.)

Macrophages can also do it

Tissue macrophages also play a crucial role in acute inflammatory reactions. They may be activated by the direct action of C5a or certain bacterial toxins such as the lipopolysaccharides (LPS), or by the phagocytosis of C3b-opsonized microbes. Following activation the macrophages will secrete a variety of soluble mediators which amplify the acute inflammatory response (figure 1.11). These include cytokines such as interleukin 1 and tumor necrosis factor, which upregulate the expression of adhesion molecules for neutrophils on the surface of endothelial cells, increase capillary permeability and promote the chemotaxis and activation of the polymorphonuclear neutrophils themselves. Thus, under the stimulus of complement activation, the macrophage provides a pattern of cellular events which reinforces acute inflammation.

HUMORAL MECHANISMS PROVIDE A SECOND DEFENSIVE STRATEGY

Turning now to those defense systems which are mediated entirely by soluble factors, we recollect that many microbes activate the complement system and may be lysed by the insertion of the membrane attack complex. The spread of infection may be limited by enzymes released through tissue injury which activate the clotting system. Of the soluble bactericidal substances elaborated by the body, perhaps the most abundant and widespread is the enzyme lysozyme, a muramidase which splits the exposed peptidoglycan wall of susceptible bacteria. Interferons are a family of broad-spectrum anti-viral agents which are induced by viruses and act to limit proliferation and spread of the infection. α-Interferons (IFNα) are produced by leukocytes, while fibroblasts, and probably all cell types, synthesize IFNβ.

Acute phase proteins increase in response to infection

During an infection, microbial products such as endotoxins stimulate macrophages to release interleukin-1 (IL-1), which is an endogenous pyrogen (incidentally capable of improving our general defenses by raising the body temperature), and IL-6. These in turn act on the liver to increase the synthesis and secretion of a number of plasma proteins collectively termed acute phase proteins. These include C-reactive protein (CRP, the plasma concentration of which may increase 1000-fold), mannose-binding protein and serum amyloid P component (Table 1.1). Other acute phase proteins showing a more modest rise in concentration

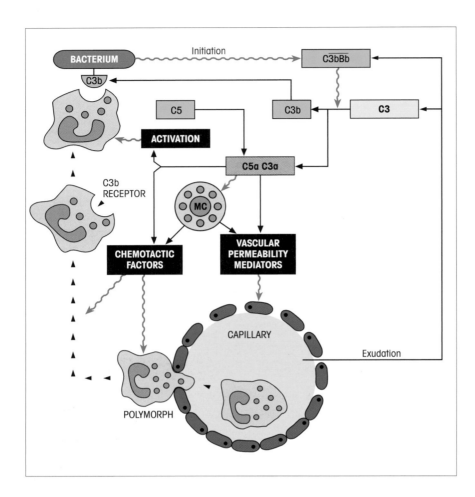

Figure 1.10 The defensive strategy of the acute inflammatory reaction initiated by bacterial activation of the alternative complement pathway. Directions: start with the activation of the $\overline{C3bBb}$ C3 convertase by the bacterium, notice the generation of C3b (which binds to the bacterium), C3a and C5a, and recruitment of mast cell mediators; follow their effect on capillary dilatation and exudation of plasma proteins and their chemotactic attraction of polymorphs to the C3b-coated bacterium and triumph in their adherence and final activation for the kill.

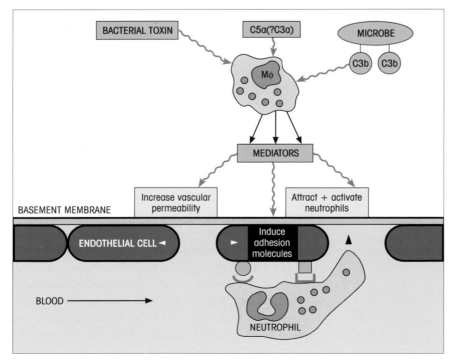

Figure 1.11 Stimulation by complement components induces macrophage secretion of mediators of the acute inflammatory response. Blood neutrophils stick to the adhesion molecules on the endothelial cell and use this to provide traction as they force their way between the cells, through the basement membrane (with the help of secreted elastase) and up the chemotactic gradient.

Table 1.1 Acute phase proteins.

Acute phase reactant	Role
Dramatic increases in concentration:	
C-reactive protein	Fixes complement, opsonizes
Mannose binding protein	Fixes complement, opsonizes
α_1-acid glycoprotein	Transport protein
Serum amyloid P component	Amyloid component precursor
Moderate increases in concentration:	
α_1-proteinase inhibitors	Inhibit bacterial proteases
α_1-antichymotrypsin	Inhibit bacterial proteases
C3, C9, factor B	Increase complement function
Ceruloplasmin	$\cdot O_2^-$ scavenger
Fibrinogen	Coagulation
Angiotensin	Blood pressure
Haptoglobin	Bind hemoglobin
Fibronectin	Cell attachment

include α_1-antitrypsin, fibrinogen, ceruloplasmin, C9 and factor B. Overall, it seems likely that the acute phase response achieves a beneficial effect through enhancing host resistance, minimizing tissue injury and promoting the resolution and repair of the inflammatory lesion. For example CRP can bind to numerous microorganisms forming a complex which may activate the complement pathway (by the classical pathway, not the alternative pathway with which we are at present familiar). This results in the deposition of C3b on the surface of the microbe which thus becomes **opsonized** (i.e. 'made ready for the table') for adherence to phagocytes. Measurement of CRP is a useful laboratory test to assess the activity of inflammatory disease.

EXTRACELLULAR KILLING

Natural killer (NK) cells

Viruses lack the apparatus for self-renewal so it is essential for them to penetrate the cells of the infected host in order to take over its replicative machinery. It is clearly in the interest of the host to find a way to kill such infected cells before the virus has had a chance to reproduce. NK cells appear to do just that.

They resemble large granular lymphocytes (figure 2.4a)

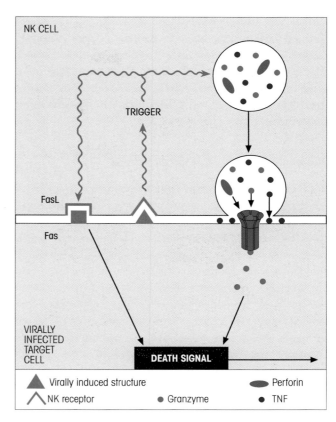

Figure 1.12 **Extracellular killing of virally infected cell by natural killer (NK) cell.** Binding of the NK receptors to the surface of the virally infected cell triggers the extracellular release of perforin molecules from the granules; these polymerize to form transmembrane channels which may facilitate lysis of the target by permitting entry of granzymes, tumor necrosis factor (TNF) and other potentially cytotoxic factors derived from the granules. (Model resembling that proposed by Hudig D., Ewoldt G.R. & Woodward S.L. (1993) *Current Opinion in Immunology* **5**, 90.) Engagement of the NK receptor also activates a parallel killing mechanism which is mediated through the binding of the Fas ligand (FasL) on the effector to the Fas receptor on the target cell thereby delivering a signal for apoptosis.

with a characteristic morphology. They are thought to recognize structures on high-molecular-weight glycoproteins which appear on the surface of virally infected cells and which allow them to be differentiated from normal cells. This recognition probably occurs through receptors on the NK cell surface which bring killer and target into close opposition (figure 1.12). Activation of the NK cell ensues and leads to polarization of granules between nucleus and target within minutes and extracellular release of their contents into the space between the two cells.

Perhaps the most important of these granule contents is a **perforin** or cytolysin bearing some structural homology to C9; like that protein, but without any help other than from

Ca^{2+} it can insert itself into the membrane of the target forming a transmembrane pore with an annular structure, comparable to the complement membrane attack complex (figure 1.8). In addition to perforin, the granules contain lymphotoxin α and a family of serine proteases termed **granzymes**, one of which, granzyme B, can function as an NK cytotoxic factor.

Target cells are told to commit suicide

NK cells may also kill by activating **apoptosis** (programmed cell death), a mechanism present in every cell which leads to self-immolation. Very rapid nuclear fragmentation effected by a Ca-dependent endonuclease which acts on the vulnerable DNA between nucleosomes can be detected. This killing may involve engagement of the Fas receptor molecules on the target cell surface by the Fas-ligand (FasL) on the effector NK cell, a process which induces an apoptotic signal in the unlucky target. It is likely that following exocytosis of the granules, apoptosis may also be effected by binding of TNF to receptors on the target cell and by the entry of granzyme B via the induced perforin membrane pore.

Eosinophils

Large parasites such as helminths (worms) cannot physically be phagocytosed and extracellular killing by eosinophils would seem to have evolved to help cope with this situation. These polymorphonuclear 'cousins' of the neutrophil have distinctive granules which stain avidly with acid dyes (figure 1.2b) and have a characteristic appearance in the electron microscope. They have surface receptors for C3b and on activation produce a particularly impressive respiratory burst with concomitant generation of active oxygen metabolites. Not satisfied with that, nature has also armed the cell with granule proteins capable of producing a transmembrane plug in the target membrane like C9 and the NK perforin—quite a nasty cell.

Most helminths can activate the alternative complement pathway, but although resistant to C9 attack, their coating with C3b allows adherence of eosinophils through their C3b receptors. If this contact should lead to activation, the eosinophil will launch its extracellular attack, which includes the release of major basic protein (MBP) present in the eosinophil granules and a cationic protein which damages the parasite membrane.

REVISION

See the accompanying website (www.roitt.com) for multiple choice questions.

A wide range of innate immune mechanisms operate which do not improve with repeated exposure to infection.

Barriers against infection
• Microorganisms are kept out of the body by the skin, the secretion of mucus, ciliary action, the lavaging action of bactericidal fluids (e.g. tears), gastric acid and microbial antagonism.
• If penetration occurs, bacteria are destroyed by soluble factors such as lysozyme and by phagocytosis with intracellular digestion.

Phagocytic cells kill microorganisms
• The main phagocytic cells are polymorphonuclear neutrophils and macrophages. Organisms adhere to their surface, activate the engulfment process and are taken inside the cell where they fuse with cytoplasmic granules.
• A formidable array of microbicidal mechanisms then

come into play: the conversion of O_2 to reactive oxygen intermediates, the synthesis of nitric oxide and the release of multiple oxygen-independent factors from the granules.

Complement facilitates phagocytosis
• The complement system, a multicomponent triggered enzyme cascade, is used to attract phagocytic cells to the microbes and engulf them.
• The most abundant component, C3, is split by a convertase enzyme to form C3b, which binds to adjacent microorganisms.
• The next component, C5, is activated yielding a small peptide, C5a; the residual C5b binds to the surface and assembles the terminal components C6–9 into a membrane attack complex, which is freely permeable to solutes and can lead to osmotic lysis.
• C3a and C5a are potent chemotactic agents for polymorphs and greatly increase capillary permeability.

• C3a and C5a act on mast cells causing the release of further mediators such as histamine, leukotriene B$_4$ and tumor necrosis factor (TNF) with effects on capillary permeability and adhesiveness, and neutrophil chemotaxis; they also activate neutrophils.

The complement-mediated acute inflammatory reaction

• Following the activation of complement with the ensuing attraction and stimulation of neutrophils, the activated phagocytes bind to the C3b-coated microbes by their surface C3b receptors and may then ingest them. The influx of polymorphs and the increase in vascular permeability constitute the potent antimicrobial **acute inflammatory response**.

• Inflammation can also be initiated by tissue macrophages, which can be activated by C5a or by bacterial products such as endotoxin, to secrete cytokines including IL-1 and TNFα which increase the adhesiveness of endothelial cells thereby bringing more cells to the site of inflammation.

Humoral mechanisms provide a second defensive strategy

• In addition to lysozyme and the complement system, other humoral defenses involve the acute phase proteins such as C-reactive and mannose-binding proteins whose synthesis is greatly augmented by infection. Mannose-binding protein is a member of the collectin family, including conglutinin and surfactants SP-A and SP-D, notable for their ability to distinguish microbial from 'self' surface carbohydrate groups.

• Recovery from viral infections can be effected by the interferons, which block viral replication.

Extracellular killing

• Virally infected cells can be killed by large granular lymphocytes with NK activity through a perforin/granzyme and a separate Fas-mediated pathway leading to programmed cell death (apoptosis).

• Extracellular killing by C3b-bound eosinophils may be responsible for the failure of many large parasites to establish a foothold in potential hosts.

FURTHER READING

Carroll M.C. & Janeway C.A. (eds) (1999) Section on 'Innate Immunity'. *Current Opinion in Immunology* **11** (1).

Gregory S.H. & Wing E.J. (1998) Neutrophil-Kupffer cell interaction in host defenses to systemic infections. *Immunology Today* **19** (11), 507.

Mollinedo F., Borregaard N. & Boxer L.A. (1999) Novel trends in neutrophil structure, function and development. *Immunology Today* **20** (12), 535.

Revillard J.-P., Adorini L., Goldman M., Kabelitz D. & Waldmann H. (1998) Apoptosis: potential for disease therapies. *Immunology Today* **19** (7), 291.

Website www.roitt.com (linked to *Roitt's Essential Immunology* and this book) Four hundred multiple-choice questions with teaching comments on every answer, further reading, immunology update, and facility for downloading the figures.

CHAPTER 2

Specific acquired immunity

THE NEED FOR SPECIFIC IMMUNE MECHANISMS

Our microbial adversaries have tremendous opportunities through mutation to evolve strategies which evade our innate immune defenses, and many organisms may shape their exteriors so as to avoid complement activation completely. The body obviously needed to 'devise' defense mechanisms which could be dovetailed individually to each of these organisms no matter how many there were. In other words *a very large number* of **specific immune defenses** needed to be at the body's disposal. Quite a tall order!

ANTIBODY—THE SPECIFIC ADAPTOR

Evolutionary processes came up with what can only be described as a brilliant solution. This was to fashion an adaptor molecule which was intrinsically capable not only of activating the complement system *and* of stimulating phagocytic cells, but also of sticking to the offending microbe. The adaptor thus had three main regions, two concerned with communicating with complement and the phagocytes (the biological functions) and one devoted to binding to an individual microorganism (the external recognition function). This latter portion would be complementary in shape to some microorganism to which it could then bind reasonably firmly. Although the part of the adaptor with biological function would be constant, a special recognition portion would be needed for each of the hundreds and thousands of different organisms. The adaptor is of course the molecule we know affectionately as **antibody** (figure 2.1).

Antibody initiates a new complement pathway ('classical')

Antibody, when bound to a microbe, will link to C1q, the first molecule in the so-called **classical complement sequence**. C1q consists of a central collagen-like stem branching into six peptide chains each tipped by an antibody-binding subunit (resembling the blooms on a bouquet of flowers). Changes in C1q consequent upon binding the antigen–antibody complex bring about the sequential activation of proteolytic activity in two other molecules, C1r and then C1s, and this forms a Ca^{2+}-stabilized trimolecular C1 complex which dutifully plays its role in an amplifying cascade by acting on components C4 and C2 to generate many molecules of $C\overline{4b2b}$, a new **C3-splitting enzyme** (figure 2.2).

The next component in the chain, C4 (unfortunately components were numbered before the sequence was established), now binds to C1 and is cleaved enzymically by $C\overline{1s}$. As expected in a multienzyme cascade, several molecules of C4 undergo cleavage into two fragments, C4a and C4b. Note that C4a, like C5a and C3a, has anaphylatoxin activity, although feeble, and C4b resembles C3b in its opsonic activity. In the presence of Mg^{2+}, C2 can complex with the $C\overline{4b}$ to become a new substrate for the $C\overline{1s}$ the resulting product, $C\overline{4b2b}$, now has the vital C3 convertase activity required to cleave C3.

This classical pathway C3 convertase has the same specificity as the $C\overline{3bBb}$ generated by the alternative pathway, likewise producing the same C3a and C3b fragments. Activation of a single C1 complex can bring about the proteolysis of literally thousands of C3 molecules. From then on things march along exactly in parallel to the post-C3 pathway, with one molecule of C3b added to the $C\overline{4b2b}$ to make it into a C5-splitting enzyme with eventual production of the **membrane attack complex** (figures 1.8 & 2.3).

The similarities between the two pathways are set out in figure 2.2 and show how antibody can supplement and even

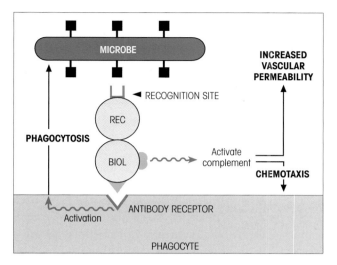

Figure 2.1 The antibody adaptor molecule. The constant part with biological function (BIOL) activates complement and the phagocyte. The portion with the recognition unit for the foreign microbe (REC) varies from one antibody to another.

improve on the ability of the innate immune system to initiate **acute inflammatory reactions**.

CELLULAR BASIS OF ANTIBODY PRODUCTION

Antigen selects the lymphocytes which make antibody

The majority of resting **lymphocytes** are small cells with a darkly staining nucleus due to condensed chromatin and relatively little cytoplasm containing the odd mitochondrion required for basic energy provision (figure 2.4a). Each lymphocyte of a subset called the **B-lymphocytes**—because they differentiate in the *bone marrow*—is programmed to make one, and only one, antibody and it places this antibody on its outer surface to act as a receptor. This can be detected by using fluorescent probes, and in figure 2.4c one can see the molecules of antibody on the surface of a human B-lymphocyte stained with a fluorescent rabbit antiserum raised against a preparation of human antibodies. Each lymphocyte has of the order of 10^5 identical antibody molecules on its surface.

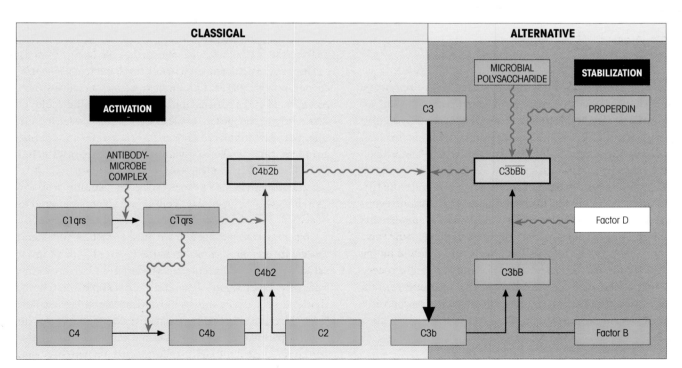

Figure 2.2 Comparison of the alternative and classical complement pathways. The classical pathway is antibody dependent, the alternative pathway is not. The molecular units with protease activity are highlighted. Beware confusion with nomenclature; the large C2 fragment which forms the C3 convertase is often labeled as C2a but to be consistent with C4b, C3b and C5b, it seems more logical to call it C2b.

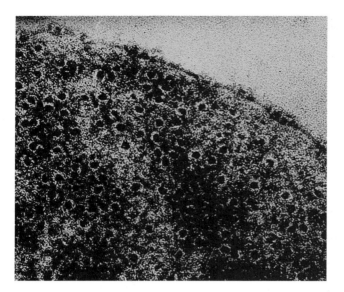

Figure 2.3 Multiple lesions in cell wall of *Escherichia coli* bacterium caused by interaction with IgM antibody and complement. (Human antibodies are divided into five main classes: immunoglobulin M (shortened to IgM), IgG, IgA, IgE and IgD, which differ in the specialization of their 'rear ends' for different biological functions such as complement activation or mast cell sensitization.) Each lesion is caused by a single IgM molecule and shows as a 'dark pit' due to penetration by the 'negative stain'. This is somewhat of an illusion since in reality these 'pits' are like volcano craters standing proud of the surface, and are each single 'membrane attack' complexes (×400 000). (Kindly supplied by Drs R. Dourmashkin and J.H. Humphrey.)

The molecules in the microorganisms which evoke and react with antibodies are called **antigens** (**gen**erates **anti**bodies). When an antigen enters the body, it is confronted by a dazzling array of lymphocytes all bearing different antibodies each with its own individual recognition site. The antigen will only bind to those receptors with which it makes a good fit. Lymphocytes whose receptors have bound antigen receive a triggering signal causing them to enlarge, proliferate (figure 2.4b) and develop into antibody-forming plasma cells (figures 2.4d & 2.5) and since the lymphocytes are programmed to make only one antibody, that secreted by the plasma cell will be identical with that originally acting as the lymphocyte receptor, i.e. it will bind well to the antigen. In this way, antigen selects for the antibodies which recognize it effectively (figure 2.6).

The need for clonal expansion means humoral immunity must be acquired

Because we can make hundreds of thousands, maybe even millions, of different antibody molecules, it is not feasible for

us to have too many lymphocytes producing each type of antibody; there just would not be enough room in the body to accommodate them. To compensate for this, lymphocytes which are triggered by contact with antigen undergo successive waves of proliferation (figure 2.4b) to build up a large clone of plasma cells which will be making antibody of the kind for which the parent lymphocyte was programmed. By this system of **clonal selection**, large enough concentrations of antibody can be produced to combat infection effectively (figure 2.6).

Because it takes time for the proliferating clone to build up its numbers sufficiently, it is usually several days before antibodies are detectable in the serum following primary contact with antigen. The newly formed antibodies are a consequence of antigen exposure and it is for this reason that we speak of the **acquired immune response**.

ACQUIRED MEMORY

When we make an antibody response to a given infectious agent, by definition that microorganism must exist in our environment and we are likely to meet it again. It would make sense then for the immune mechanisms alerted by the first contact with antigen to leave behind some memory system which would enable the response to any subsequent exposure to be faster and greater in magnitude.

Our experience of many common infections tells us that this must be so. We rarely suffer twice from such diseases as measles, mumps, chickenpox, whooping cough and so forth. The first contact clearly imprints some information, imparts some **memory**, so that the body is effectively prepared to repel any later invasion by that organism and a state of immunity is established.

Secondary antibody responses are better

By following the production of antibody on the first and second contacts with antigen we can see the basis for the development of immunity. For example, when we immunize a child with a bacterial product such as tetanus toxoid, several days elapse before antibodies can be detected in the blood; these reach a peak and then fall (figure 2.7). If at a later stage we give a second injection of toxoid, the course of events is dramatically altered. Within 2–3 days the antibody level in the blood rises steeply to reach much higher values than were observed in the **primary response**. This **secondary response** then is characterized by a more rapid and more abundant production of antibody

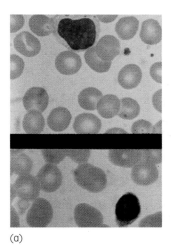
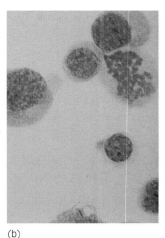
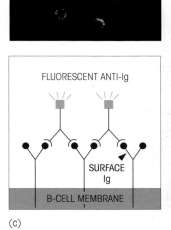
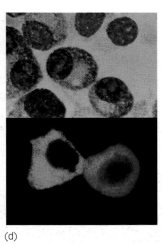

(a)   (b)   (c)   (d)

Figure 2.4 Cells involved in the acquired immune response. (a) Small lymphocytes. Condensed chromatin gives rise to heavy staining of the nucleus. The bottom cell is a typical resting agranular T-cell with a thin rim of cytoplasm. The upper nucleated cell is a large granular lymphocyte (LGL); it has more cytoplasm and azurophilic granules are evident. B-lymphocytes range from small to intermediate in size and lack granules. (Giemsa stain.) (b) Transformed lymphocytes (lymphoblasts) following stimulation of lymphocytes in culture with a polyclonal activator. The large lymphoblasts with their relatively high ratio of cytoplasm to nucleus may be compared in size with the isolated small lymphocyte. One cell is in mitosis. (May–Grünwald–Giemsa.) (c) Immunofluorescent staining of B-lymphocyte surface immunoglobulin using fluorescein-conjugated (▇) anti-Ig. Provided the reaction is carried out in the cold to prevent pinocytosis, the labeled antibody cannot penetrate to the interior of the viable lymphocytes and reacts only with surface components. Patches of aggregated surface Ig are seen which are beginning to form a cap in the right-hand lymphocyte. During cap formation, submembranous myosin becomes redistributed in association with the surface Ig and induces locomotion of the previously sessile cell in a direction away from the cap. (d) (*upper*) Plasma cells. The nucleus is eccentric. The cytoplasm is strongly basophilic due to high RNA content. The juxtanuclear lightly stained zone corresponds with the Golgi region. (May–Grünwald–Giemsa.) (*lower*) Plasma cells stained to show intracellular immunoglobulin using a fluorescein-labeled anti-IgG (green) and a rhodamine-conjugated anti-IgM (red). (Material for (a) was kindly supplied by Mr M. Watts, (b) and (c) by Dr P. Lydyard, and (d) by Professor C. Grossi.)

resulting from the 'tuning up' or priming of the antibody-forming system.

The higher response given by a primed lymphocyte population can be ascribed mainly to an expansion of the numbers of cells capable of being stimulated by the antigen, although we shall see later that there are also some qualitative differences in these memory cells.

ACQUIRED IMMUNITY HAS ANTIGEN SPECIFICITY

Discrimination between different antigens

The establishment of memory or immunity by one organism does not confer protection against another unrelated organism. After an attack of measles we are immune to further infection but are susceptible to other agents such as the polio or mumps viruses. Acquired immunity then shows speci-ficity and the immune system can differentiate specifically between the two organisms. The basis for this lies of course in the ability of the recognition sites of the antibody molecules to distinguish between antigens.

Discrimination between self and nonself

This ability to recognize one antigen and distinguish it from another goes even further. The individual must also recognize what is foreign, i.e. what is 'nonself'. The failure to discriminate between **self** and **nonself** could lead to the synthesis of antibodies directed against components of the subject's own body (**autoantibodies**), which in principle could prove to be highly embarrassing. The body must therefore develop some mechanism whereby 'self' and 'nonself' can be distinguished. As we shall see later those circulating body components which are able to reach the developing lymphoid system in the perinatal period will thereafter be regarded as 'self'. A permanent unresponsiveness or **toler-**

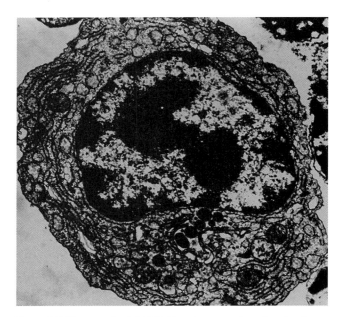

Figure 2.5 Plasma cell (×10 000). Prominent rough-surfaced endoplasmic reticulum associated with the synthesis and secretion of Ig.

ance is then created so that as immunologic maturity is reached there is normally an inability to respond to 'self' components.

VACCINATION DEPENDS ON ACQUIRED MEMORY

Nearly 200 years ago, Edward Jenner carried out the remarkable studies which mark the beginning of immunology as a systematic subject. Noting the pretty pox-free skin of the milkmaids, he reasoned that deliberate exposure to the pox virus of the cow, which is not virulent for the human, might confer protection against the related human smallpox organism. Accordingly, he inoculated a small boy with cowpox and was delighted—and presumably relieved—to observe that the child was now protected against a subsequent exposure to smallpox. By injecting a harmless form of a disease organism, Jenner had utilized the specificity and memory of the acquired immune response to lay the foundations for modern **vaccination** (Latin *vacca*, cow).

The essential strategy is to prepare an innocuous form of the infectious organism or its toxins which still substantially retains the antigens responsible for establishing protective immunity. This has been done by using killed or live attenu-

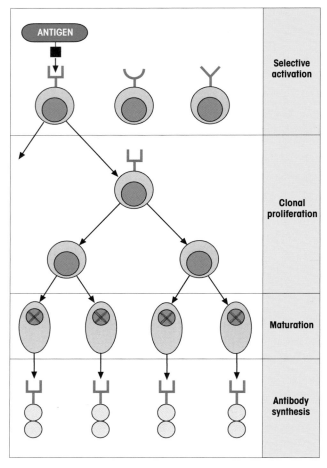

Figure 2.6 Clonal selection. The cell selected by antigen undergoes many divisions during the clonal proliferation and the progeny mature to give an expanded population of antibody-forming cells.

ated organisms, purified microbial components or chemically modified antigens (figure 2.7).

CELL-MEDIATED IMMUNITY PROTECTS AGAINST INTRACELLULAR ORGANISMS

Many microorganisms live inside host cells where it is impossible for humoral antibody to reach them. Obligate intracellular parasites like viruses have to replicate inside cells; facultative intracellular parasites like *mycobacteria* and *leishmania* can replicate within cells, particularly macrophages, but do not have to; they like the intracellular life because of the protection it affords. A totally separate acquired immunity system has evolved to deal with this situation based on a distinct lymphocyte subpopulation made

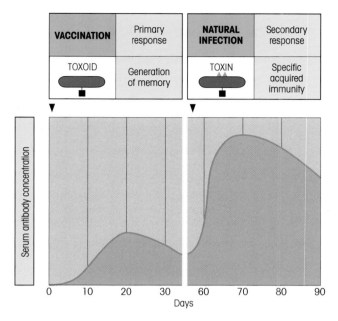

Figure 2.7 The basis of vaccination is illustrated by the response to tetanus toxoid. Formed by treatment of the bacterial toxin with formaldehyde which destroys its toxicity (associated with ▲▲) but retains antigenicity. The antibody response on the second contact with antigen is more rapid and more intense. Thus, exposure to toxin in a subsequent natural infection boosts the memory cells, rapidly producing high levels of neutralizing antibody which are protective.

up of **T-cells** (figure 2.4a), designated thus because, unlike the B-lymphocytes, they differentiate within the milieu of the **thymus gland**. Because they are specialized to operate against cells bearing intracellular organisms, T-cells only recognize antigen when it is on the surface of a body cell. Accordingly, the **T-cell surface receptors**, which are different from the antibody molecules used by B-lymphocytes, recognize antigen plus a surface marker which informs the T-lymphocyte that it is making contact with another cell. These cell markers belong to an important group of molecules known as the **major histocompatibility complex (MHC)**, identified originally through their ability to evoke powerful transplantation reactions in other members of the same species.

Cytokine-producing T-cells help macrophages to kill intracellular parasites

Intracellular organisms only survive inside macrophages through their ability to subvert the innate killing mecha-

nisms of these cells. Nonetheless, they cannot prevent the macrophage from processing small antigenic fragments (possibly of organisms which have spontaneously died) and placing them on the host cell surface. A subpopulation of T-lymphocytes called **T-helper cells**, if primed to that antigen, will recognize and bind to the combination of antigen with so-called class II MHC molecules on the macrophage surface and produce a variety of soluble factors termed **cytokines**, which include the interleukins (IL-2, etc.; see pp. 70,72). Different cytokines can be made by various cell types and generally act at a short range on neighboring cells. Some T-cell cytokines help B-cells to make antibodies while others such as γ-interferon (IFNγ) act as **macrophage activating factors**, which switch on the previously subverted microbicidal mechanisms of the macrophage and bring about the death of the intracellular microorganisms (figure 2.8).

Virally infected cells can be killed by cytotoxic T-cells and ADCC

We have already discussed the advantage to the host of killing virally infected cells before the virus begins to replicate and have seen that large granular lymphocytes with natural killer (NK) activity can subserve a cytotoxic function. However, NK cells have a limited range of specificities and in order to improve their efficacy, this range needs to be expanded.

One way in which this can be achieved is by coating the target cell with antibodies specific for the virally coded surface antigens because NK cells have receptors for the constant part of the antibody molecule, rather like phagocytic cells. Thus antibodies will bring the NK cell very close to the target by forming a bridge, and the NK cell being activated by the complexed antibody molecules is able to kill the virally infected cell by its extracellular mechanisms (figure 2.9). This system is termed **antibody-dependent cell-mediated cytotoxicity (ADCC)**.

Virally infected cells can also be controlled by a subset of **cytotoxic T-cells** which like the T-helpers have a very wide range of antigen specificities because they clonally express a large number of different surface receptors similar to, but not identical with, the surface antibody receptors on the B-lymphocytes. Again, each lymphocyte is programmed to make only one receptor and, again like the T-helper cell, recognizes antigen only in association with a cell marker, in this case the class I MHC molecule (figure 2.9). Through this recognition of surface antigen, the cytotoxic cell comes into intimate contact with its target and administers the 'kiss of apoptotic death'.

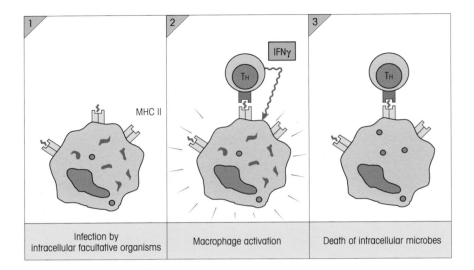

Figure 2.8 Intracellular killing of microorganisms by macrophages. (1) Surface antigen (ζ) derived from the intracellular microbes is complexed with class II MHC molecules (⊟). (2) The T-helper binds to this surface complex and is triggered to release the cytokine γ-interferon (IFNγ). This activates microbicidal mechanisms in the macrophage. (3) The infectious agent meets a timely death.

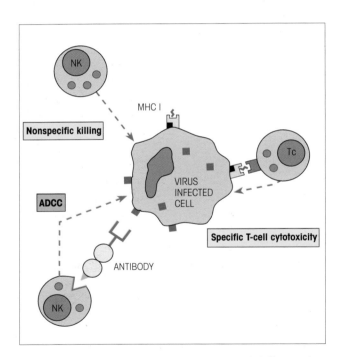

Figure 2.9 Killing virally infected cells. The nonspecific killing mechanism of the NK cell can be focused on the target by antibody to produce antibody-dependent cell-mediated cytotoxicity (ADCC). The cytotoxic T-cell homes onto its target specifically through receptor recognition of surface antigen in association with MHC class I molecules.

In an entirely analogous fashion to the B-cell, T-cells are selected and activated by combination with antigen, expanded by clonal proliferation and mature to give T-helper and cytotoxic T-effectors, together with an enlarged popula-tion of memory cells. Thus both T- and B-cells provide **specific acquired immunity** with a variety of mechanisms, which in most cases operate to extend the range of effectiveness of innate immunity and confer the valuable advantage that a first infection prepares us to withstand further contact with the same microorganism.

IMMUNOPATHOLOGY

The immune system is clearly 'a good thing', but like mercenary armies, it can turn to bite the hand that feeds it, and cause damage to the host.

Thus where there is an especially heightened response or persistent exposure to exogenous antigens, tissue-damaging or **hypersensitivity** reactions may result. Examples are allergy to grass pollens, blood dyscrasias associated with certain drugs, immune complex glomerulonephritis occur-ring after streptococcal infection, and chronic granulomas produced during tuberculosis or schistosomiasis.

In other cases, hypersensitivity to autoantigens may arise through a breakdown in the mechanisms which control self-tolerance, and a wide variety of **autoimmune diseases** such as thyrotoxicosis, myasthenia gravis and many of the rheumatologic disorders have now been recognized.

Another immunopathologic reaction of some consequence is **transplant rejection**, where the MHC antigens on the donor graft may well provoke a fierce reaction. Lastly, one should consider the by no means infrequent occurrence of inadequate functioning of the immune system—**immunodeficiency**.

REVISION

See the accompanying website (www.roitt.com) for multiple choice questions.

Antibody—the specific adaptor

The antibody molecule evolved as a specific adaptor to attach to microorganisms which either fail to activate the alternative complement pathway or prevent activation of the phagocytic cells.

• The antibody fixes to the antigen by its specific recognition site and its constant structure regions activate complement through the classical pathway (binding C1 and generating a $\overline{C4b2b}$; convertase to split C3) and phagocytes through their antibody receptors.

Cellular basis of antibody production

• Antibodies are made by plasma cells derived from B-lymphocytes, each of which is programmed to make only one antibody, which is placed on the cell surface as a receptor.

• Antigen binds to the cell with a complementary antibody, activates it and causes clonal proliferation and finally maturation to antibody-forming cells and memory cells. Thus the antigen brings about clonal selection of the cells making antibody to itself.

Acquired memory and vaccination

• The increase in memory cells after priming means that the acquired secondary response is faster and greater, providing the basis for vaccination using a harmless form of the infective agent for the initial injection.

Acquired immunity has antigen specificity

• Antibodies differentiate between antigens because recognition is based on molecular shape complementarity. Thus memory induced by one antigen will not extend to another unrelated antigen.

• The immune system differentiates self components from foreign antigens by making immature self-reacting lymphocytes unresponsive through contact with host molecules; lymphocytes reacting with foreign antigens are unaffected since they only make contact after reaching maturity.

Cell-mediated immunity protects against intracellular organisms

• Another class of lymphocyte, the T-cell, is concerned with control of intracellular infections. Like the B-cell, each T-cell has its individual antigen receptor (although it differs structurally from antibody) which recognizes antigen and undergoes clonal expansion to form effector and memory cells providing specific acquired immunity.

• The T-cell recognizes cell surface antigens in association with molecules of the MHC.

• T-helper cells which see antigen with class II MHC on the surface of macrophages, release cytokines which in some cases can help B-cells to make antibody and in others, activate macrophages and enable them to kill intracellular parasites.

• Cytotoxic T-cells have the ability to recognize specific antigen plus class I MHC on the surface of virally infected cells, which are killed before the virus replicates. They also release γ-interferon, which can make surrounding cells resistant to viral spread (figure 2.10).

• NK cells have lectin-like 'nonspecific' receptors for cells infected by viruses but do not have antigen-specific receptors; however, they can recognize antibody-coated virally infected cells through their Fcγ receptors and kill the target by antibody-dependent cell-mediated cytotoxicity (ADCC).

• Although the innate mechanisms do not improve with repeated exposure to infection as do the acquired, they play a vital role since they are intimately linked to the acquired systems by **two different pathways** which all but **encapsulate the whole of immunology**. Antibody, complement and polymorphs give protection against most extracellular organisms, while T-cells, soluble cytokines, macrophages and NK cells deal with intracellular infections (figure 2.11).

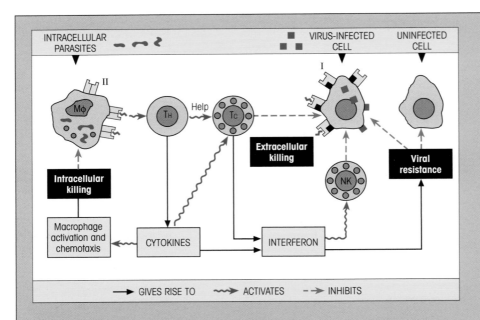

Figure 2.10 **T-cells link with the innate immune system to resist intracellular infection.** Class I (▨) and class II (▨) major histocompatibility molecules are important for T-cell recognition of surface antigen. The T-helper cells (TH) cooperate in the development of cytotoxic T-cells (Tc) from precursors. The macrophage (Mφ) microbicidal mechanisms are switched on by macrophage-activating lymphokines. Interferon inhibits viral replication and stimulates NK cells which together with Tc kill virus-infected cells.

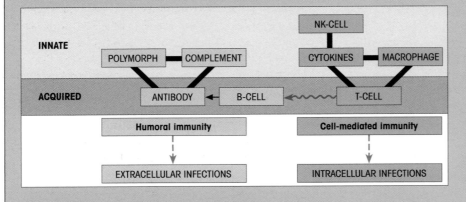

Figure 2.11 **The two pathways linking innate and acquired immunity** which provide the basis for humoral and cell-mediated immunity respectively.

Immunopathology

• Immunopathologically mediated tissue damage to the host can occur as a result of: inappropriate hypersensitivity reactions to exogenous antigens; loss of tolerance to self giving autoimmune disease; reaction to foreign grafts.

• Immunodeficiency leaves the individual susceptible to infection.

FURTHER READING

Alt F. & Marrack P. (eds) (6 issues per year) *Current Opinion in Immunology*. Current Science, London.

Immunology Today. Elsevier Science Publications, Amsterdam. [The immunologist's 'newspaper'. Excellent.]

New England Journal of Medicine Series of general articles on immunology published during the year 2000.

Roitt I.M. & Delves P.J. (eds) (1998) *Encyclopedia of Immunology*, 2nd edn. Academic Press, London. [Covers virtually all aspects of the subject and describes immune responses to most infections.]

Schwaeble W.J. & Reid K.B.M. (1999) Does properdin crosslink the cellular and the humoral immune response? *Immunology Today* **20** (1), 17.

The Immunologist. Hogrefe & Huber Publishers, Seattle. [Official organ of the International Union of Immunological Societies—IUIS. Excellent, didactic and compact articles on current trends in immunology.]

Website www.roitt.com (linked to *Roitt's Essential Immunology* and this book) Four hundred multiple-choice questions with teaching comments on every answer, further reading, immunology update, and facility for downloading the figures.

CHAPTER 3

Antibodies

THE BASIC STRUCTURE IS A FOUR-PEPTIDE UNIT

The antibody molecule is made up of two identical heavy and two identical light chains held together by interchain disulfide bonds. These chains can be separated by reduction of the S–S bonds and acidification. In the most abundant type of antibody, **immunoglobulin G**, the exposed hinge region is extended in structure due to the high proline content and is therefore vulnerable to proteolytic attack; thus the molecule is split by papain to yield two identical **Fab** fragments, each with a single combining site for antigen, and a third fragment, **Fc**, which lacks the ability to bind antigen. Pepsin strikes at a different point and cleaves the Fc from the remainder of the molecule to leave a large 5S fragment, which is formulated as $F(ab')_2$ since it is still divalent with respect to antigen binding just like the parent antibody (figure 3.1).

AMINO ACID SEQUENCES REVEAL VARIATIONS IN IMMUNOGLOBULIN STRUCTURE

For good reasons, the antibody population in any given individual is incredibly heterogeneous, and this has meant that determination of amino acid sequences was utterly useless until it proved possible to obtain the homogeneous product of a single clone. The opportunity to do this first came from the study of **myeloma proteins**.

In the human disease known as multiple myeloma, one cell making one particular individual immunoglobulin divides over and over again in the uncontrolled way a cancer cell does, without regard for the overall requirement of the host. The patient then possesses enormous numbers of identical cells derived as a clone from the original cell and they all synthesize the same immunoglobulin—the myeloma protein, or M-protein—which appears in the serum, some-

times in very high concentrations. By purification of the myeloma protein we can obtain a preparation of an immunoglobulin having a unique structure. **Monoclonal antibodies** can also be obtained by fusing individual antibody-forming cells with a B-cell tumor to produce a constantly dividing clone of cells dedicated to making the one antibody.

The sequencing of a number of such proteins has revealed that the N-terminal portions of both heavy and light chains show considerable variability, whereas the remaining parts of the chains are relatively constant, being grouped into a restricted number of structures. It is conventional to speak of variable and constant regions of both heavy and light chains (figure 3.2).

Certain sequences in the variable regions show quite remarkable diversity, and systematic analysis localizes these hypervariable sequences to three segments on the light chain and three on the heavy chain (figure 3.3).

IMMUNOGLOBULIN GENES

Immunoglobulins are encoded by multiple gene segments

Clusters of genes on three different chromosomes code for κ, λ and heavy chains respectively. Since a wide range of antibodies with differing amino acid sequences can be produced, there must be corresponding nucleotide sequences to encode them. However, the complete gene encoding each heavy and light chain is not present as such in the germ-line DNA, but is created during early development of the B-cell by the joining together of minisegments of the gene. Take the human κ light chain, for example; the variable region is encoded by two gene segments, a large V_κ and a small J_κ, while a single gene encodes the constant region (figure 3.4). There is a cluster of some 70 or more V_κ genes and just five functional J genes. In the immature B-cell, a translocation event leads to the joining of one of the V_κ genes to one

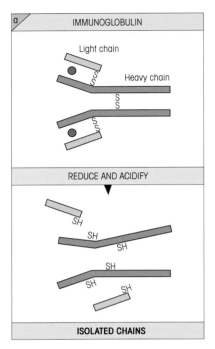
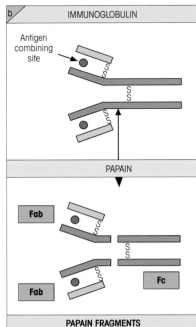
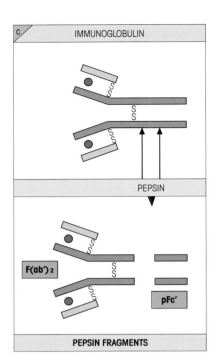

Figure 3.1 The antibody basic unit consisting of two identical heavy and two identical light chains held together by interchain disulfide bonds, can be broken down into its constituent peptide chains and to proteolytic fragments, the pepsin F(ab′)$_2$ retaining two binding sites for antigen and the papain Fab with one. After pepsin digestion the pFc′ fragment representing the C-terminal half of the Fc region is formed and is held together by noncovalent bonds. The portion of the heavy chain in the Fab fragment is given the symbol Fd. The N-terminal residue is on the left for each chain.

of the *J* segments. Each *V* segment has its own leader sequence and a number of upstream promoter sites including a characteristic octamer sequence, to which regulatory elements bind. When the Ig gene is transcribed, splicing of the nuclear RNA brings the V$_\kappa$J sequence into contiguity with the constant region C$_\kappa$ transcript, the whole being read off as a continuous κ chain peptide within the endoplasmic reticulum.

The same general principles apply to the arrangement of λ and heavy chain genes, although the latter constellation shows additional features: the subclass constant region genes form a single cluster and there is a group of four highly variable *D* segments inserted between the *V* and *J* regions (figure 3.5). The *D* and *J* segments together encode almost the entire third hypervariable region, the first two being contributed by the *V* sequence.

A special mechanism effects *VDJ* recombination

In essence, the translocation involves the mutual recognition of conserved heptamer–spacer–nonamer recombina-tion signal sequences which flank each germ-line *V*, *D* and *J* segment. Recombinase activation genes *RAG-1* and *RAG-2* catalyse the introduction of double-strand breaks between the elements to be joined and their respective flanking sequences. At this stage, nucleotides may either be deleted or inserted between the *VD*, *DJ* or *VJ* joining elements before they are ultimately ligated.

STRUCTURAL VARIANTS OF THE BASIC IMMUNOGLOBULIN MOLECULE

Isotypes

Based upon the structure of their heavy chain constant regions, immunoglobulins are divided into major groups termed **classes**, which may be further subdivided into **subclasses**. In the human, there are five classes: immunoglobulin G (IgG), IgA, IgM, IgD and IgE. Since all the heavy chain constant region (C$_H$) structures which give rise to classes and subclasses are expressed together in the serum of a

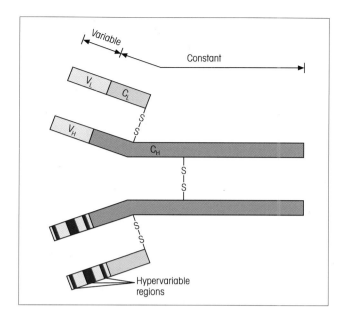

Figure 3.2 Amino acid sequence variability in the antibody molecule.
The terms 'V region' and 'C region' are used to designate the variable and constant regions respectively, 'V_L' and 'C_L' are generic terms for these regions on the light chain and 'V_H' and 'C_H' specify variable and constant regions on the heavy chain. Certain segments of the variable region are hypervariable but adjacent framework regions are more conserved. As stressed previously, each pair of heavy chains is identical, as is each pair of light chains.

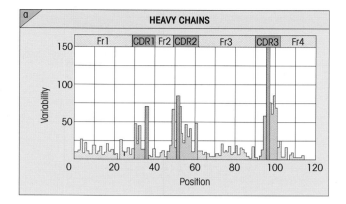

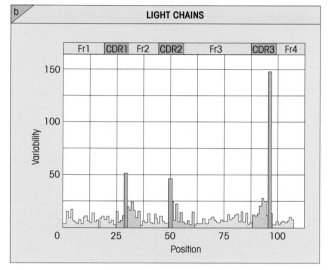

Figure 3.3 Wu and Kabat plot of amino acid variability in the variable region of immunoglobulin heavy and light chains.
The sequences of chains from a large number of myeloma monoclonal proteins are compared and variability at each position is computed as the number of different amino acids found divided by the frequency of the most common amino acid. Obviously, the higher the number the greater the variability; for a residue at which all 20 amino acids occur randomly, the number will be 400 (20 / 0.05) and at a completely invariant residue, the figure will be 1 (1 / 1). The three hypervariable regions (darker blue) in the (a) heavy and (b) light chains, usually referred to as **complementarity-determining regions (CDR)**, are clearly defined. The intervening peptide sequences (gray) are termed framework regions (Fr1–4). (Courtesy of Professor E.A. Kabat.)

normal subject, they are termed **isotypic variants** (table 3.1). Likewise, the light chain constant regions (C_L) exist in isotypic forms known as κ and λ which are associated with all heavy chain isotypes. Because the light chains in a given antibody are identical, immunoglobulins are either κ or λ but never mixed (unless specially engineered in the laboratory). Thus IgG exists as IgGκ or IgGλ, IgM as IgMκ or IgMλ, and so on.

Allotypes

This type of variation depends upon the existence of allelic forms (encoded by alleles or alternative genes at a single locus) which therefore provide genetic markers (table 3.1). In somewhat the same way as the red cells in genetically different individuals can differ in terms of the blood group antigen system ABO, so the Ig heavy chains differ in the expression of their allotypic groups. Typical allotypes are the **Gm specificities** on IgG (Gm = *marker* on IgG). Allotypic differences at a given Gm locus usually involve one or two amino acids in the peptide chain. Take, for example, the G1m(a) locus on IgG1. An individual with this allotype would have the peptide sequence Asp.Glu.Leu.Thr.Lys on each of his IgG1 molecules. Another person whose IgG1 was a-negative would have the sequence Glu.Glu.Met.Thr. Lys, i.e. two amino acids different. To date, 25 Gm groups have been found on the γ-heavy chains and a further three on the κ constant region.

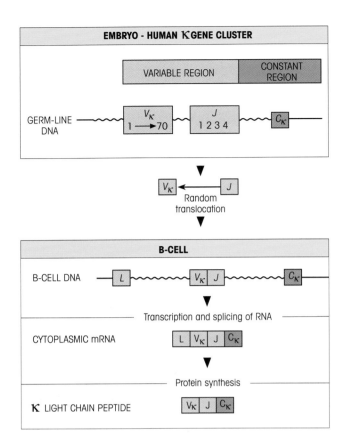

Figure 3.4 Genetic basis for synthesis of human κ chains. The V_κ genes are arranged in a series of families or sets of a closely related sequence. Each V_κ gene has its own leader sequence (L). As the cell becomes immunocompetent, the variable region is formed by the random combination of a V_κ with a joining segment J, a translocation process facilitated by base sequences in the intron following the 3′ end of the V_κ segment pairing up with sequences in the intron 5′ to J. The final joining occurs when the intervening intron sequence is spliced out of the RNA transcript. By convention, the genes are represented in italics and the antigens they encode in normal type.

Idiotypes

We have seen that it is possible to obtain antibodies that recognize isotypic and allotypic variants; one can also raise antiserums which are specific for individual antibody molecules and discriminate between one monoclonal antibody and another independently of isotypic or allotypic structures. Such antiserums define the individual determinants characteristic of each antibody, collectively termed the **idiotype**. Not surprisingly, it turns out that the idiotypic determinants are located in the variable part of the antibody associated with the hypervariable regions. The reader will (or should) be startled to learn that it is possible to raise autoanti-idiotypic sera since this means that individuals can make antibodies to their own idiotypes.

IMMUNOGLOBULINS ARE FOLDED INTO GLOBULAR DOMAINS WHICH SUBSERVE DIFFERENT FUNCTIONS

Immunoglobulin domains have a characteristic structure

In addition to the *interchain* disulfide bonds which bridge heavy and light chains, there are internal, *intrachain* disulfide links which form loops in the peptide chain. These loops are compactly folded to form globular **domains** which have a characteristic β-pleated sheet protein structure.

Significantly, the hypervariable sequences appear at one end of the variable domain where they form parts of the β-turn loops and are clustered close to each other in space (figure 3.6).

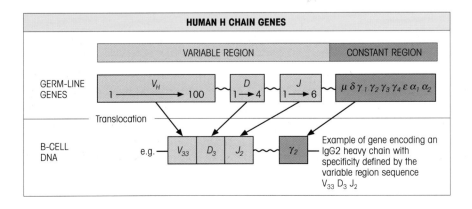

Figure 3.5 Human V-region genes shuffled by translocation to generate the single heavy chain specificity characteristic of each B-cell. Note the additional *D*-segment minigenes.

Table 3.1 Summary of immunoglobulin variants.

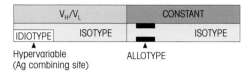

TYPE OF VARIATION	DISTRIBUTION	VARIANT	LOCATION	EXAMPLES
ISOTYPIC	All variants present in serum of a normal individual	Classes Subclasses Types Subgroups Subgroups	C_H C_H C_L C_L V_H/V_L	IgM, IgE IgA1, IgA2 κ, λ $\lambda Oz^+, \lambda Oz^-$ $V_{\kappa I}\ V_{\kappa II}\ V_{\kappa III}$ $V_{HI}\ V_{HII}\ V_{HIII}$
ALLOTYPIC	Alternative forms: genetically controlled so not present in all individuals	Allotypes	Mainly C_H/C_L sometimes V_H/V_L	Gm groups (human) b4, b5, b6, b9 (rabbit light chains) Igh-1^a, Igh-1^b (mouse γ_{2a} heavy chains)
IDIOTYPIC	Individually specific to each immuno-globulin molecule	Idiotypes	Variable regions	Probably one or more hypervariable regions forming the antigen-combining site

The variable domain binds antigen

The clustering of the hypervariable loops at the tips of the variable regions where the antigen binding site is localized makes them the obvious candidates to subserve the function of antigen recognition (figures 3.6 & 3.7), and this has been confirmed by X-ray crystallographic analysis of complexes formed between the Fab fragments of monoclonal antibodies and their respective antigens. The sequence heterogeneity of the three heavy and three light chain hypervariable loops ensures tremendous diversity in combining specificity for antigen through variation in the shape and nature of the surface they create. Thus each hypervariable region may be looked upon as an independent structure contributing to the complementarity of the binding site for antigen, and one speaks of **complementarity determining regions (CDR)**.

Constant region domains determine secondary biological function

The classes of antibody differ from each other in many respects: in their half-life, their distribution throughout the body, their ability to fix complement and their binding to cell surface Fc receptors. Since the classes all have the same κ and λ light chains, and heavy and light variable region domains, these differences must lie in the heavy chain constant regions.

A model of the IgG molecule is presented in figure 3.8 which indicates the spatial disposition and interaction of the domains in IgG and ascribes the various biological functions to the relevant structures. In principle, the V-region domains form the recognition unit and the constant-region domains mediate the secondary biological functions.

IMMUNOGLOBULIN CLASSES AND SUBCLASSES

The physical and biological characteristics of the five major immunoglobulin classes in the human are summarized in tables 3.2 and 3.3. The following comments are intended to supplement this information.

Immunoglobulin G has major but varied roles in extracellular defenses

Its relative abundance, its ability to develop high-affinity binding for antigen and its wide spectrum of secondary biological properties, make IgG appear as the prime workhorse of the Ig stable. During the secondary response IgG is probably the major immunoglobulin to be synthesized. IgG diffuses more readily than the other immunoglobulins into the extravascular body spaces where, as the predominant species, it carries the major burden of neutralizing bacterial toxins and of binding to microorganisms to enhance their phagocytosis.

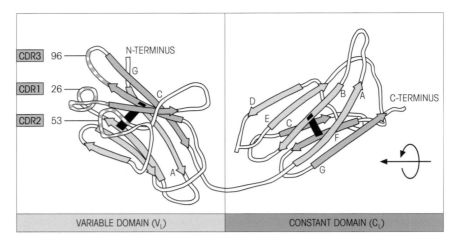

Figure 3.6 Ig domain structure. Structure of the globular domains of a light chain (from X-ray crystallographic studies of a Bence-Jones protein by Schiffler *et al.* (1973) *Biochemistry* **12**, 4620). One surface of each domain is composed essentially of four chains (light blue arrows) arranged in an antiparallel β-pleated structure stabilized by interchain H bonds between the amide CO· and NH· groups running along the peptide backbone, and the other surface of three such chains (darker blue arrows); the black bar represents the intrachain disulfide bond. This structure is characteristic of all immunoglobulin domains. Of particular interest is the location of the hypervariable regions (▪ ▪ ▪ ▪) in three separate loops which are closely disposed relative to each other and form the light chain contribution to the antigen binding site. One numbered residue from each complementarity determinant is identified.

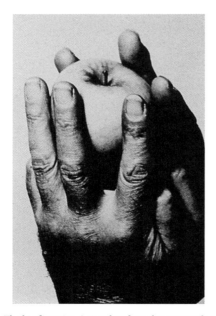

Figure 3.7 The binding site. A simulated combining site for the reactive surface of a single antigenic epitope (such as a hapten, cf. figure 5.1) formed by apposing the three middle fingers of each hand, each finger representing a hypervariable loop. With protein epitopes the area of contact is usually greater and tends to involve more superficial residues. (Cf. figure 5.3; photograph by B.N.A. Rice; inspired by A. Munro!)

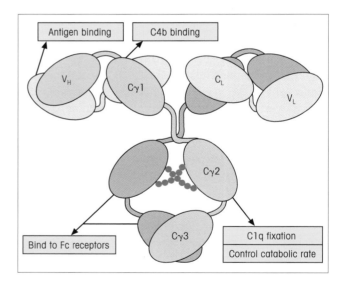

Figure 3.8 Location of biological function. The combined Cγ2 and Cγ3 domains bind to Fc receptors on phagocytic cells, NK cells and placental syncytiotrophoblast; also to staphylococcal protein A. (Note the IgG heavy chain is designated γ and the constant region domains Cγ1, Cγ2 and Cγ3.)

Table 3.2 Physical properties of major human immunoglobulin classes.

DESIGNATION	IgG	IgA	IgM	IgD	IgE
Sedimentation coefficient	7S	7S,9S,11S*	19S	7S	8S
Molecular weight	150 000	160 000 and dimer	900 000	185 000	200 000
Number of basic four-peptide units	1	1,2*	5	1	1
Heavy chains	γ	α	μ	δ	ε
Light chains $\kappa + \lambda$	$\kappa + \lambda$	$\kappa + \lambda$	$\kappa + \lambda$	$\kappa + \lambda$	$\kappa + \lambda$
Molecular formula†	$\gamma_2\kappa_2, \gamma_2\lambda_2$	$(\alpha_2\kappa_2)_{1-2}$ $(\alpha_2\lambda_2)_{1-2}$ $(\alpha_2\kappa_2)_2 S*$ $(\alpha_2\lambda_2)_2 S*$	$(\mu_2\kappa_2)_5$ $(\mu_2\lambda_2)_5$	$\delta_2\kappa_2(\delta_2\lambda_2?)$	$\varepsilon_2\kappa_2, \varepsilon_2\lambda_2$
Valency for antigen binding	2	2,4	5(10)	2	2
Concentration range in normal serum	8-16 mg/ml	1.4-4 mg/ml	0.5-2 mg/ml	0-0.4 mg/ml	17-450 ng/ml‡
% Total immunoglobulin	80	13	6	0-1	0.002
% Carbohydrate content	3	8	12	13	12

*Dimer in external secretions carries secretory component—S
†IgA dimer and IgM contain J-chain
‡ng=10^{-9}g

Table 3.3 Biological properties of major immunoglobulin classes in the human.

	IgG	IgA	IgM	IgD	IgE
Major characteristics	Most abundant Ig of internal body fluids particularly extravascular where it combats micro-organisms and their toxins	Major Ig in sero-mucous secretions where it defends external body surfaces	Very effective agglutinator; produced early in immune response – effective first-line defence vs. bacteremia	Most, if not all present on lymphocyte surface	Protection of external body surfaces. Recruits anti-microbial agents. Raised in parasitic infections. Responsible for symptoms of atopic allergy
Complement fixation Classical Alternative	++ –	– +	+++ –	– –	– –
Cross placenta	++	–	–	–	–
Fix to homologous mast cells and basophils	–	–	–	–	+++
Binding to macrophages and polymorphs	+++	+	–	–	+

Activation of the classical complement pathway

Complexes of bacteria with IgG antibody trigger the C1 complex when a minimum of two Fcγ regions in the complex bind C1q. Activation of the next component, C4, produces attachment of C4b to the Cγ1 domain. Thereafter, one observes C3 convertase formation, covalent coupling of C3b to the bacteria and release of C3a and C5a leading to the chemotactic attraction of our friendly polymorpho-nuclear phagocytic cells. These adhere to the bacteria through surface receptors for complement and the Fc portion of IgG (Fcγ) and then ingest the microorganisms through phagocytosis. In a similar way, the extracellular killing of target cells coated with IgG antibody is mediated largely through recognition of the surface Fcγ by NK cells bearing the appropriate receptors (cf. pp. 11,20). The thesis that the **biological individuality of different immunoglobulin classes is dependent on the heavy chain constant regions, particularly the Fc**, is amply borne out in relationship to activities such as transplacental passage, complement fixation and binding to various cell types, where function has been shown to be mediated by the Fc part of the molecule.

Opsonization by IgG

All phagocytic cells have the ability to phagocytose microorganisms, a process which can be considerably enhanced by coating the invaders with IgG antibody. This binds to specific epitopes on the microbe via its Fab fragment and to Fcγ receptors on the phagocytic cells by its Fc portion, allowing the phagocytic cell to attach itself firmly to the microbe and provoking much greater phagocytic activity.

Transplacental passage of IgG

Alone of the Ig classes, IgG possesses the crucially important ability to cross the human placenta so that it can provide a major line of defense for the first few weeks of a baby's life. This may be further reinforced by the transfer of colostral IgG across the gut mucosa in the neonate. These transport processes involve translocation of IgG across the cell barrier by complexing to an Fcγ receptor.

Immunoglobulin A guards the mucosal surfaces

IgA appears selectively in the seromucous secretions such as saliva, tears, nasal fluids, sweat, colostrum, and secretions of the lung, genitourinary and gastrointestinal tracts, where it has the job of defending the exposed external surfaces of the body against attack by microorganisms. The IgA is synthesized locally by plasma cells and is dimerized intracellularly together with a cysteine-rich polypeptide called J-chain. The dimeric IgA binds strongly through its J-chain to a receptor for polymeric Ig present in the membrane of mucosal epithelial cells. The complex is then actively endocytosed, transported across the cytoplasm and secreted into the external body fluids after cleavage of the poly Ig receptor peptide chain. The fragment of the receptor remaining bound to the IgA is termed secretory piece, and the whole molecule is called **secretory IgA** (figure 3.9).

The function of the secretory piece may be to protect the IgA hinge from bacterial proteases. It would also be nice to think that it acted as a molecular Teflon to endow the IgA dimer with 'nonstick' potential, since IgA antibodies function by inhibiting the adherence of coated microorganisms to the surface of mucosal cells, thereby preventing entry into the body tissues. They will also combine with the myriad soluble antigens of dietary and microbial origin to block their access to the body.

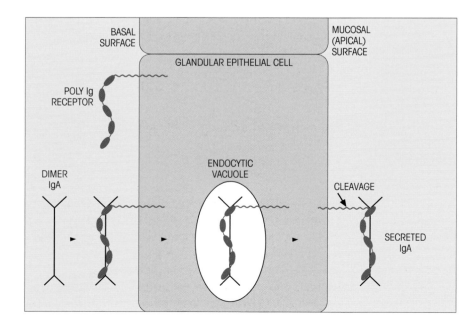

Figure 3.9 Secretory IgA. The mechanism of IgA secretion at the mucosal surface. The mucosal cell synthesizes a receptor for polymeric Ig which is inserted into the basal membrane. Dimeric IgA binds to this receptor and is transported via an endocytic vacuole to the apical surface. Cleavage of the receptor releases secretory IgA still attached to part of the receptor, termed secretory piece. Note how the receptor cleavage introduces an asymmetry which drives the transport of IgA dimers to the mucosal surface.

Immunoglobulin M provides a defense against bacteremia

Often referred to as the macroglobulin antibodies because of their high molecular weight, IgM molecules are polymers of five four-peptide subunits each bearing an extra C_H domain. As with IgA, a single J-chain is incorporated into the pentamer. IgM antibodies tend to be of relatively low affinity as measured against single determinants (haptens) but, because of their high valency, they bind with quite respectable avidity to antigens with multiple epitopes. For the same reason, these antibodies are extremely efficient agglutinating and cytolytic agents and since they appear early in the response to infection and are largely confined to the bloodstream, it is likely that they play a role of particular importance in cases of bacteremia. The isohemagglutinins (anti-A, anti-B) and many of the 'natural' antibodies to microorganisms are usually IgM.

Monomeric IgM (i.e. a single four-peptide unit) anchored in the cell membrane, is the major antibody receptor used by B-lymphocytes to recognize antigen.

Immunoglobulin D is a cell surface receptor

This class was recognized through the discovery of a myeloma protein which did not have the antigenic specificity of IgG, A or M, although it reacted with antibodies to immunoglobulin light chains and had the basic four-peptide structure. The hinge region is particularly extended and although protected to some degree by carbohydrate, it may be this feature which makes IgD, among the different immunoglobulin classes, uniquely susceptible to proteolytic degradation, and accounts for its short half-life in plasma (2.8 days). An exciting development has been the demonstration that nearly all the IgD is present together with IgM on the surface of a proportion of B-lymphocytes, where it seems likely that the two immunoglobins may operate as mutually interacting antigen receptors for the control of lymphocyte activation and suppression.

Immunoglobulin E triggers inflammatory reactions

Only very low concentrations of IgE are present in serum and only a very small proportion of the plasma cells in the body are synthesizing this immunoglobulin. It is not surprising, therefore, that so far only a handful of IgE myelomas have been recognized compared with tens of thousands of IgG paraproteinemias. IgE antibodies remain firmly fixed for an extended period when they are bound with high affinity to the FcεRI receptor on mast cells. Contact with antigen leads to degranulation of the mast cells with release of preformed vasoactive amines and cytokines, and the synthesis of a variety of inflammatory mediators derived from arachidonic acid. This process is responsible for the symptoms of hay fever and of extrinsic asthma when patients with atopic allergy come into contact with the allergen, for example grass pollen.

The main *physiological* role of IgE would appear to be protection of anatomical sites susceptible to trauma and pathogen entry, by local recruitment of plasma factors and effector cells through **triggering an acute inflammatory reaction**. Infectious agents penetrating the IgA defenses would combine with specific IgE on the mast cell surface and trigger the release of vasoactive agents and factors chemotactic for granulocytes, so leading to an influx of plasma IgG, complement, polymorphs and eosinophils.

Immunoglobulins are further subdivided into subclasses

Antigenic analysis of IgG myelomas revealed further variation and showed that they could be grouped into four isotypic **subclasses** now termed IgG1, IgG2, IgG3 and IgG4. The differences all lie in the heavy chains, which have been labeled γ1, γ2, γ3 and γ4, respectively. These heavy chains show considerable homology and have certain structures in common with each other—the ones which react with specific anti-IgG antisera—but each has one or more additional structures characteristic of its own subclass arising from differences in primary amino acid composition and in interchain disulfide bridging. These give rise to differences in biological behaviour, which are summarized in table 3.4.

Two subclasses of IgA have also been found, of which IgA1 constitutes 80–90% of the total.

MAKING ANTIBODIES TO ORDER

The monoclonal antibody revolution

First in rodents

A fantastic technological breakthrough was achieved by Milstein and Kohler who devised a technique for the production of 'immortal' clones of cells making single antibody specificities, by fusing normal antibody-forming cells with an appropriate B-cell tumor line. These so-called 'hybridomas' can be grown up either in the ascitic form in mice, when quite prodigious titers of monoclonal antibody can be attained, or propagated in large-scale culture. It must be

	IgG1	IgG2	IgG3	IgG4
% Total IgG in normal serum	65	23	8	4
Electrophoretic mobility	slow	slow	slow	slow
Spontaneous aggregation	−	−	+++	−
Gm allotypes	a,z,f,x	n	b0,b1,b3 g,s,t,etc.	
Ga site reacting with rheumatoid factor*	+++	+++	−	+++
Combination with staphylococcal A protein	+++	+++	−	+++
Binding to staphylococcal protein G	+++	+++	+++	+++
Cross placenta	++	±	++	++
Complement fixation (C1 pathway)**	+++	++	++++	±
Binding to monocytes	+++	+	+++	±
Binding to heterologous skin	++	−	++	++
Blocking IgE binding	−	−	−	+
Antibody dominance	Anti-Rh	Anti-dextran Anti-levan	Anti-Rh	Anti-Factor VIII

Table 3.4 Comparison of human IgG subclasses.

*Other rheumatoid factors apparently react with Gm-specific sites.
**The very poor complement-fixing ability of IgG4 cannot be ascribed to its rigid hinge region since substitution of serine 331 with proline (as in IgG1 and IgG3) endows the molecule with excellent C1q binding and C-mediated lytic capability. Intriguingly, substitution of proline 331 with serine in IgG1 maintains C1q binding but grossly diminishes lytic activity, a puzzle still to be resolved.

clear that we have in our hands a really powerful technique whose applications are truly legion. Some of these are touched upon in table 3.5 to give the reader an inkling of what is possible, but the potential defies the imagination: the separation of individual cell types with specific surface markers (lymphocyte subpopulations, neural cells, etc.), diagnosis of lymphoid and myeloid malignancies, radioimmunoassay, serotyping of microorganisms, immunologic intervention with passive antibody, anti-idiotype inhibition or 'magic bullet' therapy with cytotoxic agents coupled to antitumor-specific antibody—these and many other areas have been transformed by hybridoma technology.

Human monoclonals can be made

Mouse monoclonals injected into human subjects for therapeutic purposes are highly immunogenic and may lead to immune-complex mediated disease. It would be useful to remove the xenogeneic (foreign) portions of the monoclonal antibody and replace those portions with human Ig structures using recombinant DNA technology. Chimeric constructs, in which the V_H and V_L mouse domains are spliced onto human C_H and C_L genes (figure 3.10a), are far less immunogenic in humans. Such antibodies can now be produced in 'humanized' mice immunized by conventional antigens. One initiative involved the replacement of the mouse Cγ1 gene by its human counterpart in embryonic stem cells. The resulting mutant mice were crossed with animals expressing human in place of murine $C_κ$ chains and mice homozygous for both mutants produced humanized IgG1κ antibodies

Yet another approach is to graft the six complementarity-determining regions (CDR) of a high-affinity rodent monoclonal onto a completely human Ig framework without loss of specific reactivity (figure 3.10b). This is not a trivial exercise, however, and the objective of fusing human B-cells to make hybridomas is still appealing. A major restriction arises because the peripheral blood B-cells, which are the only B-cells readily available in the human, are not normally regarded as a good source of antibody-forming cells. Notwithstanding the difficulties in finding good fusion partners, large numbers of human monoclonals have been established and are awaiting the go-ahead for clinical use; one can cite IgG anti-RhD for the prevention of rhesus disease of the newborn (see p. 130), and highly potent monoclonals for protection against varicella zoster, cytomegalovirus, group B streptococci and lipopolysaccharide endotoxins of Gram-negative bacteria.

Engineering antibodies

There are other ways around the problems associated with the production of human monoclonals which exploit the wiles of modern molecular biology. Reference has already

Table 3.5 Some applications of monoclonal antibodies.

ENUMERATION OF HUMAN LYMPHOCYTE SUBPOPULATIONS	Anti-CD3 identifies all mature T-cells Anti-CD4 identifies subset containing T-helpers Anti-CD8 identifies cytotoxic-suppressor T-cells
CELL DEPLETION	Cocktail of anti-CD3 monoclonals + complement kills T-cells in human bone marrow to prevent graft-vs-host reaction
CELL ISOLATION	Enrichment of bone marrow stem cells by anti-CD34 in the FACS
IMMUNOSUPPRESSION	Anti-CD3 depresses T-cell function Anti-CD4 induces tolerance
PASSIVE IMMUNIZATION	High titer antimicrobial human monoclonals can give passive protection
PROBING FUNCTION OF CELL SURFACE MOLECULES	Anti-CD8 inhibits killing by cytotoxic T-cells Anti-class II MHC monoclonal inhibits T-cell response to macrophage-processed Ag
BLOOD GROUPING	Anti-A monoclonal provides more reliable standard reagent than conventional antisera
DIAGNOSIS IN CANCER	Monoclonal anti T-ALL allows differentiation from non T-ALL Follicle center cell lymphoma identified by peroxidase-labeled anticommon ALL in tissue sections
IMAGING	Radioactive anti-carcinoembryonic antigen used to localize colonic tumors or secondaries by scanning
NEPHELOMETRIC ASSAY	Routine estimation of individual soluble serum proteins e.g. IgG
SOLID-PHASE IMMUNOASSAY	Good discrimination for noncompetitive assay of antigen by monoclonals to more than one site
ANALYSIS OF COMPLEX ANTIGEN MIXTURES	Identification of the 'protective' antigen in parasite suitable for vaccine production Identification of antigenic 'patch' on acetyl-choline receptor involved in experimental myasthenia gravis
PURIFICATION OF ANTIGEN	Isolate from mixtures by monoclonal on affinity column
ANALYSIS OF EMBRYOLOGICAL RELATIONSHIPS	Separate monoclonals to neurons of neural tube and neural crest origin help to define embryological derivation of cells in nervous system
MONOCLONAL MUTANTS	Mutants lacking Fc structures used for in vivo neutralization of toxic drugs e.g. digoxin overdose, or for defining biological roles of Fc domains
GENETICALLY ENGINEERED ANTIBODIES	Transfer mouse CDRs to human Ig framework Change Fc isotype to improve particular function
FUSED HYBRIDOMAS	Producing antibodies with dual specificity
ANALYSIS OF IMMUNE RESPONSE	Hybridomas made during an immune response give data on repertoire and on mutation events (the original reason for developing the hybridoma technology)
ARTIFICIAL ENZYMES (CATALYTIC ANTIBODIES)	Monoclonal antibodies which recognize the transitional state of the reactants in a reversible reaction can simulate an enzyme – early days but big potential

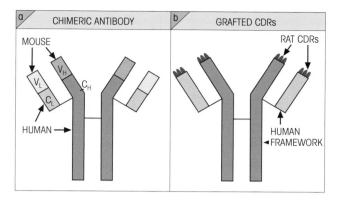

Figure 3.10 **Genetically engineering rodent antibody specificities into the human.** (a) Chimeric antibody with mouse variable regions fused to human Ig constant region. (b) 'Humanized' rat monoclonal in which gene segments coding for all six CDRs are grafted onto a human Ig framework.

the light- and heavy-chain genes are allowed to combine randomly in tandem with the bacteriophage pIII gene. This **combinatorial library** containing most random pairings of heavy- and light-chain genes encodes a huge repertoire of antibodies (or their fragments) expressed as fusion proteins with the filamentous coat protein pIII on the bacteriophage surface. The extremely high number of phages can now be panned on solid-phase antigen to select those bearing the highest affinity antibodies attached to their surface. Because the genes which encode these highest affinity antibodies are already present within the selected phage, they can readily be cloned and the antibody expressed in bulk. It should be recognized that this **selection** procedure has an enormous advantage over techniques which employ **screening** because the number of phages which can be examined is several logs higher.

Although a 'test-tube' operation, this approach to the generation of specific antibodies does resemble the affinity maturation of the immune response *in vivo* (see p. 78) in the sense that antigen is the determining factor in selecting out the highest affinity responders.

Fields of antibodies

Not only can the products of genes for a monoclonal antibody be obtained in bulk in the milk of lactating animals but plants can also be exploited for this purpose. So-called 'plantibodies' have been expressed in bananas, potatoes and tobacco plants. One can imagine a high-tech farmer drawing the attention of a bemused visitor to one field

been made to the 'humanizing' of rodent antibodies (figure 3.10), but an important new strategy based upon bacteriophage expression and **selection** has achieved a prominent position. In essence, mRNA from primed human B-cells is converted to cDNA and the antibody genes, or fragments therefrom, expanded by the polymerase chain reaction (PCR). Single constructs are then made in which

growing anti-tetanus toxoid, another anti-meningococcal polysaccharide, and so on. Multifunctional plants might be quite profitable with, say, the root being harvested as a food crop and the leaves expressing some desirable gene product. At this rate there may not be much left for science fiction authors to write about!

REVISION

See the accompanying website (www.roitt.com) for multiple choice questions.

The basic immunoglobulin structure is a four-peptide unit

• Immunoglobulins (Ig) have a basic four-peptide structure of two identical heavy and two identical light chains joined by interchain disulfide links.
• Papain splits the molecule at the exposed flexible hinge region to give two identical univalent antigen-binding fragments (Fab) and a further fragment (Fc). Pepsin proteolysis gives a divalent antigen-binding fragment F(ab′)$_2$ lacking the Fc.

Amino acid sequences reveal variations in immunoglobulin structure

• There are perhaps 10^8 or more different Ig molecules in normal serum.
• Analysis of myeloma proteins, which are homogeneous Ig produced by single clones of malignant plasma cells, has shown the N-terminal region of heavy and light chains to have a variable amino acid structure and the remainder to be relatively constant in structure.

Immunoglobulin genes

• Clusters of genes on three different chromosomes encode κ, λ and heavy Ig chains respectively. In each cluster there are approximately 100 or more variable region (V) genes and around five small J minisegments. Heavy chain clusters in addition contain of the order of four D minigenes. There is a single gene encoding each constant region.
• A special splicing mechanism involving mutual recognition of 5′ and 3′ flanking sequences, catalysed by recombinase enzymes, effects the VD, VJ and DJ translocations.

Structural variants of the basic Ig molecule

• Isotypes are Ig variants based on different heavy chain constant structures, all of which are present in each individual; examples are the Ig classes IgG, IgA, etc.
• Allotypes are heavy chain variants encoded by allelic (alternative) genes at single loci and are therefore genetically distributed; examples are Gm groups.

• An idiotype is the collection of antigenic determinants on an antibody, usually associated with the hypervariable regions, recognized by other antigen-specific receptors, either antibody (the anti-idiotype) or T-cell receptors.
• The variable region domains bind antigen, and three hypervariable loops on the heavy chain, termed complementarity-determining regions, and three on the light chain, form the antigen-binding site.
• The constant region domains of the heavy chain (particularly the Fc) carry out a secondary biological function after the binding of antigen, e.g. complement fixation and macrophage binding.

Immunoglobulin classes and subclasses

• In the human there are five major types of heavy chain giving five classes of Ig. IgG is the most abundant Ig, particularly in the extravascular fluids where it neutralizes toxins and combats microorganisms by fixing complement via the C1 pathway, and facilitating the binding to phagocytic cells by receptors for C3b and Fcγ. It crosses the placenta in late pregnancy and the intestine in the neonate.
• IgA exists mainly as a monomer (basic four-peptide unit) in plasma, but in the seromucous secretions, where it is the major Ig concerned in the defense of the external body surfaces, it is present as a dimer linked to a secretory component.
• IgM is basically a pentameric molecule although a minor fraction may be hexameric. It is essentially intravascular and is produced early in the immune response. Because of its high valency it is a very effective bacterial agglutinator and mediator of complement-dependent cytolysis and is therefore a powerful first-line defense against bacteremia.
• IgD is largely present on the lymphocyte and probably functions as an antigen receptor.
• IgE binds firmly to mast cells and contact with antigen leads to local recruitment of antimicrobial agents through degranulation of the mast cells and release of inflammatory mediators. IgE is of importance in certain parasitic

infections and is responsible for the symptoms of atopic allergy.

• Further diversity of function is possible through subdivision of classes into subclasses based on structural differences in heavy chains all present in each normal individual.

Making antibodies to order

• Immortal hybridoma cell lines making monoclonal antibodies provide powerful immunologic reagents and insights into the immune response. Applications include enumeration of lymphocyte subpopulations, cell depletion, immunoassay, cancer diagnosis and imaging, purification of antigen from complex mixtures, and recently the use of monoclonals as artificial enzymes (abzymes).

• Mouse monoclonal antibodies are immunogenic in humans. Chimeric constructs can be produced by splicing mouse *V* genes onto human *C* genes.

• Genetically engineered human antibody fragments can be derived by expanding the V_H and V_L genes from unimmunized, but preferably immunized, donors and expressing them as completely randomized combinatorial libraries on the surface of bacteriophage.

FURTHER READING

Cedar H. & Bergman Y. (1999) Developmental regulation of immune system gene rearrangement. *Current Opinion in Immunology* 11 (1), 64.

Reddy P.S. & Corley R.B. (1999) The contribution of ER quality control to the biologic functions of secretory IgM. *Immunology Today* 20 (12), 582.

Roitt I.M. & Delves P.J. (eds) (1992) *Encyclopedia of Immunology*. Academic Press, London. [Articles on IgG, IgA, IgM, IgD and IgE and immunoglobulin function and domains.]

Zola H. (1994) *Monoclonal Antibodies: the Second Generation*. Bios Scientific Publishers, Oxford. [New approaches including phage display combinatorial libraries.]

CHAPTER 4

Membrane receptors for antigen

THE B-CELL SURFACE RECEPTOR FOR ANTIGEN

The B-cell inserts a transmembrane immunoglobulin into its surface

In Chapter 2 we discussed the cunning system by which an antigen can be led inexorably to its doom by selecting the lymphocytes capable of making antibodies complementary in shape to itself through its ability to combine with a copy of the antibody molecule on the lymphocyte surface. It will be recalled that combination with the surface receptor can activate the cell to proliferate before maturing into a clone of plasma cells secreting antibody specific for the inciting antigen (cf. figure 2.6)

Immunofluorescent staining of live B-cells with labeled anti-Ig (e.g. figure 2.4c) reveals the earliest membrane Ig to be of the IgM class. The cell is committed to the production of just one antibody specificity and so transcribes its individual rearranged VJC_κ (or λ) and $VDJC\mu$ genes. The solution to the problem of secreting antibody with the same specificity as that present on the cell surface as a membrane Ig is found in a **differential splicing** mechanism. The initial nuclear μ-chain RNA transcript includes sequences coding for **hydrophobic transmembrane regions** which enable the IgM to sit in the membrane as a receptor, but if these are spliced out, the antibody molecules can be secreted in a soluble form (figure 4.1).

As the B-cell matures, it coexpresses surface IgD with the same specificity. This phenotype is abundant in the mantle zone lymphocytes of secondary lymphoid follicles (cf. figure 6.7c & d) and is achieved by differential splicing of a single transcript containing VDJ, Cμ and Cδ segments producing either membrane IgM or IgD . As the B-cell matures further, other isotypes such as IgG may be expressed.

The surface immunoglobulin is complexed with associated membrane proteins

The cytoplasmic tail of the surface IgM is a miserable three amino acids long. In no way could this accommodate the structural motifs required for interaction with intracellular protein tyrosine kinases or G proteins which mediate the activation of signal transduction cascades. However, it seems most likely that the surface Ig transduces signals through associated membrane proteins. These consist of two glycoprotein chains called Ig-α and Ig-β which interact with the immunoglobulin receptor and are involved in cell activation. In this regard their relationship to the immunoglobulin receptor is similar to that of the CD3 molecule and the T-cell receptor.

THE T-CELL SURFACE RECEPTOR FOR ANTIGEN

The receptor for antigen is a transmembrane heterodimer

The antigen-specific **T-cell receptor** is a membrane-bound molecule composed of two disulfide-linked chains, α and β. Each chain folds into two Ig-like domains, one having a relatively invariant structure, the other exhibiting a high degree of variability rather like an Ig Fab fragment.

There are two classes of T-cell receptors

Not long after the breakthrough in identifying the αβ T-cell receptor, came reports of the existence of a second type of receptor composed of γ and δ chains. This TCRγδ appears earlier in thymic ontogeny than the TCRαβ.

In the human, γδ cells make up only 0.5–15% of the T-cells in peripheral blood but they show greater dominance in the intestinal epithelium and in skin.

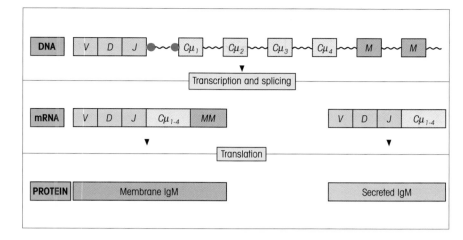

Figure 4.1 Splicing mechanism for the switch from the membrane to the secreted form of IgM. The hydrophobic sequence encoded by the exons *M–M* which anchors the receptor IgM to the membrane is spliced out in the secreted form. For simplicity, the leader sequence has been omitted. ∿ = introns.

The encoding of T-cell receptors is similar to that of immunoglobulins

The gene segments encoding the T-cell receptor β chains follow a similar arrangement of *V, D, J* and constant segments to those described for the immunoglobulins. Similarly, as an immunocompetent T-cell is formed, rearrangement of *V, D* and *J* genes occurs to form a continuous *VDJ* sequence. The firmest evidence that B- and T-cells use similar recombination mechanisms comes from mice with severe combined immunodeficiency (SCID) due to a single autosomal recessive defect preventing successful linkage of *V, D* and *J* segments. Homozygous mutants fail to develop immunocompetent B- and T-cells and identical sequence defects in *VDJ* joint formation are seen in both pre-B- and pre-T-cell lines.

Looking first at the β-chain cluster, one of the large number of *Vβ* genes translocates to a preformed $D\beta_1J\beta_1$ or $D\beta_2J\beta_2$ segment. **Variability in junction formation** and the **random insertion of nucleotides** at the N region of *D* and *J* segment joins, parallels the same phenomenon seen with Ig gene rearrangements. Sequence analysis emphasizes the analogy with the antibody molecule; each *V* segment contains two hypervariable regions, while the *DJ* **sequence** provides a **very hypervariable** structure, making a total of six potential complementarity-determining regions for antigen binding in each TCR. As in the synthesis of antibody, the intron between *VDJ* and *C* is spliced out of the mRNA before translation with the restriction that $V\beta D\beta_2J\beta_2$ can only link to $C\beta_2$.

All the other chains are encoded by genes formed through similar translocations. The α-chain gene pool lacks *D* segments but more than makes up for it with a prodigious number of *J* segments. The number of *Vγ* and *Vδ* genes is very small in comparison with *Vα* and *Vβ*. Like the α-chain pool, the γ chain cluster has no *D* segments.

The CD3 complex is an integral part of the T-cell receptor

The T-cell antigen recognition complex and its B-cell counterpart, can be likened to specialized army platoons whose job is to send out a signal when the enemy has been sighted. When the TCR 'sights the enemy', i.e. ligates antigen, it relays a signal through an associated complex of transmembrane peptides (**CD3**) to the interior of the T-lymphocyte, instructing it to awaken from its slumbering G0 state and do something useful—like becoming an effector cell. In all immunocompetent T-cells, the antigen receptor is noncovalently but still intimately linked with CD3 in a complex, which contains two heterodimeric TCR$\alpha\beta$ or $\gamma\delta$ recognition units closely apposed to the invariant CD3 peptide chains γ, δ, ε plus the disulfide-linked ζ–ζ dimer. Either or both of the ζ chains can be replaced by η. The total complex has the structure $TCR_2CD3\gamma\delta\varepsilon_2\zeta_2$ (figure 4.2).

THE GENERATION OF DIVERSITY FOR ANTIGEN RECOGNITION

We know that the immune system has to be capable of recognizing virtually any pathogen that has arisen or might arise. The extravagant genetic solution to this problem of anticipating an unpredictable future involves the generation of millions of different specific antigen receptors, probably vastly more than the lifetime needs of the individual. Since this is likely to exceed the number of genes in the body, there must be some clever ways to generate all this diversity, partic-

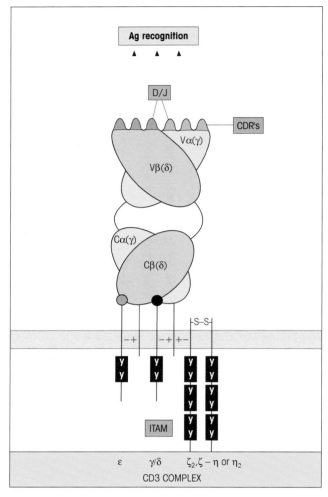

Figure 4.2 The T-cell receptor/CD3 complex. The TCR resembles the immunoglobulin Fab antigen-binding fragment in structure. The TCRs are probably expressed as dimeric structures linked to the CD3 complex. Negative charges on transmembrane segments of the five invariant chains of the CD3 complex contact the opposite charges on the TCR Cα and Cβ chains. The cytoplasmic domains of the CD3 peptide chains, shown in black, contact protein tyrosine kinases which activate cellular transcription factors.

ularly since the number of genes coding for antibodies and T-cell receptors is only of the order of 1000. We can now profitably examine the mechanisms which have evolved to generate tremendous diversity from such limited gene pools.

Intrachain amplification of diversity

Random VDJ combination increases diversity geometrically

Just as we can use a relatively small number of different building units in a child's construction set to create a rich variety of architectural masterpieces, so the individual receptor gene segments can be viewed as building blocks to fashion a multiplicity of antigen-specific receptors for both B- and T-cells.

Take, for example, the immunoglobulin heavy-chain genes (table 4.1). There are 30 D and 6 J functional segments. If there were entirely **random joining** of any one D to any one J segment (cf. figure 3.5), we would have the possibility of generating 180 DJ combinations (30×6). Let us go to the next stage. Since each of these 180 DJ segments could join with any one of the 51 V_H functional sequences, the net potential repertoire of VDJ genes encoding the heavy-chain variable region would be 51×180= 9180. In other words, just taking our V, D and J genes, which add up arithmetically to 87, we have produced a range of some 9000 different variable regions by **geometric recombination** of the basic elements. But that is only the beginning.

Playing with the junctions

Another ploy to squeeze more variation out of the germ-line repertoire involves variable boundary recombinations of V, D and J to produce different junctional sequences.

Further diversity arises from the insertion of nucleotides at the N region of the D and J segments, a process associated with the expression of terminal deoxynucleotidyl transferase. This maneuver greatly increases the repertoire of T-receptor γ and δ genes which are otherwise rather limited in number.

Just to make sure that we are really impressed, it transpires that even after a $V_H D J_H$ rearrangement has occurred, an interchange with a quite different 5′ V_H gene can still take place; since the process is not precise, bases can be lost and/or added at the region joining the new V_H to the N-terminal end of the D sequence. This V_H 'swapping' may prevent bias in the development of the heavy-chain V-region repertoire because the earliest differentiating B-cells utilize the V_H segments most proximal to D with high frequency to form their $V_H D J_H$ rearrangements. Yet additional mechanisms work on the D regions: in some cases the D segment can be read in three different reading frames and in others DD combinations may be formed.

Interchain amplification

The immune system took an ingenious step forward when two different types of chain were utilized for the recognition

Table 4.1 Calculations of human V gene diversity. The minimum number of specificities generated by straightforward random combination of germ-line segments are calculated. These will be increased by the further mechanisms listed.

	TCR1		TCR2		Ig		
					H	L	
	γ	δ	α	β		κ	λ
V gene segments	8	3	50	57	51	~70	25
D gene segments	-	3	-	1,1	30	-	-
J gene segments	3,2	3	70	6,7	6	5	8
Random Combinatorial joining (without junctional diversity)	$V \times J$ 8 × 5	$V \times D \times J$ 3 × 3 × 3	$V \times J$ 50 × 70	$V \times D \times J$ 57(13+7)	$V \times D \times J$ 51 × 30 × 6	$V \times J$ 70 × 5	$V \times J$ 25 × 8
Total	40	27	3500	1140	9000	350	200
Combinatorial heterodimers	40 × 27		3500 × 1140		9000 × 350	9000 × 200	
Total (rounded)	10^3		4×10^6		3.2×10^6	1.8×10^6	
Other mechanisms: D's in 3 reading frames, junctional diversity, N region insertion;* x 10^3	10^6		4×10^9		3.2×10^9	1.8×10^9	
Somatic mutation	–		–		+++	+++	

*minimal assumption of approximately 10 variants for chains lacking D segments and 100 for chains with D segments. The calculation for the T-cell receptor β-chain requires further explanation. The first of the two D segments, $D_{\beta 1}$ can combine with 57 V genes and all 13 $J_{\beta 1}$ and $J_{\beta 2}$ genes. $D_{\beta 2}$ behaves similarly but can only combine with the seven downstream $J_{\beta 2}$ genes.

molecules because the combination produces not only a larger combining site with potentially greater affinity, but also new variability. Thus when one heavy chain is paired with different light chains the specificity of the final antibody is altered.

This random association between TCR γ and δ chains, TCR α and β chains, and Ig heavy and light chains yields a further geometric increase in diversity. From table 4.1 it can be seen that approximately 200 T-cell receptor and 200 Ig germ-line segments can give rise to 4 million and 5 million different combinations respectively, by straightforward associations *without* taking into account all of the fancy additional *D/J* mechanisms described above. Hats off to evolution!

Somatic hypermutation

There is inescapable evidence that immunoglobulin *V*-region genes can undergo significant **somatic mutation**.

A number of features of this somatic diversification phenomenon deserve mention. The mutations are the result of single nucleotide substitutions, they are restricted to the variable as distinct from the constant region, and occur in both framework and hypervariable regions. The mutation rate is remarkably high, between 2 and 4% for V_H genes as compared with a value of less than 0.0001% for a nonimmunologic lymphocyte gene. It is likely that somatic mutation does not add to the repertoire available in the early phases of the primary response,

but occurs during the generation of memory and is probably responsible for tuning the response towards higher affinity.

T-cell receptor genes, on the other hand, **do not appear to undergo serious somatic mutation.** This is fortunate since T-cells are so close to recognizing self, that mutations could readily encourage the emergence of high affinity autoreactive receptors and resulting autoimmunity.

THE MAJOR HISTOCOMPATIBILITY COMPLEX (MHC)

Molecules expressed by genes which constitute this complex chromosomal region were originally defined by their ability to provoke vigorous rejection of grafts exchanged between different members of a species. In Chapter 2, brief mention was made of the necessity for cell-surface antigens to be associated with class I or class II MHC molecules so that they can be recognized by T-lymphocytes. The intention now is to give more insight into the nature of these molecules.

Class I and class II molecules are membrane-bound heterodimers

MHC class I

Class I molecules consist of a heavy peptide chain of 43 kDa noncovalently linked to a smaller 11 kDa peptide called **β₂-microglobulin**. The largest part of the heavy chain is organized into three globular domains (α_1, α_2 and α_3; figure 4.3a) which protrude from the cell surface; a hydrophobic section anchors the molecule in the membrane and a short hydrophilic sequence carries the C-terminus into the cytoplasm.

X-ray analysis of crystals of a human class I molecule has provided an exciting leap forwards in our understanding of MHC function. Both β₂-microglobulin and the α_3 region resemble classic Ig domains in their folding pattern. However, the α_1 and α_2 domains which are most distal to the membrane, form an utterly surprising structure composed of two extended α-helices above a floor created by peptide strands held together in a β-pleated sheet, the whole forming an undeniable **cavity** (figure 4.3b,c). Another curious feature emerged. The cavity was occupied by a linear molecule, now known to be a peptide, which had cocrystallized with the class I protein. The significance of these unique findings for T-cell recognition of antigen will be revealed in Chapter 5.

MHC class II

Class II MHC molecules are also transmembrane glycoproteins, in this case consisting of α and β polypeptide chains of molecular weight 34 kDa and 28 kDa respectively.

There is considerable sequence homology with class I, and structural studies have shown that the α_2 and β_2 domains, the ones nearest to the cell membrane, assume the characteristic Ig fold, while the α_1 and β_1 domains mimic the class I α_1 and α_2 in forming a groove bounded by two α-helices and a β-pleated sheet floor (figure 4.3a).

Complement genes contribute to the remaining class III region of the MHC

A variety of other genes which congregate within the MHC chromosome region are grouped under the heading of class III. Broadly, one could say that many are directly or indirectly related to immune defense functions. A notable cluster are the genes coding for two C4 isotypes and the two complement proteins, C2 and factor B, which each carry an active site for C3 convertase. Tumor necrosis factors TNFα and TNFβ (also known as lymphotoxin α) are also encoded under the class III umbrella.

Gene map of the MHC

An overall view of the main clusters of class I, II and III

genes in the human MHC (HLA system) may be gained from figure 4.4. A number of silent or pseudogenes have been omitted from these gene maps in the interest of simplicity.

The genes of the MHC display remarkable polymorphism

Unlike the immunoglobulin system where, as we have seen, variability is achieved in each individual by a **multigenic** system, the MHC has evolved in terms of variability between individuals with a highly **polymorphic** (literally 'many-shaped') system based on **multiple alleles** (i.e. alternative genes at each locus). These were initially defined serologically by the antibodies arising in grafted individuals. The amino acid changes responsible for these polymorphisms are restricted to the α_1 and α_2 domains of class I and to the α_1 and β_1 domains of class II. It is of enormous significance that they occur essentially in the β-sheet floor and the inner surfaces of the α-helices which line the central cavity (figure 4.3) and also on the upper surface of the helices.

The tissue distribution of MHC molecules

Essentially, all nucleated cells carry classical class I molecules. These are abundantly expressed on lymphoid cells, less so on liver, lung and kidney, and only sparsely on brain and skeletal muscle. In the human, the surface of the villous trophoblast lacks HLA-A, B or C components; instead it bears HLA-G, which does not appear on any other body cells in nonpregnant females. Class II molecules are also restricted, being especially associated with antigen-presenting cells such as B-cells, dendritic cells and macrophages; however, when activated by agents such as γ-interferon, capillary endothelia and many epithelial cells can develop surface class II and increased expression of class I.

Under normal circumstances, a soluble form of HLA is present in serum; the level rises markedly during the course of a viral infection, presumably due to an increase in HLA synthesis mediated by endogenous production of interferons and other cytokines.

MHC functions

Although originally discovered through transplantation reactions, the MHC molecules are utilized for vital biological functions by the host. Their function as cell surface markers enabling infected cells to signal cytotoxic and helper T-cells will be explored in depth in subsequent chap-

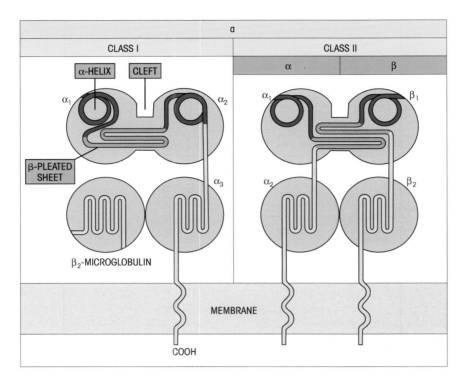

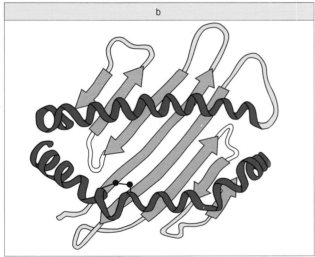

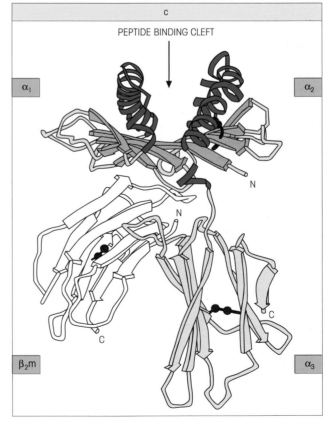

Figure 4.3 Class I and class II MHC molecules. (a) Diagram showing domains and transmembrane segments; the α-helices and β-sheets are viewed end on. (b) Schematic bird's eye representation of top surface of human class I molecule (HLA-A2) based on X-ray crystallographic structure. The strands making the β-pleated sheet are shown as thick gray arrows in the amino to carboxy direction, α-helices are represented as dark-red helical ribbons. The inside-facing surfaces of the two helices and the upper surface of the β-sheet form a cleft which binds and presents the T-cell epitope. The two black spheres represent an intrachain disulfide bond. (c) Side view of the same molecule clearly showing the anatomy of the cleft and the typical Ig folding of the α_3- and β_2-microglobulin domains (four antiparallel β-strands on one face and three on the other). (Reproduced from Bjorkman P.J. *et al.* (1987) *Nature* **329**, 506, with permission.)

The major histocompatibility complex														
MHC class	II				III						I			
HLA	DP	LMP & TAP	DQ	DR	C4	FB	C2	HSP70	TNF	B	C	E	A	G

Figure 4.4 **Main genetic regions of the human major histocompatibility complex** (HLA-human lymphocyte antigen).

ters. There is no doubt that this role in immune responsiveness is immensely important, and in this respect the rich **polymorphism of the MHC** region would represent a species response to **maximize protection against diverse microorganisms**.

REVISION

See the accompanying website (www.roitt.com) for multiple choice questions.

The B-cell surface receptor for antigen

• The B-cell inserts its Ig gene product containing a transmembrane segment into its surface where it acts as a specific receptor for antigen.

• The surface Ig is complexed with the membrane proteins Ig-α and Ig-β which become phosphorylated on cell activation and presumably transduce signals received through the Ig antigen receptor.

The T-cell surface receptor for antigen

• The receptor for antigen is a transmembrane dimer, each chain consisting of two Ig-like domains.

• The outer domains are variable in structure, the inner ones constant, rather like a membrane-bound Fab.

• Both chains are required for antigen recognition.

• Most T-cells express a receptor (TCR) with α and β chains. A separate lineage bearing γδ receptors is transcribed strongly in early thymic ontogeny but is associated mainly with epithelial tissues in the adult.

• The encoding of the TCR is similar to that of immunoglobulins. The variable region coding sequence in the differentiating T-cell is formed by random translocation from clusters of V, D (in most cases) and J segments to form a single recombinant $V(D)J$ sequence for each chain.

• Like the Ig chains, each variable region has three hypervariable sequences which are presumed to function in antigen recognition.

• The CD3 complex, composed of γ, δ, ε and either ζ_2, ζη or η_2 covalently linked dimers, forms an intimate part of the receptor and probably has a signal transducing role following ligand binding by the TCR.

The generation of antibody diversity for antigen recognition

• The individual receptor gene segments can be viewed as building blocks to produce very large numbers of antigen-specific T- or B-cell receptors.

• Further diversity is introduced at the junctions between V, D and J segments by variable recombination as they are spliced together by recombinase enzymes.

• In addition, after a primary response, B-cells but not T-cells undergo high rate somatic mutation affecting the V regions.

MHC

• Each vertebrate species has an MHC identified originally through its ability to evoke very powerful transplantation rejection.

• Each contains three classes of genes. Class I encodes peptides associated at the cell surface with β_2-microglobulin. Class II molecules are transmembrane heterodimers. Class III products are heterogeneous but include complement components and tumor necrosis factors.

• The genes display remarkable polymorphism. A given MHC gene cluster is referred to as a 'haplotype' and is usually inherited *en bloc* as a single Mendelian trait.

• Classical class I molecules are present on virtually all nucleated cells in the body and signal cytotoxic T-cells.

• Class II molecules are particularly associated with B-cells and macrophages but can be induced on capillary endothelial cells and epithelial cells by γ-interferon. They signal T-helpers for B-cells and macrophages.

• Structural analysis indicates that the two domains distal to the cell membrane form a cavity bounded by two parallel α-helices sitting on a floor of β-sheet peptide strands; the walls and floor of the cavity and the upper surface of the helices are the sites of maximum polymorphic amino acid substitutions.

• Class III gene products are associated with innate recognition of and defense against danger such as infection.

FURTHER READING

Campbell K.S. (1999) Signal transduction from the B-cell antigen-receptor. *Current Opinion in Immunology* **11** (3), 256.

Campbell R.D. & Trowsdale J. (1993) Map of the human MHC. *Immunology Today* **14**, 349.

Campbell R.D. & Trowsdale J. (1997) Map of the human major histo-compatibility complex. *Immunology Today* **18** (1) pullout.

Howard J.C. (1991) Disease and evolution. *Nature* **352**, 565.

Hughes A.L., Yeager M., Ten Elshof A.E. & Chorney M.J. (1999) A new taxonomy of mammalian MHC class I molecules. *Immunology Today* **20** (1), 22.

CHAPTER 5

The primary interaction with antigen

WHAT IS AN ANTIGEN?

A man cannot be a husband without a wife and a molecule cannot be an antigen without a corresponding antiserum or antibody or T-cell receptor. The term **antigen** is used in two senses, the first to describe a molecule which *gen*erates an immune response (also called an **immunogen**), and the second a molecule which reacts with antibodies or primed T-cells. **Haptens** are small well-defined chemical groupings, such as dinitrophenyl (DNP) or *m*-aminobenzene sulfonate, which are not immunogenic on their own but will react with preformed antibodies induced by injection of the hapten linked to a 'carrier' molecule which is itself an immunogen (figure 5.1).

The part of the hypervariable regions on the antibody which contacts the antigen is termed the **paratope** and the part of the antigen which is in contact with the paratope is designated the **epitope** or **antigenic determinant**. It is important to be aware that each antigen usually bears several determinants on its surface, which may well be structurally distinct from each other; thus a monoclonal antibody reacting with one determinant will usually not react with any other determinants on the same antigen (figure 5.2). To get some idea of size, if the antigen is a linear peptide or carbohydrate, the combining site can usually accommodate up to five or six amino acid residues or hexose units. With a globular protein as many as 16 or so amino acid side-chains may be in contact with an antibody (cf. figure 5.3).

The structure of antigens

In general, large proteins, because they have more potential determinants, are better antigens than small ones. Furthermore, the more foreign an antigen, that is the less similar to self-configurations, the more effective it is in provoking an immune response. Although antibodies can be produced to almost any part of a foreign protein, certain areas of the antigen are more immunogenic and are called the immunodominant regions of the antigen. These sites of high epitope density are often those parts of the peptide chains which protrude significantly from the globular surface.

ANTIGEN AND ANTIBODY INTERACTIONS

Antigen and antibody interact due to complementarity in shape over a wide area of contact (figure 5.3), not so much as inflexible entities which fit together precisely in a 'lock and key' manner but rather as mutually deformable surfaces—more like clouds than rocks. The interaction depends upon weak van der Waals, electrostatic, hydrophobic and hydrogen bonding forces which only become of significant magnitude when the interacting molecules are very close together. Thus, the more snugly the paratope and epitope fit together, the stronger the strength of binding, termed the **affinity**. This is defined as the equilibrium constant (K_a) of the reversible association of antibody with a single epitope (e.g. a hapten, figure 5.1), represented by the equation:

$$Ab + Hp \rightleftharpoons AbHp$$

Obviously a high affinity betokens strong binding. Usually, we are concerned with the interaction of an antiserum, i.e. the serum from an immunized individual with a multivalent antigen where the binding is geometrically increased relative to a monovalent hapten or single antigenic epitope. The term employed to express this binding is avidity, which being a measure of the functional affinity of an antiserum for the whole antigen is of obvious relevance to the reaction with antigen in the body. High avidity is superior to low for a wide variety of functions *in vivo*, including immune elimination of antigen, virus neutralization and the protective role against bacteria and other organisms.

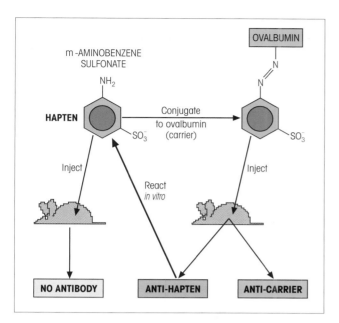

Figure 5.1 A hapten on its own will not induce antibodies. However, it will react *in vitro* with antibodies formed to a conjugate of the hapten with an immunogenic carrier.

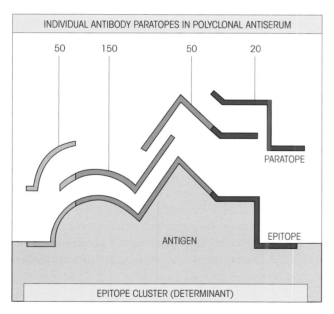

Figure 5.2 A globular protein antigen usually bears a mosaic of determinants (dominant epitope clusters) on its surface, defined by the heterogeneous population of antibody molecules in a given antiserum. This highly idealized diagram illustrates the idea that individual antibodies in a polyclonal antiserum with different combining sites (paratopes) can react with overlapping epitopes forming a determinant on the surface of the antigen. The numbers refer to the imagined relative frequency of each antibody specificity.

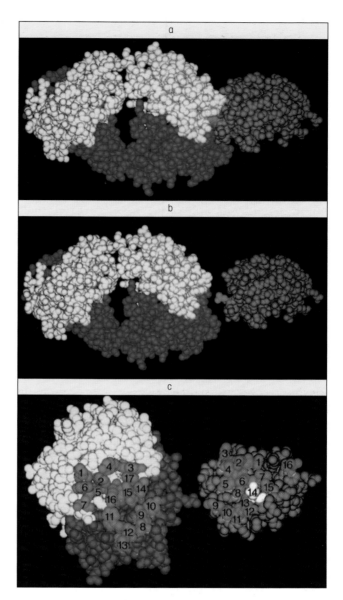

Figure 5.3 Structure of the contact regions between a monoclonal Fab antilysozyme and lysozyme. (a) Space-filling model showing Fab and lysozyme molecules fitting snugly together. Antibody heavy chain, blue; light chain, yellow; lysozyme, green with its glutamine-121 in red. (b) Fab and lysozyme models pulled apart to show how the protuberances and depressions of each are complementary to each other. (c) End-on views of antibody combining site (*left*) and the lysozyme epitope (*right*) obtained from (b) by rotating each molecule 90° about a vertical axis. (Reproduced with permission from Amit A. *et al.* (1986) *Science* **233**, 747–753. Copyright 1986 by the AAAS.)

THE SPECIFICITY OF ANTIGEN RECOGNITION BY ANTIBODY IS NOT ABSOLUTE

The strength of an antigen–antibody reaction can be quantified by the affinity or avidity of the antibody to that specific antigen. In so far as we recognize that an antiserum may have a relatively greater avidity for one antigen than another, by the same token we are saying that the antiserum is displaying relative rather than absolute specificity; in practice we speak of degrees of **cross-reactivity**. An antiserum raised against a given antigen can cross-react with a partially related antigen which bears one or more identical or similar determinants. In figure 5.4 it can be seen that an antiserum to antigen$_1$ (Ag$_1$) will react less strongly with Ag$_2$, which bears just one identical determinant, because only certain of the antibodies in the serum can bind. Ag$_3$, which possesses a similar but not identical determinant, will not fit as well with the antibody, and hence the binding is even weaker. Ag$_4$, which has no structural similarity at all, will not react significantly with the antibody. Thus, based upon stereochemical considerations, we can see why the avidity of the antiserum for Ag$_2$ and Ag$_3$ is less than for the homologous antigen, while for the unrelated Ag$_4$ it is negligible. It would be customary to describe the antiserum as being highly specific for Ag$_1$ in relation to Ag$_4$ but cross-reacting with Ag$_2$ and Ag$_3$ to different extents. These principles have significance in human autoimmune diseases since an antibody may react not only with the antigen which stimulated its production, but also with some possibly quite unrelated molecules.

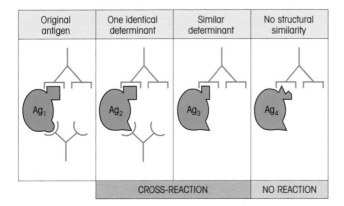

Original antigen	One identical determinant	Similar determinant	No structural similarity
Ag$_1$	Ag$_2$	Ag$_3$	Ag$_4$
	CROSS-REACTION		NO REACTION

Figure 5.4 Specificity and cross-reaction. The avidity of the serum antibodies ⊢ and ⊱ for Ag$_1$ > Ag$_2$ > Ag$_3$ ≫ Ag$_4$.

IN VITRO ANTIGEN–ANTIBODY REACTIONS

The specificity of antigen–antibody reactions enables us to detect the presence of specific antibody in serum or other fluid by combining it with the known antigen under strict laboratory conditions. Not only will positive reactions tell us that specific antibodies are present but by testing a series of antibody dilutions, we can get an idea of the quantity, or titer, of specific antibody in the fluid. To take an example, a serum might be diluted 10 000 times and still just give a positive reaction. This titer of 1 : 10 000 enables comparison to be made with another much weaker serum which has a titer of, say, 1 : 100, i.e. it can only be diluted out 100 times before the test becomes negative. The titer is of crucial importance in interpreting the significance of antibodies in patients with clinical disease. Many normal individuals, for example, may have low titer antibodies to cytomegalovirus resulting from previous, perhaps subclinical, infection. In active infection titers may be high and increasing.

Numerous techniques are available to detect the presence and the titer of an antibody

Precipitation

When an antigen solution is added progressively to a potent antiserum, antigen–antibody precipitates are formed which can be detected by a variety of laboratory techniques. Such precipitation reactions are useful for detecting antibodies.

Nonprecipitating antibodies can be detected by nephelometry

The small aggregates formed when dilute solutions of antigen and antibody are mixed create a cloudiness or turbidity which can be measured by forward angle scattering of an incident light source (nephelometry). Greater sensitivity can be obtained by using monochromatic light from a laser.

Enhancement of precipitation by countercurrent immunoelectrophoresis

Antigen and antiserum are placed in wells punched in an agar gel and a current applied. The antigen migrates steadily into the antibody zone and forms a precipitin line which provides a fairly sensitive and rapid test that has been applied to the detection of antibodies (and by the same means, antigen) to hepatitis B antigen, DNA antibodies in systemic lupus erythematosus (SLE) (see p. 171), autoantibodies to soluble nuclear antigens in mixed connective tissue disease, and *Aspergillus* precipitins in cases with allergic bronchopulmonary aspergillosis.

Agglutination of antigen-coated particles

Whereas the cross-linking of multivalent protein antigens by antibody leads to precipitation, cross-linking of cells or large particles by antibody directed against surface antigens leads to agglutination.

Agglutination reactions are used to identify bacteria and to type red cells.

Immunoassay for antibody using solid-phase antigen

The antibody content of a serum can be assessed by its ability to bind to antigen which has been insolubilized by physical adsorption to a plastic tube or microagglutination tray with multiple wells; the bound immunoglobulin may then be estimated by addition of a labeled anti-Ig raised in another species (figure 5.5). Consider, for example, the determination of DNA autoantibodies in SLE. When a patient's serum is added to a microwell coated with antigen (in this case DNA), the autoantibodies will bind to the plastic and remaining serum proteins can be readily washed away. Bound antibody can now be estimated by addition of enzyme-labeled purified rabbit anti-human IgG. After rinsing out excess unbound reagent, the enzyme activity of the tube will clearly be a measure of the autoantibody content of the patient's serum. The diagnostic radioallergosorbent test (RAST) measures specific IgE antibodies in a patient's serum binding to solid phase allergen. Enzymes such as horseradish peroxidase and phosphatase, which give a colored soluble reaction product, are widely employed in these enzyme-linked immunosorbent assays (ELISA).

Identification and measurement of antigen

Antigens can be readily identified and quantitated *in vitro*, provided that specific antibody is available in the reaction mixture. Laboratory techniques similar to those employed to detect antibodies can be used to detect antigens. For example, precipitation reactions can be carried out in gels to detect an abnormal protein in serum or urine secreted by a B-cell or plasma cell tumor. The monoclonal paraprotein localizes as a dense compact 'M' band of defined electrophoretic mobility and its antigenic identity is then revealed by immunofixation with specific precipitating antiserums applied in paper strips overlying parallel lanes in the electrophoresis gel.

The nephelometric assay for antigen

If antigen is added to a solution of excess antibody, the amount of complex which can be assessed by forward light scatter in a nephelometer is linearly related to the concentration of antigen. With the ready availability of a wide range of monoclonal antibodies which facilitate the standardization of the method, nephelometry is commonly used to detect a wide array of serum proteins including immunoglobulins, C3, C4, haptoglobin, ceruloplasmin and CRP.

WHAT THE T-CELL SEES

We have on several occasions alluded to the fact that the T-cell receptor sees antigen on the surface of cells associated with an MHC class I or II molecule. Now is the time for us to go into the nuts and bolts of this relationship.

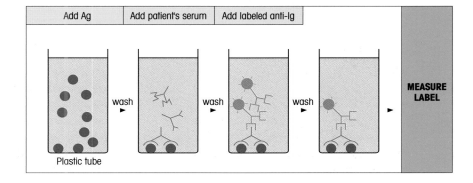

Figure 5.5 Solid-phase immunoassay for antibody. The anti-immunoglobulin may be labeled by radioactive iodine or, more usually, by an enzyme which gives a soluble colored or chemiluminescent reaction product.

Haplotype restriction reveals the need for MHC participation

It has been established that T-cells bearing $\alpha\beta$ receptors, with some exceptions, only respond when the antigen-presenting cells express the same MHC haplotype as the host from which the T-cells were derived. This **haplotype restriction** on T-cell recognition tells us unequivocally that MHC molecules are intimately and necessarily involved in the interaction of the antigen-bearing cell with its corresponding antigen-specific T-lymphocyte. We also learn that cytotoxic T-cells recognize antigen in the context of class I MHC, and helper T-cells respond when the antigen is associated with class II molecules on antigen-presenting cells.

One of the seminal observations which helped to elucidate the role of the MHC was the dramatic Nobel Prize-winning revelation by Peter Doherty and Rolf Zinkernagel that cytotoxic T-cells taken from an individual recovering from a viral infection will only kill virally infected cells which share an MHC haplotype with the host. For example, on recovery from influenza, individuals bearing the MHC haplotype HLA-A2 have cytolytic T-cells which kill HLA-A2 target cells infected with influenza virus but not cells of a different HLA-A tissue-type specificity.

T-cells recognize a linear peptide sequence from the antigen

With any complex antigen only certain peptides can be recognized by polyclonal T-cells. These can therefore be regarded as T-cell epitopes. When clones of identical specificity are derived from these T-cells, each clone reacts with only one of the peptides; in other words, like B-cell clones, each clone is specific for one corresponding epitope. Therefore when either cytotoxic or helper T-cell clones are stimulated by antigen-presenting cells to which certain peptides derived from the original antigen had been added, the clones can be activated. By synthesizing a series of such peptides, the T-cell epitope can be mapped with some precision.

The conclusion is that the **T-cell recognizes both MHC and peptide** and we now know that the peptide which acts as a T-cell epitope lies along the groove formed by the α-helices and the β-sheet floor of the class I and class II outermost domains. Just how does it get there?

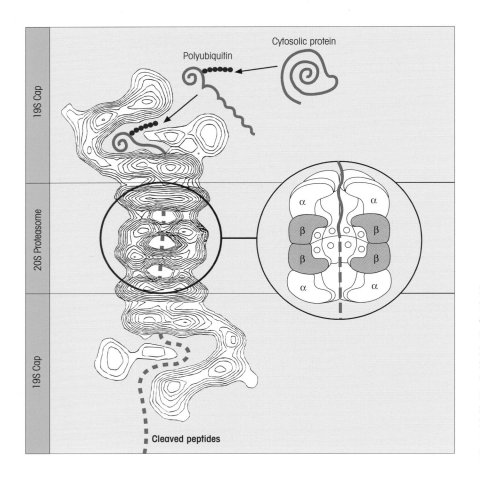

Figure 5.6 Cleavage of cytosolic proteins by the proteasome. The whole 26S protease complex consisting of the 20S proteasome with twin 19S caps is displayed as a contour plot derived from electron microscopy and image analysis. The cross-section of the proteasome reveals the sites of peptidase activity (o) within the inner core of the seven-membered rings of β-subunits. (Based on Peters J.-M. *et al.* (1993) *Journal of Molecular Biology* **234**, 932; and Rubin D.M. & Finley D. (1995) *Current Biology* **5**, 854.)

PROCESSING OF INTRACELLULAR ANTIGEN FOR PRESENTATION BY CLASS I MHC

Cytosolic proteins are degraded to peptides via a ubiquitin-sensitive pathway, by an ATP-dependent complex of peptidases termed a **proteasome** (figure 5.6). This structure contains two MHC-associated low molecular weight proteins, LMP2 and 7, which are polymorphic and may serve to optimize delivery of the peptides to the TAP1/TAP2 membrane-spanning transporter mechanism responsible for translocation of the peptides into the endoplasmic reticulum (ER) (figure 5.7). Now within the lumen of the ER, the peptides complex with the membrane-bound class I MHC molecules thereby releasing them from their association with the TAP transporter. Thence, the complex traverses the Golgi stack, presumably picking up carbohydrate side-chains en route, and reaches the surface where it is a sitting target for the cytotoxic T-cell.

PROCESSING OF ANTIGEN FOR CLASS II MHC PRESENTATION FOLLOWS A DIFFERENT PATHWAY

Class II MHC complexes with antigenic peptide are generated by a fundamentally different intracellular mechanism, since the antigen-presenting cells which interact with T-helper cells need to sample the antigen from both the *extra*cellular and *intra*cellular compartments. In essence, a trans-Golgi vesicle containing class II has to intersect with a late endosome containing exogenous protein antigen taken into the cell by an endocytic mechanism.

First let us consider the class II molecules themselves. These are assembled from α- and β-chains in the endoplasmic reticulum in association with the transmembrane **invariant chain** (figure 5.8), which has several functions. It acts as a dedicated chaperone to ensure correct folding of the nascent class II molecule and it inhibits the precocious binding of peptides in the ER before the class II reaches the endocytic compartment containing antigen. Its combination with the αβ class II heterodimer inactivates a retention signal and allows transport through the Golgi to the late endosomal compartment.

Meanwhile, exogenous protein is taken up by endocytosis and is subjected to partial degradation as the early endosome undergoes progressive acidification. The late endosome, having many of the characteristics of a lysosomal granule, now fuses with the vacuole containing the class II-

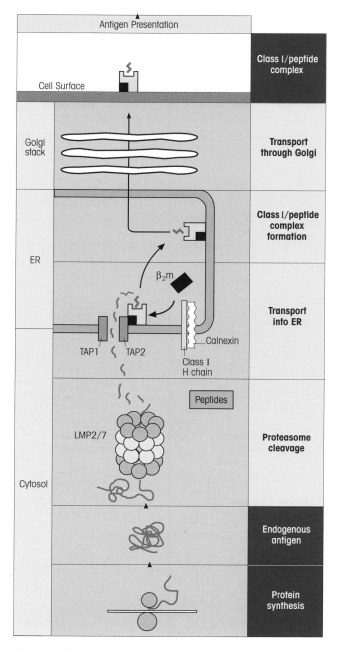

Figure 5.7 Processing and presentation of endogenous antigen by class I MHC. Cytosolic proteins are degraded by the proteasome complex into peptides which are transported into the endoplasmic reticulum (ER). There, they bind to membrane-bound class I MHC formed by β_2-microglobulin (β_2m)-induced dissociation of nascent class I heavy chains from their calnexin chaperone. The peptide/MHC complex is now released from its association with the TAP transporter, traverses the Golgi system, and appears on the cell surface ready for presentation to the T-cell receptor.

invariant chain complex. Under the acidic conditions within this MHC class II-enriched compartment the invariant chain is degraded, after which the complexes are transported to the membrane for presentation to T-helper cells.

Processing of antigens for class II presentation is not confined to soluble proteins taken up from the exterior but can also encompass proteins and peptides within the ER and microorganisms whose antigens reach the lysosomal

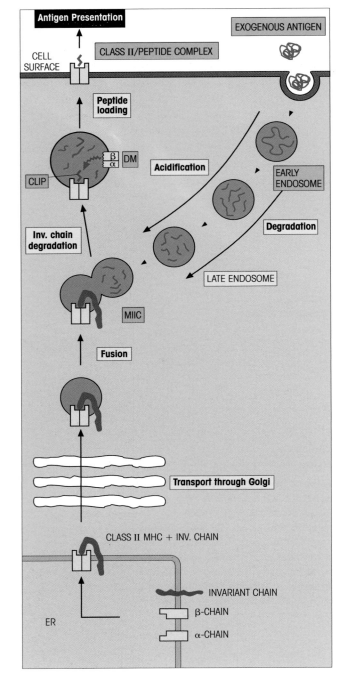

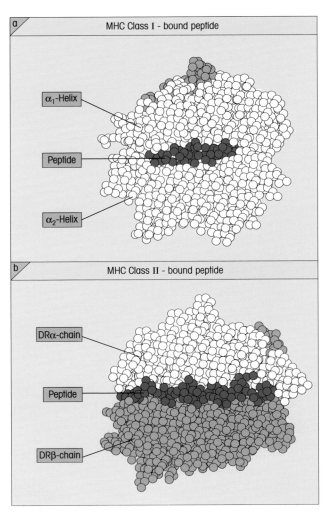

Figure 5.9 Binding of peptides to the MHC cleft. T-cell receptor 'view' looking down on the α-helices lining the cleft represented in space-filling models. (a) Peptide 309–317 from HIV-1 reverse transcriptase bound tightly within the class I HLA-A2 cleft. (b) Influenza hemagglutinin 306–318 lying in the class II HLA-DR1 cleft. In contrast with class I, the peptide extends out of both ends of the binding groove. (Based on Vignali D.A.A. & Strominger J.L. (1994) *The Immunologist* **2**, 112, with permission of the authors and publisher.)

Figure 5.8 Processing and presentation of exogenous antigen by class II MHC. Class II molecules with invariant chain are assembled in the endoplasmic reticulum (ER) and transported through the Golgi to the trans-Golgi reticulum. There they are sorted to a late endosomal vesicle with lysosomal characteristics known as MIIC (meaning MHC class II enriched compartment) containing partially degraded protein derived from the endocytic uptake of exogenous antigen. Degradation of invariant chains leaves the CLIP (class II-associated invariant chain peptide) peptides lying in the groove but under the influence of the MCH-related dimeric molecule (DM), they are replaced by other peptides in the vesicle including those derived from exogenous antigen, and the complexes are transported to the cell surface for presentation to T-helper cells.

structures, either after direct phagocytosis or prolonged intracellular cohabitation.

Binding to MHC class I

Except in the case of viral infection, the natural class I ligands will be self-peptides derived from proteins endogenously synthesized by the cell, histones, heat-shock proteins, enzymes, leader signal sequences and so on. It turns out that 75% or so of these peptides originate in the cytosol.

Binding to MHC class II

The open nature of the class II groove places no constraint on the length of the peptide, which can dangle nonchalantly from each end of the groove, quite unlike the straitjacket of the class I ligand site (figure 5.9). Thus, each class II molecule binds a collection of peptides with a spectrum of lengths ranging from 10 to 34 mers.

SUPERANTIGENS STIMULATE WHOLE FAMILIES OF LYMPHOCYTE RECEPTORS

Bacterial toxins represent one major group of T-cell superantigens

Whereas an individual peptide complexed to MHC will react

with antigen-specific T-cells, which represent a relatively small percentage of the T-cell pool, molecules have been identified which stimulate that proportion of the total T-cell population which express the same TCR Vβ family structure irrespective of their antigen specificity. They have been described as **superantigens** and include *Staphylococcus aureus* enterotoxins (SEA, SEB and several others), which are single-chain proteins responsible for food poisoning. They are strongly mitogenic for T-cells expressing particular Vβ families in the presence of MHC class II accessory cells. SEA must be one of the most potent T-cell mitogens known, causing marked T-cell proliferation. Another example of superantigen-induced disease is the toxic shock syndrome, a multisystem febrile illness caused by staphylococci or Group A streptococci. This disease is seen more often in menstruating women using tampons and is due to bacterial toxins acting as superantigens, inducing sustained release of cytokines from T-cells and macrophages.

Superantigens are not processed by the antigen-presenting cell but cross-link the class II and Vβ independently of direct interaction between MHC and TCR molecules.

REVISION

See the accompanying website (www.roitt.com) for multiple choice questions.

The nature of antigens
• An antigen is defined by its antibody. The contact area with an antibody is called an **epitope** and the corresponding area on an antibody is a **paratope**.
• Antisera recognize a series of dominant epitope clusters on the surface of an antigen; each cluster is called a determinant.

Antigens and antibodies interact by spatial complementarity, not by covalent binding
• The forces of interaction include electrostatic, hydrogen-bonding, hydrophobic and van der Waals.
• Antigen–antibody bonds are readily **reversible**.
• Antigens and antibodies are mutually deformable.

• The strength of binding to a single antibody combining site is measured by the **affinity**.
• The reaction of multivalent antigens with the heterogeneous mixture of antibodies in an antiserum is defined by **avidity (functional affinity)**.
• **Specificity** of antibodies is not absolute and they may cross-react with other antigens to different extents measured by their relative avidities.

In vitro antigen–antibody reactions
• Antibody can be detected in serum or other fluids by its ability to bind to specific antigens.
• The level of antibodies in a solution is called the antibody titer.

Numerous techniques are available for the estimation of antibody

- Antibody in solution can be assayed by the formation of frank precipitates which can be enhanced by countercurrent electrophoresis in gels.
- Nonprecipitating antibodies can be measured by laser nephelometry.
- Antibodies can also be detected by macroscopic agglutination of antigen-coated particles, and by one of the most important methods, ELISA, a two-stage procedure in which antibody bound to solid-phase antigen is detected by an enzyme-linked anti-Ig.

Identification and measurement of antigen

- Antigens can be quantified by their reaction in gels with antibody using single radial immunodiffusion.
- Higher concentrations of antigens are frequently estimated by nephelometry.

T-cell recognition

- Most T-cells see antigen in association with MHC molecules.
- They are restricted to the haplotype of the cell which first primed the T-cell.
- Protein antigens are processed by antigen-presenting cells to form small linear peptides which associate with the MHC molecules, binding to the central groove formed by the α-helices and the β-sheet floor.

Processing of antigen for presentation by class I MHC

- Endogenous cytosolic antigens such as viral proteins are cleaved by **proteasomes** and the peptides so-formed **transported** to the ER by the TAP1/2 system.

- The peptide then cooperates with β_2-microglobulin to combine with newly synthesized class I MHC heavy chain to form a stable heterotrimer which dissociates from TAP1/2.
- This **peptide–MHC complex** is then transported to the surface for presentation to cytotoxic T-cells.

Processing of antigen for presentation by class II MHC

- The **αβ class II molecule** is synthesized in the ER and complexes with membrane-bound **invariant chain**.
- This facilitates transport of the vesicles containing class II across the Golgi and directs it to the late endosomal compartment.
- The antigen is degraded to peptides which bind to class II now free of invariant chain.
- The **class II-peptide** complex now appears on the cell surface for presentation to T-helper cells.

The nature of the peptide

- Class I peptides are held in extended conformation within the MHC groove.
- They are usually 9–11 residues in length.
- Class II peptides are between 10 and 34 residues long and extend beyond the groove.

Superantigens

- These are potent mitogens which stimulate whole T-cell subpopulations sharing the same TCR Vβ family independently of antigen specificity.
- *Staphylococcus aureus* enterotoxins are powerful human superantigens which cause food poisoning and toxic-shock syndrome.
- They are not processed but cross-link MHC class II and TCR Vβ independently of their direct interaction.

FURTHER READING

Cresswell P. & Howard J. (eds) (1999) Section on Antigen Recognition. *Current Opinion in Immunology* **11** (1).

Karush F. (1976) Multivalent binding and functional affinity. In: *Contemporary Topics in Molecular Immunology*, Vol. 5 (ed. F.P. Inman), p. 217. Plenum Press, New York. [Bonus effect of multivalency.]

Lindahl K.F. & Rammensee H.-G. (eds) (1996) Antigen recognition. *Current Opinion in Immunology* **8**, 1. [Regular series of articulate and coherent reviews with extensive citation of key supporting experimental work.]

Moss D.J. & Khanna R. (1999) Major histocompatibility complex: from genes to function. *Immunology Today* **20** (4), 165.

Nisonoff A. & Pressman D. (1957) Closeness of fit and forces involved in the reactions of antibody homologous to the p-(p'-N-azophenylazo)-benzoate ion group. *Journal of the American Chemical Society* **79**, 1616.

Sekaly R.-P. (ed.) (1993) Bacterial superantigens. *Seminars in Immunology* **5**, 1.

CHAPTER 6

The anatomy of the immune response

THE SURFACE MARKERS OF CELLS IN THE IMMUNE SYSTEM

In order to discuss the events which occur in the operation of the immune system as a whole, it is imperative to establish a nomenclature which identifies the surface markers on the cells involved since these are used for communication and are usually functional molecules reflecting the state of cellular differentiation. The nomenclature system is established as follows. Immunologists from the far corners of the world who have produced monoclonal antibodies directed to surface molecules on B- and T-cells, macrophages, neutrophils and natural killer (NK) cells and so on, get together every so often, to compare the specificities of their reagents in international workshops. Where a cluster of monoclonals are found to react with the same polypeptide, they clearly represent a series of reagents defining a given marker and we label it with a CD (**cluster of differentiation**) number. The number of CD specificities on leukocytes is well over the 100s and some of them are shown in table 6.1.

Detection of surface markers

Because fluorescent dyes such as fluorescein and rhodamine can be coupled to antibodies without destroying their specificity, the conjugates can combine with antigen present in a tissue section and be visualized in the fluorescence microscope (figure 6.1a). In this way the distribution of antigen throughout a tissue and within cells can be demonstrated.

In place of fluorescent markers, other workers have evolved methods in which enzymes such as alkaline phosphatase or peroxidase are coupled to antibodies and these can be visualized by conventional histochemical methods at the level of both the light microscope (figure 6.1b) and the electron microscope.

When enumerating cells in suspensions such as in blood or other fluids, surface antigens can be detected by the use of labeled antibodies. It is now possible to stain single cells with up to four different fluorochromes and analyse the cells in individual droplets as they flow past a laser beam in a flow cytometer. The laser light excites the fluorochrome and the intensity of the fluorescence is displayed on an oscilloscope. With the impressive number of monoclonal antibodies to hand, highly detailed phenotypic analysis of single-cell populations is now a practical proposition. Of the ever-growing number of applications, the contribution to diagnosis of leukemia (cf. p. 152) is quite notable.

THE NEED FOR ORGANIZED LYMPHOID TISSUE

For an effective immune response an intricate series of cellular events must occur. Antigen must bind and if necessary be processed by antigen-presenting cells, which must then make contact with and activate T- and B-cells. In addition T-helper cells must assist certain B-cells and cytotoxic T-cell precursors to perform their functions, which include amplification of the numbers of potential effector cells by proliferation and the generation of the mediators of humoral and cellular immunity. In addition, memory cells for secondary responses must be formed and the whole response controlled so that it is adequate but not excessive and is appropriate to the type of infection being dealt with. The integration of the complex cellular interactions which form the basis of the immune response takes place within the organized architecture of peripheral, or secondary, lymphoid tissue, which includes the lymph glands, spleen and unencapsulated tissue lining the respiratory, alimentary and genitourinary tracts.

These tissues become populated by cells of reticular origin and by macrophages and lymphocytes derived from bone marrow stem cells, the T-cells first differentiating into immunocompetent cells by a high-pressure training period in the thymus, the B-cells undergoing their education in the

Table 6.1 Some of the major cluster of differentiation (CD) markers on human cells.

CD	Main cellular association	Membrane component
CD2	T	Receptor for LFA-3 and sheep rbc
CD2R	act. T	Ab's activate through these epitopes
CD3	T	Transducing elements of T-cell receptor
CD4	T-helper	MHC class II and HIV receptor
CD5	T, B subset	Ab increases second messenger pool
CD8	T-cytotoxic	MHC class I receptor
CD18	Leukocytes	Integrin β_2-chain
CD19	B	Pan B-cell marker associated with CD21
CD21	B subset	CR2, C3dg/EBV receptor
CD23	B subset, act. M, Eo	FcεRII
CD25	act. T, B, M	IL-2R β-chain
CD28	T-cells	Receptor for B7 costimulator
CD29	Leukocytes	VLA β, integrin β_1-chain
CD34	Bone marrow	Stem cell marker
CD40	B-cells	Receptor for CD40L costimulator
CD44	Leukocytes	Homing receptor
CD45	Leukocytes	Leukocyte common antigen
CD45 RA	T subset, B, G, M	Resting (naive?) T-cells
CD45 RO	T subset, B, G, M	Activated (memory?) T-cells

M = macrophage; G = granulocyte; Eo = eosinophil.

bone marrow itself (figure 6.3). In essence, the lymph nodes filter off and, if necessary, respond to foreign material draining body tissues, the spleen monitors the blood, and the unencapsulated lymphoid tissue is strategically integrated into mucosal surfaces of the body as a forward defensive system based on IgA secretion.

Communication between these tissues and the rest of the body is maintained by a pool of recirculating lymphocytes which pass from the blood into the lymph nodes, spleen and other tissues and back to the blood by the major lymphatic channels such as the thoracic duct (figure 6.4).

LYMPHOCYTES TRAFFIC BETWEEN LYMPHOID TISSUES

This traffic of lymphocytes between the tissues, the bloodstream and the lymph glands enables antigen-sensitive cells to seek the antigen and to be recruited to sites at which a response is occurring, while the dissemination of memory cells enables a more widespread response to be organized throughout the lymphoid system. Thus, antigen-reactive cells are depleted from the circulating pool of lymphocytes within 24 hours of antigen first localizing in the lymph nodes or spleen; several days later, after proliferation at the site of antigen localization, a peak of activated cells appears in the thoracic duct.

Lymphocytes home to their specific tissues

Naive lymphocytes enter a lymph node through the afferent

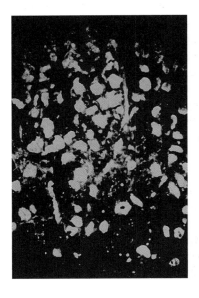
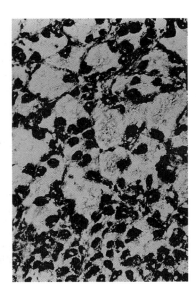

Figure 6.1 Staining of gastric parietal cells by (a) fluorescein (white cells) and (b) peroxidase-linked antibody (black cells). The sections were sequentially treated with human parietal cell autoantibodies and then with the conjugated rabbit anti-human IgG. The enzyme was visualized by the peroxidase reaction. (Courtesy of Miss V. Petts.)

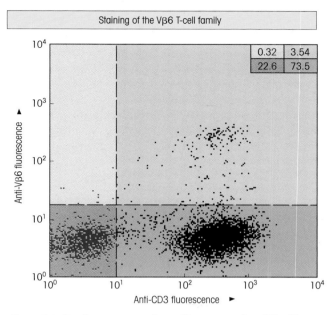

Figure 6.2 **Cytofluorimetric analysis of human peripheral blood lymphocytes.** Cells stained with fluoresceinated anti-TCR Vβ6 and phycoerythrin conjugated anti-CD3. Each dot represents an individual lymphocyte and the numbers refer to the percentage of lymphocytes lying within the four quadrants formed by the two gating levels arbitrarily used to segregate positive from negative values. Virtually no lymphocytes bearing the T-cell receptors belonging to the Vβ6 family lack CD3, while 4.6% (3.5 out of 77.0) of the mature T-cells express Vβ6. (Data kindly provided by D. Morrison.)

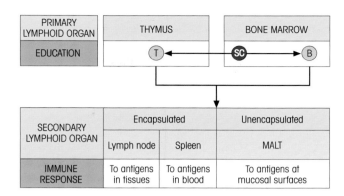

Figure 6.3 **The functional organization of lymphoid tissue.** Stem cells (SC) arising in the bone marrow differentiate into immunocompetent T- and B-cells in the primary lymphoid organs and then colonize the secondary lymphoid tissues where immune responses are organized. The mucosal-associated lymphoid tissue which produces the antibodies for mucosal secretions is often referred to as the MALT system.

lymphatics and by guided passage across the specialized **high-walled endothelial cells of the postcapillary venules (HEV)** (figure 6.5). Comparable endothelial cells offer transit to Peyer's patches of cells concerned in mucosal immunity. In other cases involving migration into normal and inflamed tissues, the lymphocytes bind to and cross nonspecialized flatter endothelia in response to locally produced mediators.

This highly organized traffic is orchestrated by directing the relevant lymphocytes to different parts of the lymphoid system and the various other tissues by a series of **homing receptors** which recognize their complementary ligands, termed **vascular addressins**, on the surface of the appropriate endothelial cells of the blood vessels. These act as selective gateways which allow lymphocytes access to the tissue in question.

Transmigration

Lymphocytes normally travel in the fast lane down the centre of the blood vessels. However, for the lymphocyte to become attached to the endothelial cell it has to overcome the shear forces that this creates. This is effected by a force of attraction between **selectins** and their ligands on the lymphocyte and vessel wall which operates through microvilli on the leukocyte surface. After this tethering process, the lymphocyte rolls along the endothelial cell, partly through the selectin interactions but now increasingly through the binding of various **integrins** to their respective ligands.

This process leads to activation and recruitment of members of the β_2 integrin family to the nonvillous surface of the lymphocyte. In particular, molecules such as LFA-1 (lymphocyte functional antigen-1) bind very strongly to ICAM-1 and 2 (intercellular adhesion molecule-1 and 2) on the endothelial cell, the intimate contact causing the lymphocyte to flatten (figure 6.6, step 4). The flattened lymphocyte may now elbow its way between the endothelial cells and into the tissue (figure 6.6, step 5)

Homing of either previously activated or memory lymphocytes to sites of inflammation provoked by infectious agents makes a great deal of sense. The same may be said for the mechanisms which enable lymphocytes bearing receptors for mucosal-associated lymphoid tissue (MALT) to circulate within and between the collections of lymphoid tissue guarding the external body surfaces (see figure 6.10).

ENCAPSULATED LYMPH NODES

The encapsulated tissue of the lymph node contains a meshwork of reticular cells and their fibers organized into sinuses. These act as a filter for lymph draining the body

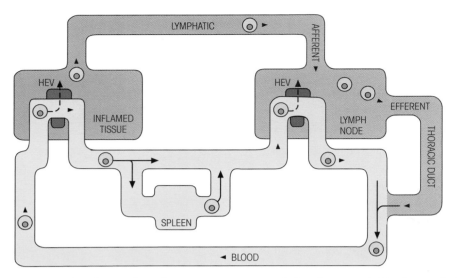

Figure 6.4 Traffic and recirculation of lymphocytes through encapsulated lymphoid tissue and sites of inflammation. Blood-borne lymphocytes enter the tissues and lymph nodes passing through the high-walled endothelium of the postcapillary venules (HEV) and leave via the draining lymphatics. The efferent lymphatics, finally emerging from the last node in each chain, join to form the thoracic duct, which returns the lymphocytes to the bloodstream. In the spleen, lymphocytes enter the lymphoid area (white pulp) from the arterioles, pass to the sinusoids of the erythroid area (red pulp) and leave by the splenic vein. Traffic through the mucosal immune system is elaborated in figure 6.10.

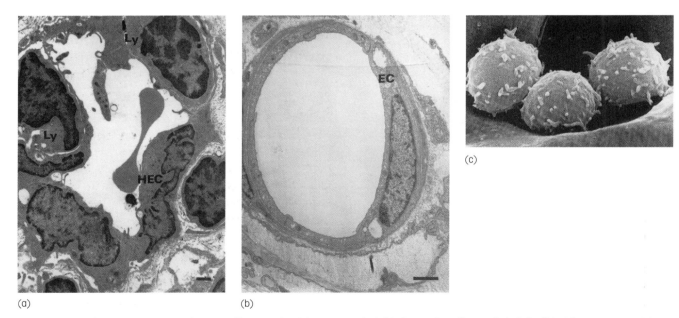

(a)   (b)

Figure 6.5 Lymphocyte association with postcapillary venules. (a) High-walled endothelial cells (HEC) of postcapillary venules in rat cervical lymph nodes showing intimate association with lymphocytes (Ly). (b) Flattened capillary endothelial cell (EC) for comparison. (c) Lymphocytes adhering to HEC (scanning electron micrograph). ((a) and (b) kindly provided by Dr Ann Ager and (c) by Dr W. van Ewijk.)

tissues and possibly bearing foreign antigens; this lymph enters the subcapsular sinus by the afferent vessels and diffuses past the lymphocytes in the cortex to reach the macrophages of the medullary sinuses (figure 6.7a,c) and thence the efferent lymphatics. What is so striking about the organization of the lymph node is that the T- and B-lymphocytes are very largely separated into different anatomical compartments.

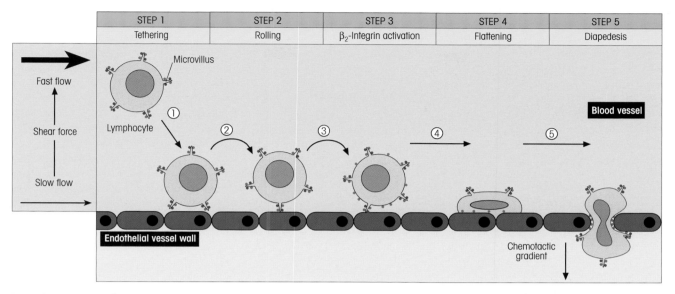

STEP 1	STEP 2	STEP 3	STEP 4	STEP 5
Tethering	Rolling	β_2-Integrin activation	Flattening	Diapedesis

Figure 6.6 Homing and transmigration of lymphocytes. Fast-moving lymphocytes are tethered (Step 1) to the vessel walls of the tissue they are being guided to enter through an interaction between specific homing receptors and their ligands. After rolling along the surface of the endothelial cells making up the vessel wall, activation of β_2 integrins occurs (Step 3) which leads to firm binding, cell flattening and (Step 5) migration of the lymphocyte between adjacent endothelial cells.

B-cell areas

The follicular aggregations of B-lymphocytes are a prominent feature of the outer cortex. In the unstimulated node they are present as spherical collections of cells termed **primary follicles** (figure 6.7f), which are composed of a mesh of follicular dendritic cells (FDC) whose spaces are filled with recirculating but resting small B-lymphocytes. After antigenic challenge they form **secondary follicles** which consist of a corona or mantle of concentrically packed, resting, small B-lymphocytes possessing both IgM and IgD on their surface surrounding a pale-staining **germinal center** (figure 6.7b,c). This contains large, usually proliferating, B-blasts and a tight network of specialized follicular dendritic cells. Germinal centers are greatly enlarged in secondary antibody responses (figure 6.7d) and they are regarded as important sites of B-cell maturation and the generation of B-cell memory.

A proportion of the B-cells which are shunted down the **memory** cell pathway take up residence in the mantle zone population, the remainder joining the recirculating B-cell pool. Other cells differentiate into plasmablasts, with a well-defined endoplasmic reticulum, prominent Golgi apparatus and cytoplasmic Ig; these migrate to become plasma cells in the medullary cords of lymphoid cells which project between the medullary sinuses. This maturation of antibody-forming cells at a site distant from that at which antigen triggering has occurred is also seen in the spleen, where plasma cells are found predominantly in the marginal zone. The remainder of the outer cortex is also essentially a B-cell area with scattered T-cells.

T-cell areas

T-cells are mainly confined to a region referred to as the paracortical (or thymus-dependent) area (figure 6.7a); in nodes taken from children with selective T-cell deficiency (figure 13.5) or neonatally thymectomized mice the para-cortical region is seen to be virtually devoid of lymphocytes (figure 6.7f). Furthermore, when a T-cell-mediated response is elicited, say by a skin graft or by exposure to poison ivy which induces contact hypersensitivity, there is a marked proliferation of cells in the thymus-dependent area and typical lymphoblasts are evident (figure 6.7e). In contrast, stimulation of antibody formation by thymus-independent antigens leads to proliferation in the cortical lymphoid follicles with development of germinal centers, while the paracortical region remains inactive (figure 6.7d). As expected, nodes taken from children with congenital hypogammaglobulinemia associated with failure of B-cell development conspicuously lack primary and secondary follicles.

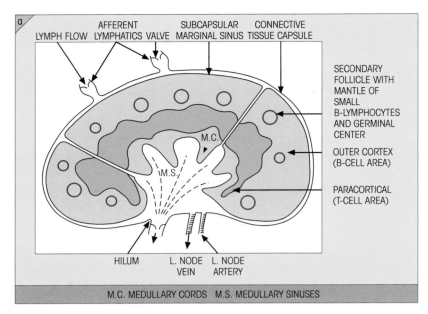

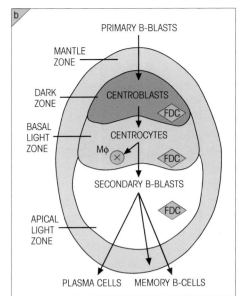

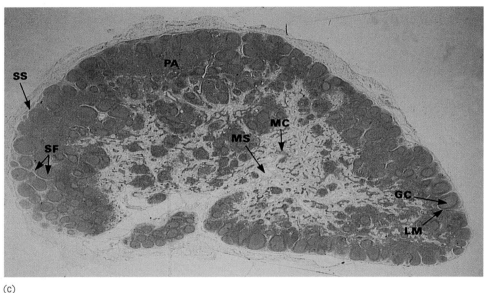

(c)

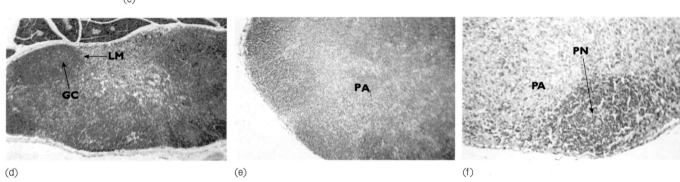

(d)   (e)   (f)

Figure 6.7 Lymph node. (a) Diagrammatic representation of section through a whole node. (b) Diagram showing differentiation of B-cells during passage through different regions of an active germinal center. FDC = follicular dendritic cell; Mφ = macrophage; × = apoptotic B-cell. (c) Human lymph node, low-power view. (d) Secondary lymphoid follicle showing germinal center in a mouse immunized with the thymus-independent antigen, pneumococcus polysaccharide SIII, revealing prominent stimulation of secondary follicles with germinal centers. (e) Methyl Green/Pyronin stain of lymph node draining site of skin painted with the contact sensitizer oxazolone, highlighting the generalized expansion and activation of the paracortical T-cells, the T-blasts being strongly basophilic. (f) The same study in a neonatally thymectomized mouse shows a lonely primary nodule (follicle) with complete lack of cellular response in the paracortical area. SS = subcapsular sinus; PN = primary nodule; SF = secondary follicle; LM = lymphocyte mantle of SF; GC = germinal center; PA = paracortical area; MC = medullary cords; MS = medullary sinus; ((d–f) courtesy of Dr M. de Sousa and Professor D.M.V. Parrott.)

SPLEEN

On a fresh section of spleen, the lymphoid tissue forming the white pulp is seen as circular or elongated gray areas (figure 6.8b,c) within the erythrocyte-filled red pulp consisting of splenic cords lined with macrophages and venous sinusoids. As in the lymph node, T- and B-cell areas are segregated (figure 6.8a). The spleen is a very effective blood filter, removing effete red and white cells and responding actively to blood-borne antigens, the more so if particulate. Plas-

mablasts and mature plasma cells are present in the marginal zone extending into the red pulp (figure 6.8c).

MUCOSAL-ASSOCIATED LYMPHOID TISSUE (MALT)

The respiratory, alimentary and genitourinary tracts are guarded immunologically by subepithelial accumulations of lymphoid tissue which are not constrained by a connective tissue capsule (figure 6.9). These may occur as diffuse collec-

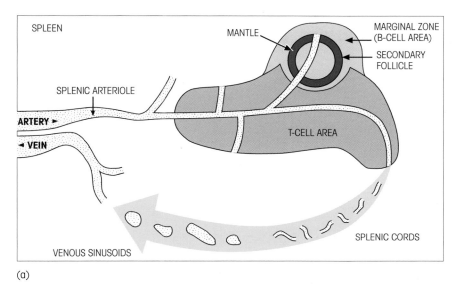

(a)

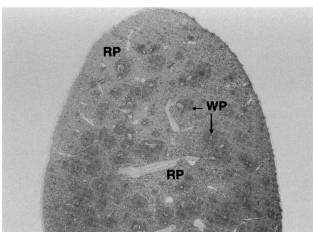

(b)

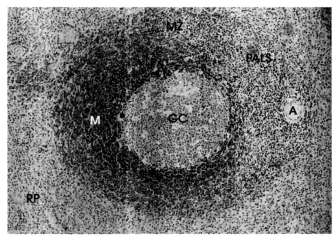

(c)

Figure 6.8 Spleen. (a) Diagrammatic representation. (b) Low-power view showing lymphoid white pulp (WP) and red pulp (RP). (c) High-power view of germinal center (GC) and lymphocyte mantle (M) surrounded by marginal zone (MZ) and red pulp (RP). Adjacent to the follicle, an arteriole (A) is surrounded by the periarteriolar lymphoid sheath (PALS) predominantly consisting of T-cells. Note that the marginal zone is only present above the secondary follicle. ((b) Photographed by Professor P.M. Lydyard and (c) by Professor Novica Milicevic.)

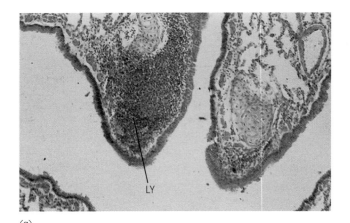

(a)

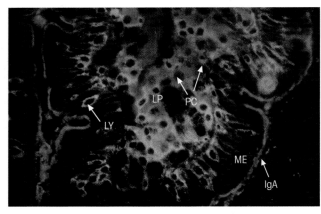

(b)

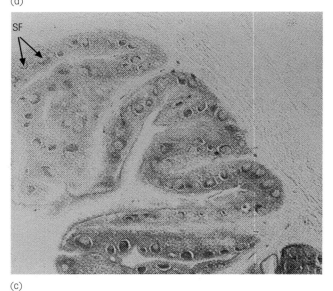

(c)

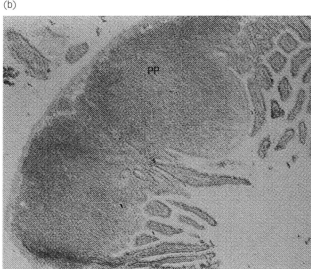

(d)

Figure 6.9 The IgA secretory immune system (MALT). (a) Section of lung showing a diffuse accumulation of lymphocytes (LY) in the bronchial wall. (b) Section of human jejunum showing lymphoid cells (LY) stained green by a fluorescent anti-leukocyte monoclonal antibody, in the mucosal epithelium (ME) and in the lamina propria (LP). A red fluorescent anti-IgA conjugate stains the cytoplasm of plasma cells (PC) in the lamina propria and detects IgA in the surface mucus, alto-gether a super picture! (c) Low-power view of human tonsil showing the MALT with numerous secondary follicles (SF) containing germinal centers. (d) Peyer's patches (PP) in mouse ileum. The T-cell areas are stained brown by a peroxidase-labeled monoclonal antibody to Thy 1. ((a) Kindly provided by Professor P. Lydyard, (b) by Professor G. Jannosy, (c) by Mr C. Symes and (d) by Dr E. Andrew.)

tions of lymphocytes, plasma cells and phagocytes throughout the lung and the lamina propria of the intestinal wall (figure 6.9a,b) or as more clearly organized tissue with well-formed follicles. The latter includes tonsils (figure 6.9c), the small intestinal Peyer's patches (figure 6.9d) and the appendix. It is generally agreed that this MALT forms a separate interconnected secretory system within which cells committed to IgA or IgE synthesis may circulate.

In the gut, antigen enters the Peyer's patches (figure 6.9d) across specialized epithelial cells called M-cells (cf figure 6.11) and stimulates the antigen-sensitive lymphocytes. After activation these drain into the lymph and after a journey through the mesenteric lymph nodes and the thoracic duct, they pass from the bloodstream into the lamina propria (figure 6.10) where they become IgA-forming cells which, because they are now broadly distributed, protect a wide area of the bowel with protective antibody. The cells also appear in the lymphoid tissue of the lung and in other mucosal sites guided by the interactions of specific homing receptors with appropriate HEC addressins as discussed earlier.

Intestinal lymphocytes

The intestinal **lamina propria** is home to a predominantly

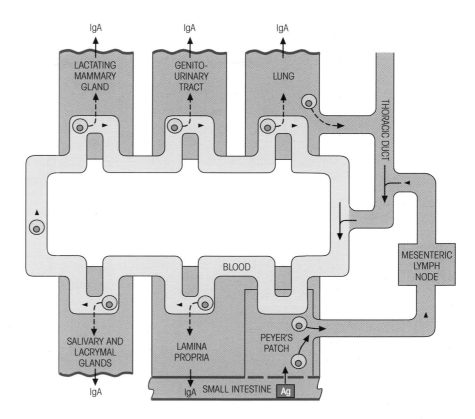

Figure 6.10 Circulation of lymphocytes within the mucosal-associated lymphoid system. Antigen-stimulated cells move from Peyer's patches (and probably lung and maybe all the mucosal member sites) to colonize the lamina propria and the other mucosal surfaces (⌇⌇⌇).

activated T-cell population comparable to that of peripheral blood lymphocytes, characterized by > 95% T-cell receptor (TCR) αβ and a CD4 : CD8 ratio of 7 : 3. There is also a generous sprinkling of activated B-blasts and plasma cells secreting IgA for transport by the poly-Ig receptor to the **intestinal lumen. Intraepithelial lymphocytes**, however, are also mostly T-cells but 10–40% are TCR γδ+ cells. This relatively high proportion of TCR γδ cells is unusual.

THE ENJOYMENT OF PRIVILEGED SITES

Certain selected parts of the body, brain, anterior chamber of the eye and testis have been designated **privileged immunologic sites**, in the sense that antigens located within them do not provoke reactions against themselves. It has long been known, for example, that foreign corneal grafts are not usually rejected even without immunosuppressive therapy.

Generally speaking, privileged sites are protected by rather strong blood–tissue barriers and low permeability to hydrophilic compounds. Functionally insignificant levels of complement reduce the threat of acute inflammatory reac-

tions and unusually high concentrations of immunomodulators, such as transforming growth factor-β (TGFβ) endow macrophages with an immunosuppressive capacity.

However, inflammatory reactions at the blood–tissue barrier can open the gates to invasion by immunologic marauders — witness the inability of corneal grafts to take in the face of a local pre-existing inflammation.

THE HANDLING OF ANTIGEN

Where does antigen go when it enters the body? If it penetrates the tissues, it will tend to finish up in the draining lymph nodes. Antigens which are encountered in the upper respiratory tract or intestine are trapped by local mucosal-associated lymphoid tissue, whereas antigens in the blood provoke a reaction in the spleen.

Macrophages are general antigen-presenting cells

It has always been recognized that antigens draining into lymphoid tissue are taken up by macrophages. They are then partially, if not completely, broken down in the lysosomes; some may escape from the cell in a soluble form to be taken up by other antigen-presenting cells and a fraction may reappear at the surface, as a processed peptide associated with class II major histocompatibility molecules. Some antigens, such as polymeric carbohydrates, cannot be degraded because the macrophages lack the enzymes required; in these instances, specialized macrophages in the marginal zone of the spleen or the lymph node subcapsular sinus, trap and present the antigen to B-cells directly, apparently without any processing or intervention from T-cells.

Interdigitating dendritic cells present antigen to T-lymphocytes

Cells other than macrophages prime T-helper cells and it is now generally accepted that these belong to the group of dendritic cells which can display the surface costimulatory molecules B7 and CD40 (cf. pp. 65 and 68) and additionally secrete interleukin-2 (IL-2), IL-4 and γ-interferon (IFNγ), which are important for lymphocyte activation. The dendritic cells have the awesome capacity to process four times their own volume of extracellular fluid in one hour thereby facilitating antigen capture and processing in their abundant intracellular MHC class II-rich compartments.

The scenario for T-cell priming appears to be as follows. Peripheral immature dendritic cells such as the Langerhans' cells, can pick up and process antigen. As maturation proceeds, they settle down as interdigitating dendritic cells (IDC) in the paracortical T-cell zone of the draining lymph node. There, its maturation complete, the IDC delivers the antigen with costimulatory signals to naive specific T-cells which take advantage of the large surface area to bind to the MHC–peptide complex on the IDC membrane. Sites of chronic T-cell inflammation seem to attract these cells, since abnormally high numbers are found closely adhering to activated T-lymphocytes in synovial tissue from patients with ongoing rheumatoid arthritis and in the glands of subjects with chronic autoimmune thyroiditis lesions.

An important take-home message is that whereas macrophages and dendritic cells at all stages of maturity can present antigen to preactivated T-cells, only mature dendritic cells are capable of priming naive T-cells.

Follicular dendritic cells stimulate B-cells in germinal centers

Secondary antibody responses can be boosted by quite small amounts of immunogen which complex with circulating antibody and fix C3 so that they localize very effectively on the surface of the follicular dendritic cells within the germinal centers of secondary follicles. These cells have very elongated processes which can make contact with numerous lymphocytes, and their surface receptors for IgG Fc and C3b enable them to trap the complexed antigen very efficiently and hold the antigen on their surface for extended periods, in keeping with the memory function of secondary follicles.

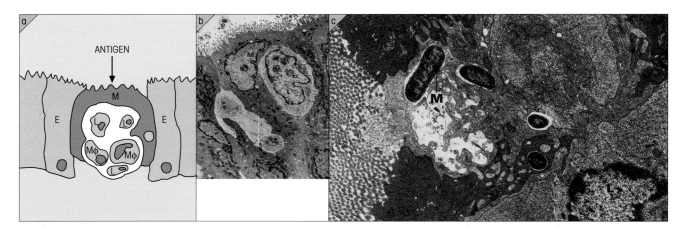

Figure 6.11 M-cell within Peyer's patch epithelium. (a) After uptake and transcellular transport by the M-cell, antigen is processed by macrophages and thence by dendritic cells which present antigen to T-cells in Peyer's patches and mesenteric lymph nodes. E = enterocyte; Mφ = macrophage; L = lymphocyte. (b) Electron photomicrograph of an M-cell (M in nucleus) with adjacent lymphocyte (L in nucleus). Note the flanking epithelial cells are both absorptive epithelial cells with a typical brush border. Lead citrate and uranyl acetate, × 1600. (c) An M-cell and an adjacent lymphocyte (L). A rod-shaped bacterium taken up from the intestinal lumen and packaged within an M-cell vesicle is indicated. Lead citrate and uranyl acetate, × 4600. ((a) Based on Sminia T. (1992) In: *Encyclopedia of Immunology* (eds Roitt I.M. & P.J. Delves), p. 107. Academic Press, London.)

M-cells provide the gateway to the mucosal lymphoid system

The mucosal surface is in the front line facing a very unfriendly sea of microbes and, for the most part, antigens are excluded by the epithelium with its tight junctions and mucous layer. Gut lymphoid tissue, such as Peyer's patches, is separated from the lumen by a single layer of columnar epithelium interspersed with M-cells; these are specialized antigen-transporting cells. They overlay intraepithelial cells and macrophage-like dendritic cells (figure 6.11). A diverse array of foreign material including bacteria is taken up by M-cells (figure 6.11) and passed on to the underlying antigen-presenting cells which, in turn, migrate to the local lymphoid tissue to stir the appropriate lymphocytes into action.

REVISION

See the accompanying website (www.roitt.com) for multiple choice questions.

The surface markers of cells in the immune system
• Individual surface molecules are assigned a cluster of differentiation (CD) number defined by a cluster of monoclonal antibodies reacting with that molecule.
• Antigens can be localized if stained by fluorescent antibodies and viewed in an appropriate microscope.
• Antibodies can be labeled by enzymes for histochemical definition of antigens.
• Cells in suspension can be labeled with fluorescent antibodies and analysed in a flow cytometer.

Organized lymphoid tissue
• The complexity of immune responses is catered for by a sophisticated structure.
• Lymph nodes filter and screen lymph flowing from the body tissues while spleen filters the blood.
• B- and T-cell areas are separated.
• B-cell structures appear in the lymph node cortex as primary nodules which become secondary follicles with germinal centers after antigen stimulation.
• Germinal centers with their meshwork of follicular dendritic cells expand B-cell blasts produced by secondary antigen challenge and direct their differentiation into memory cells and antibody-forming plasma cells.

Mucosal-associated lymphoid tissue
• Lymphoid tissue guarding the gastrointestinal tract is unencapsulated and somewhat structured (tonsils, Peyer's patches, appendix) or present as diffuse cellular collections in the lamina propria.
• Together with the subepithelial accumulations of cells lining the mucosal surfaces of the respiratory and genitourinary tracts, this lymphoid tissue forms the 'secretory immune system' which bathes the surface with protective IgA antibodies.

Other sites
• Bone marrow is a major site of antibody production.
• The brain, anterior chamber of the eye and testis are privileged sites in which antigens can be safely sequestered.

Lymphocyte traffic
• Lymphocyte recirculation between the blood and lymphoid tissues is guided by specialized homing receptors on the surface of the high-walled endothelium of the postcapillary venules.
• Lymphocytes are tethered and then roll along the surface of the selected endothelial cells through interactions between selectins and integrins and their respective ligands. Flattening of the lymphocyte and transmigration across the endothelial cell follow LFA-1 activation.
• Entry of memory T-cells into sites of inflammation is facilitated by upregulation of integrin molecules on the lymphocyte and corresponding binding ligands on the vascular endothelium

The handling of antigen
• Macrophages are general antigen-presenting cells for primed lymphocytes but cannot stimulate naive T-cells.
• T-cell stimulation is effected by dendritic cells which process antigen, migrate to the draining lymph node and settle down as interdigitating dendritic cells which powerfully initiate primary T-cell responses.
• Follicular dendritic cells in germinal centers bind immune complexes to their surface through Ig and C3b receptors. The complexes are long-lived and provide a sustained source of antigenic stimulation for B-cells.
• Specialized antigen-transporting M-cells provide the gateway for antigens to the mucosal lymphoid tissue.

FURTHER READING

Benner R., Hijmans W. & Haaijman J.J. (1981) The bone marrow: the major source of serum immunoglobulins, but still a neglected site of antibody formation. *Clinical and Experimental Immunology* **46**, 1–8.

Bradley L.M. & Watson S.R. (1996) Lymphocyte migration into tissue: the paradigm derived from CD4 subsets. *Current Opinion in Immunology* **8**, 312–320.

Brandtzaaeg P., Farstad I.N. & Haraldsen G. (1999) Regional specialization in the mucosal immune system: primed cells do not always home along the same track. *Immunology Today* **20** (6), 267.

Caligaris-Cappio F. (1992) Germinal centres. In: *Encyclopedia of Immunology* (eds I.M. Roitt & P.J. Delves), p. 613. Academic Press, London.

Girard J.-P. & Springer T.A. (1995) High endothelial (HEVs): specialized endothelium for lymphocyte migration. *Immunology Today* **16**, 449–457.

Hirsch E., Iglesias A. *et al.* (1996) Impaired migration but not differentiation of haematopoietic stem cells in the absence of β_1 integrins. *Nature* **380** (6570), 171–175.

Lane P.J.L. & Brocker T. (1999) Developmental regulation of dendritic cell function. *Current Opinion in Immunology* **11** (3), 308.

Peters J.H., Gieseler R., Thiele B. & Steinbach F. (1996) Dendritic cells: from ontogenetic orphans to myelomonocytic descendants. *Immunology Today* **17**, 273–278.

Poussier P. & Julius M. (eds) (1995) T-cell development and selection in the intestinal epithelium. *Seminars in Immunology* **7**, 289–342.

Stingl G. (1995) Dendritic cells: a major story unfolds. *Immunology Today* **16**, 330–333.

Tew J.G. (ed.) (1992) Antigen trapping and presentation. *Seminars in Immunology* **4**, 203–274.

CHAPTER 7

Lymphocyte activation

IMMUNOCOMPETENT T- AND B-CELLS DIFFER IN MANY RESPECTS

The differences between immunocompetent T- and B-cells are sharply demarcated at the cell surface (table 7.1). The most clear-cut discrimination is established by reagents which recognize anti-CD3 for T-cells and anti-CD19 or anti-CD20 for B-cells. In laboratory practice these are the markers most often used to enumerate the two lymphocyte populations. B-cells also demonstrate immunoglobulin on their surface and they express receptors for Ig, C3b and certain viruses.

Differences in the cluster of differentiation (CD) markers determined by monoclonal antibodies reflect disparate functional properties and in particular define specialized T-cell subsets. CD4 is a marker of T-helper cell populations, which promote activation and maturation of B-cells and cytotoxic T-cells, and control antigen-specific chronic inflammatory reactions through stimulation of macrophages. CD4 molecules form subsidiary links with class II MHC on antigen-presenting cells. Similarly, the CD8 molecules on cytotoxic T-cells associate with major histocompatibility complex (MHC) class I (figure 7.1).

T-LYMPHOCYTES AND ANTIGEN-PRESENTING CELLS INTERACT THROUGH SEVERAL PAIRS OF ACCESSORY MOLECULES

The affinity of an individual TCR for its specific MHC–antigen peptide complex is relatively low and a sufficiently stable association with the antigen-presenting cell (APC) can only be achieved by the interaction of complementary pairs of accessory molecules such as LFA-1/ICAM-1 and CD2/LFA-3 (figure 7.2). However, these molecular couplings are not necessarily concerned just with intercellular adhesion.

THE ACTIVATION OF T-CELLS REQUIRES TWO SIGNALS

It has been known for some time that two signals are required to induce RNA and protein synthesis in a resting T-cell (figure 7.2) and to move it from G0 into the G1 phase of the mitotic cycle. Antigen in association with MHC class II on the surface of APCs is clearly capable of fulfilling these requirements. Complex formation between the TCR, antigen and MHC provides signal 1 through the receptor–CD3 complex, and this is greatly enhanced by the coupling of CD4 with the MHC. The T-cell is now exposed to a costimulatory signal 2 from the APC in the form of the B7 molecule on the APC binding to CD28 on the T-helper cell, and also to a receptor called CTLA-4 on activated T-cells. Thus activation of resting T-cells can be blocked by anti-B7; surprisingly, this renders the T-cell **anergic**, i.e. unresponsive to any further stimulation by antigen. As we shall see in later chapters, the principle that two signals activate but one may induce anergy in an antigen-specific cell, provides a potential for targeted immunosuppressive therapy. Unlike resting T-lymphocytes, **activated T-cells proliferate in response to a *single* signal**.

Adhesion molecules such as ICAM-1, VCAM-1 (vascular cell adhesion molecule-1) and LFA-3 are not themselves costimulatory but augment the effect of other signals—an important distinction.

PROTEIN TYROSINE PHOSPHORYLATION IS AN EARLY EVENT IN T-CELL SIGNALING

The major docking forces which conjugate the APC and its T-lymphocyte counterpart come from the complementary accessory molecules such as ICAM-1, LFA-1 and LFA-3/CD2, rather than through the relatively low-affinity TCR–MHC/peptide links. Nonetheless, cognate antigen recognition by the TCR remains a *sine qua non* for T-cell

Table 7.1 Comparison of human T- and B-cells.

	T	B
% in peripheral blood	65–80	8–15
ANTIGEN RECEPTORS:		
Surface Ig	–	+ +
TCR/CD3	+ +	–
OTHER MARKERS	CD2 *4/5/*8/45	CD *5/19/23/40/45
MHC: Class I	+ +**	+ +
Class II	+ +**	+ +
POLYCLONAL ACTIVATION	anti-CD3	anti-Ig
	phytohemagglutinin (PHA)	*Staph. aureus* (str. Cowan 1)
	pokeweed mitogen (PWM)	pokeweed mitogen (PWM)
	concanavalin A	
	*superantigen (e.g. enterotoxin)	EBV

*subpopulation; **only activated cells; CD2 receptor forming sheep cell rosettes; CR1/2 complement receptors 1/2; EBV Epstein–Barr virus

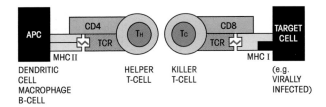

Figure 7.1 Helper and killer T-cell subsets are restricted by MHC class. CD4 on helpers contacts MHC class II; CD8 on killers associates with class I.

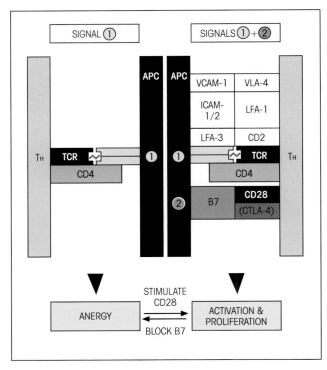

Figure 7.2 Activation of resting T-cells. Interaction of costimulatory molecules leads to activation of resting T-lymphocyte by antigen-presenting cell (APC) on engagement of the T-cell receptor (TCR) with its antigen–MHC complex. Engagement of the TCR signal 1 without accompanying costimulatory signal 2 leads to anergy. Note, a cytotoxic rather than a helper T-cell would, of course, involve coupling CD8 to MHC I. Engagement of the CTLA-4 molecule (CD152) with B7 down-regulates signal 1. LFA-1/2 = lymphocyte function associated molecule-1/2; ICAM-1/2 = intercellular adhesion molecule-1/2; VLA-4 = very late integrin antigen-4; VCAM-1 = vascular cell adhesion molecule-1. (Based on Liu Y. & Linsley P.S. (1992) *Current Opinion in Immunology* **4**, 265–270.)

activation. Interaction of the TCR with peptide bound to MHC molecules triggers a remarkable cascade of signaling events that culminates in cell cycle progression and cytokine production. This begins with phosphorylation by src-family kinases of tyrosine residues present within a tyrosine-containing structural motif (ITAM) in the cytoplasmic tails of portions of the CD3 molecule. This recruits and activates ZAP-70 (zeta chain associated protein kinase), which now becomes an active protein tyrosine kinase (PTK) (figure 7.3) capable of initiating a series of downstream biochemical events. It is now becoming clear that very large numbers of T-cell receptors interact with only a few peptide–MHC complexes, and it has been suggested that each MHC–peptide complex can serially engage up to 200 TCRs. This they do for a prolonged period of time during which the TCRs move across the surface of the APC. As they do so they undergo a sustained increase in intracellular calcium levels which is required for the induction of T-cell proliferation and cytokine production.

THE NATURE OF B-CELL ACTIVATION

B-cells are stimulated by cross-linking surface Ig

Cross-linking of B-cell surface receptors, for example by thymus independent antigens, induces the early activation events. Within one minute of surface Ig ligation, there is rapid phosphorylation of the sIg receptor chains Ig-α and Ig-β and a subsequent rise in intracellular calcium and activation of phosphokinase C.

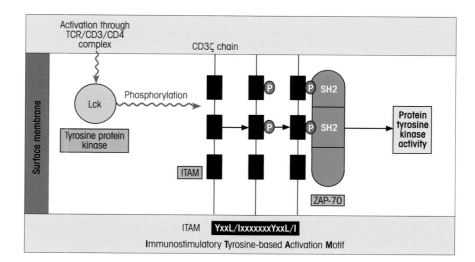

Figure 7.3 Signals through the TCR/CD3/CD4/8 complex initiate a tyrosine protein kinase (TPK) cascade. The TPK lck phosphorylates the tyrosine within the ITAM sequences of CD3 ζ-chains. These bind the ζ-associated protein (ZAP-70) through its SH2 domains and this in turn acquires TPK activity for downstream phosphorylation of later components in the chain. The other CD3 chains each bear a single ITAM.

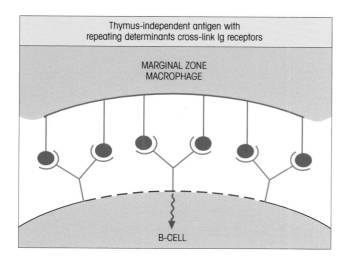

Figure 7.4 B-cell recognition of thymus-independent antigens. The complex gives a sustained signal to the B-cell because of the long half-life of this type of molecule. ∿➤ = activation signal; ⫶ = surface Ig receptor; – – – = cross-linking of receptors.

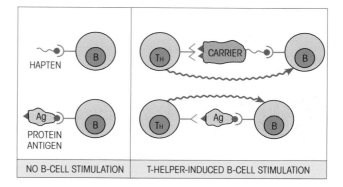

Figure 7.5 T-helper cells cooperate through protein carrier determinants to help B-cells respond to hapten or equivalent determinants on antigens by providing accessory signals. (For simplicity we are ignoring the MHC component and epitope processing in T-cell recognition, but we won't forget it.)

B-cells respond to T-independent and T-dependent antigens

Thymus-independent antigens

Certain linear antigens which are not readily degraded in the body and which have an appropriately spaced, highly repeating determinant such as the *Pneumococcus* polysaccharide, are thymus independent in their ability to stimulate B-cells directly without the need for T-cell involvement. They persist for long periods on the surface of specialized macrophages located at the subcapsular sinus of the lymph nodes and the splenic marginal zone and they bind to antigen-specific B-cells with great avidity through their multivalent attachment to the complementary Ig receptors which they cross-link (figure 7.4). This cross-linking induces early B-cell activation events. In general, the thymus-independent antigens give rise to predominantly low-affinity IgM responses, and relatively poor, if any, memory.

Thymus-dependent antigens

Many antigens are thymus-dependent in that they provoke little or no antibody response in animals which have been thymectomized at birth. Such antigens cannot fulfil the molecular requirements for direct stimulation and if they bind to B-cell receptors, they will sit on the surface just like a hapten and do nothing to trigger the B-cell (figure 7.5). Cast

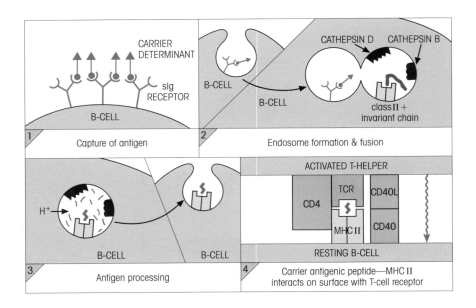

Figure 7.6 B-cell handling of a thymus-dependent antigen. Antigen captured by the surface Ig receptor is internalized within an endosome, processed and expressed on the surface with MHC class II (cf. figure 5.8). Costimulatory signals through the CD40–CD40L interaction are required for activation of the resting cell by the T-helper. ⟿ = activation signal; ⑂⑂⑂ = cross-linking of receptors.

your mind back to the definition of a hapten—a small molecule which binds to preformed antibody (e.g. the surface receptor of a specific B-cell) but fails to stimulate antibody production (i.e. stimulate the B-cell). Remember also that haptens become immunogenic when coupled to an appropriate carrier protein (see p. 44). Building on the knowledge that both T- and B-cells are necessary for antibody responses to thymus-dependent antigens, we now know that the carrier functions to stimulate T-helper cells, which cooperate with B-cells to enable them to respond to the hapten by providing accessory signals (figure 7.5). It should also be evident from figure 7.5 that while one determinant on a typical protein antigen is behaving as a hapten in binding to the B-cell, the other determinants subserve a carrier function in recruiting T-helper cells.

Primed B-cells can present antigen to T-helper cells which in turn activate B-cells

B-cells function at much lower antigen concentrations than conventional presenting cells because they can focus antigen through their surface receptors. Antigen bound to surface Ig is internalized in endosomes which then fuse with vesicles containing MHC class II molecules with their invariant chain. Processing of the protein antigen then occurs as described in Chapter 5 and the resulting antigenic peptide is then recycled to the surface in association with the class II molecules. There it is available for recognition by the TCR on a carrier-specific T-helper cell (figure 7.6). With the assistance of costimulatory signals arising from the interaction of **CD40 with its ligand CD40L**, B-cell activation is ensured.

REVISION

See the accompanying website (www.roitt.com) for multiple choice questions.

Immunocompetent T- and B-cells differ in many respects
• Markers relating to the antigen-specific receptors TCR/CD3 on T-cells and surface Ig on B-cells provide clear discrimination.
• Differences in CD markers define specialized T-cell subsets.

T-lymphocytes and antigen-presenting cells interact through pairs of accessory molecules
• The docking of T-cells and APCs depends upon strong mutual interactions between complementary molecular pairs on their surfaces: MHC II/CD4; MHC I/CD8; ICAM-1/LFA-1; LFA-3/CD2; B7/CD28 (and CTLA-4) respectively.

Activation of T-cells requires two signals
- Two signals activate T-cells, but one alone produces unresponsiveness (anergy).
- One signal is provided by the low-affinity cognate TCR/MHC–peptide interaction.
- The second costimulatory signal is mediated through ligation of CD28 by B7.

Protein tyrosine phosphorylation is an early event in T-cell signaling
- The TCR signal is transduced and amplified through a protein tyrosine kinase (PTK) enzymic cascade.
- Large numbers of T-cell receptors interact with only a few peptide–MHC complexes.

 As activation proceeds intracellular calcium levels increase.

B-cells respond to two different types of antigen
- Thymus-independent antigens are polymeric molecules which cross-link many sIg receptors and, because of their long half-lives, provide a persistent signal to the B-cell.
- Thymus-dependent antigens require the cooperation of helper T-cells to stimulate antibody production by B-cells.
- Antigen captured by specific sIg receptors is taken into the B-cell, processed, and expressed on the surface as a peptide in association with MHC II.
- This complex is recognized by the T-helper cell, which activates the resting B-cell.

The nature of B-cell activation
- Cross-linking of surface Ig receptors (e.g. thymus-independent antigens) activates B-cells.
- T-helper cells activate resting B-cells through TCR recognition of MHC II–carrier peptide complexes and costimulation through CD40L/CD40 interactions (analogous to the B7/CD28 second signal for T-cell activation).

FURTHER READING

Borst J. & Cope A. (1999) Turning the immune system on. *Immunology Today* **20** (4), 156.

Linsley P.S. & Reth M. (eds) (1999) Section on Lymphocyte Activation and Effector Functions. *Current Opinion in Immunology* **11** (3).

Swain S.L. & Cambier J.C. (eds) (1996) Lymphocyte activation and effector functions. *Current Opinion in Immunology* **8**, 309–418.

Valitutti S. *et al.* (1995) Serial triggering of many T-cell receptors by a few peptide–MHC complexes. *Nature* **375**, 148.

Ward S.G., June C.H. & Olive D. (1996) PI 3-kinase: a pivotal pathway in T-cell activation? *Immunology Today* **17**, 187.

CHAPTER 8

The production of effectors

A SUCCESSION OF GENES ARE UPREGULATED BY T-CELL ACTIVATION

We have dwelt upon the early events in lymphocyte activation consequent upon the engagement of the T-cell receptor (TCR) and the provision of an appropriate costimulatory signal. A complex series of tyrosine and serine/threonine phosphorylation reactions produces the factors which push the cell into the mitotic cycle and drive clonal proliferation and differentiation to effector cells. Within the first half hour, nuclear transcription factors which regulate interleukin-2 (IL-2) expression and the cellular proto-oncogene c-*myc* are expressed, but the next few hours see the synthesis of a range of **soluble cytokines and their receptors** (figure 8.1). Much later we see molecules like the transferrin receptor related to cell division and very late antigens such as the adhesion molecule VLA-1.

CYTOKINES ACT AS INTERCELLULAR MESSENGERS

In contrast with the initial activation of T-cells and T-dependent B-cells, which involves intimate contact with the antigen-presenting cells (APCs), subsequent proliferation and maturation of the response is orchestrated by the cytokines, which relay information between cells as soluble messengers. A list of these protein mediators is shown in table 8.1.

Cytokine action is transient and usually short range

These low molecular weight secreted proteins mediate cell growth, inflammation, immunity, differentiation and repair. They are highly potent, often acting at femtomolar (10^{-15} M) concentrations, combining with small numbers of high-affinity cell surface receptors to produce changes in the pattern of RNA and protein synthesis. Unlike endocrine hor-

mones, the majority of cytokines normally act locally in a paracrine or even autocrine fashion. Thus lymphokines, the lymphoid cytokines, rarely persist in the circulation, but nonlymphoid cells such as macrophages can be triggered by bacterial products to release cytokines which may be detected in the bloodstream, often to the detriment of the host. Certain cytokines, including interleukin-1 (IL-1) and tumor necrosis factor (TNF), also exist in membrane forms which could exert their stimulatory effects without becoming soluble.

Cytokines often have multiple effects

In general, cytokines are **pleiotropic**, i.e. with multiple effects on growth and differentiation of a variety of cell types (table 8.1), and there is considerable overlapping and redundancy between them, partially accounted for by the induction of synthesis of common proteins.

Their roles in the generation of T- and B-cell effectors, and in the regulation of chronic inflammatory reactions (figure 8.2a,b) will be discussed at length later in this chapter. We should note here the important role of cytokines in the control of hematopoiesis (figure 8.2c). Thus we now realize that the differentiation of stem cells to become the formed elements of blood within the environment of the bone marrow is carefully nurtured through production of cytokines such as GM-CSF (granulocyte macrophage-colony stimulating factor) by the stromal cells or by T-cells or macrophages. It is not surprising, therefore, that during a period of inflammation, the cytokines that are produced recruit new precursors into the hematopoietic differentiation pathway giving rise to the leukocytosis so often seen in patients with active infection.

Network interactions

The complex and integrated relationships between the different cytokines are mediated through cellular events. For example, the genes for IL-3, 4 and 5 and GM-CSF are all

ACTIVATION	0 min		
EARLY	15 min	cfos/cjun	Nuclear binding transcription factor; binds to AP-1
		c-myc	Cellular oncogene; controls G0 → G1
	30 min	Nur77	Function in TCR-mediated apoptosis in immature T-cells
		NFAT	Nuclear transcription factor of activated-T; regulates IL-2 gene
		NFκB	Nuclear binding protein; regulates expression of many genes
		IκB-α	Inhibitor of NFκB
		PAC-1	Nuclear phosphatase which inactivates ERKs
MEDIUM TERM	Several hours	IL-2/3/4/5/6	Cytokines and their receptors influencing growth and differentiation of myeloid and lymphoid cells, controlling viral growth and mediating chronic inflammatory processes
		IL-9/10/13	
		GM-CSF	
		IFNγ TGFβ	
LATE	14h	Transferrin receptor	Related to cell division
	16h	c-myb	Cellular oncogene
	3-5 days	Class II MHC	Antigen presentation
	7-14 days	VLA-1	Very late 'antigen'; adhesion molecule

Figure 8.1 Sequential gene activation on T-cell stimulation, appearance of mRNA.

tightly linked on chromosome 5 in a region containing genes for M-CSF (macrophage-colony stimulating factor) and its receptor and several other growth factors and receptors. Interaction may occur through a cascade in which one cytokine induces the production of another, through trans-modulation of the receptor for another cytokine and through synergism or antagonism of two cytokines acting on the same cell (figure 8.3). Furthermore, many cytokines share the same signaling pathways and this too may contribute to the redundancy in their effect.

DIFFERENT CD4 T-CELL SUBSETS CAN MAKE DIFFERENT CYTOKINE PATTERNS

The bipolar Tн1 /Tн2 concept

The T-helper cells can be classified into one of two subsets, either Tн1 or Tн2 , with distinct patterns of cytokine secretion. Tн1 cells, which secrete γ-interferon (IFNγ) and IL-2, promote cell-mediated immunity, especially cytotoxic and delayed hypersensitivity reactions and macrophage activa-

tion. Tн2 cells, which secrete IL-4, IL-5, IL-6 and IL-10, activate B-lymphocytes resulting in upregulation of antibody production. The characteristic cytokines produced by Tн1 and Tн2 cells have mutually inhibitory effects on the reciprocal phenotype. IFNγ will inhibit the proliferation of Tн2 cells and IL-10 will downregulate Tн1 cells. Although the factors involved in directing immune responses to these two subpopulations are not fully elucidated, it appears that the cytokine environment in which these cells develop may influence their ultimate phenotype. Therefore IL-12 produced by antigen-presenting cells will stimulate IFNγ production from NK cells, and both these cytokines will drive differentiation of Tн1 cells and inhibit Tн2 responses. On the other side of the coin, when T-helper cells are activated by antigen in the presence of IL-4 they develop into Tн2 cells (figure 8.4).

The different patterns of cytokine production by these T-cell subtypes are of importance in protection against different classes of microorganisms. Tн1 cells producing lymphokines like IFNγ would be especially effective against viruses and intracellular organisms which grow in macrophages. Tн2 cells are very good helpers for B-cells and

Table 8.1 Cytokines: their origin and function.

CYTOKINE	SOURCE	EFFECTOR FUNCTION
INTERLEUKINS		
IL-1	Mφ, fibroblasts	Proliferation activated B- & T-cells; induction PGE$_2$ & cytokines by Mφ; induction neutrophil & T-adhesion molecules on endothelial cells; induction IL-6, IFNβ1 & GM-CSF; induction fever, acute phase proteins, bone resorption by osteoclasts
IL-2	T	Growth activated T- and B-cells; activation NK cells
IL-3	T, MC	Growth & differentiation hematopoietic precursors Mast cell growth
IL-4	CD4 T, MC, BM stroma	Proliferation activated B-, T-, mast & hematopoietic precursor; induction MHC class II and FcεR on B-cells, p75 IL-2R on T-cells; isotype switch to IgG1 & IgE; Mφ APC & cytotoxic function, Mφ fusion (migration inhibition)
IL-5	CD4 T, MC	Proliferation activated B-cells; production IgM & IgA; proliferation eosinophils; expression p55 IL-2R
IL-6	CD4 T, Mφ, MC, fibroblasts	Growth & differentiation B- and T-cell effectors, & hematopoietic precursors; induction acute phase proteins
IL-7	BM stromal cells	Proliferation pre-B, CD4- CD8- T-cells & activated mature T-cells
IL-8	Monocytes	Chemotaxis & activation neutrophils
IL-9	T	Growth and proliferation T-cells
IL-10	CD4 T, B, Mφ	Inhibits IFNγ secretion; inhibits mononuclear cell inflammation
IL-11	BM stromal cells	Induction acute phase proteins
IL-12	Monocytes, Mφ	Induction of T$_{H1}$ cells
IL-13	T	Inhibits mononuclear phagocyte inflammation; proliferation and differentiation B-cells
IL-16	CD8 T, CD4 (not preformed)	Chemotaxis CD4 T-cells and eosinophils
COLONY STIMULATING FACTORS		
GM-CSF	T, Mφ, fibroblasts MC, endothelium	Growth granulocyte & Mφ colonies Activates Mφ, neutrophils, eosinophils
G-CSF	Fibroblasts, endothelium	Growth mature granulocytes
M-CSF	Fibroblasts, endothelium, epithelium	Growth macrophage colonies
Steel factor	BM stromal cells	Stem cell division (c-*kit* ligand)
TUMOR NECROSIS FACTORS		
TNFα LTα	Mφ, T T	Tumor cytotoxicity; cachexia; induction acute phase proteins; anti-viral & anti-parasitic activity; activation phagocytic cells; induction IFNγ, TNFα, IL-1, GM-CSF & IL-6; endotoxic shock
INTERFERONS		
IFNα IFNβ	Leukocytes Fibroblasts	Anti-viral; expression MHC I
IFNγ	T	Anti-viral; Mφ activation; expression MHC class I & II on Mφ & other cells; differentiation of cytotoxic T; synthesis IgG2a by activated B; antagonism several IL-4 actions
CHEMOKINES		
α e.g. IL-8, NAP-2	Mφ, T	Chemotactic for neutrophils
β e.g. MCP, MIP, RANTES	Mφ T	Chemotactic for T-cells
OTHERS		
TGFβ	T, B	Inhibition IL-2R upregulation and IL-2 dependent T- and B-cell proliferation Inhibition (by TGFβ1) of IL-3 + CSF induced hematopoiesis; isotype switch to IgA Wound repair (fibroblast chemotaxin) and angiogenesis Neoplastic transformation certain normal cells
LIF	T	Proliferation embryonic stem cells without affecting differentiation Chemoattraction & activation of eosinophils

Mφ=macrophage; MC=mast cell; BM=bone marrow; IL=interleukin; GM-CSF=granulocyte–macrophage colony-stimulating factor; LTα=lymphotoxin α; TGFβ=transforming growth factor-β; NAP=neutrophil activating peptide; MCP=membrane cofactor protein; MIP=membrane inhibitory peptide; LIF=leukemia inhibitory factor; chemokines are small basic heparin-binding polypeptides, mol.wt 8–14 kDa (see Table 11.1, p. 96, for definitions). IL-5 is chemotactic for eosinophils, IL-8 for neutrophils, and for eosinophils which have been primed with IL-5.

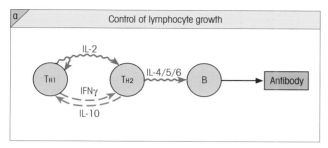

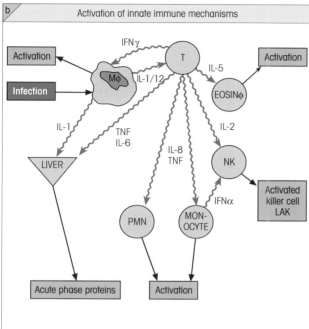

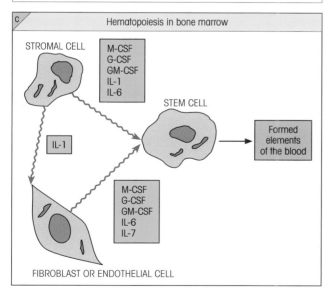

Figure 8.2 Cytokine action. A general but not entirely comprehensive guide to indicate the scope of cytokine interactions Mφ = macrophage; PMN = polymorphonuclear neutrophil; NK = natural killer cell; LAK = lymphokine activated killer; EOSINφ = eosinophil.

would seem to be adapted for defence against parasites which are vulnerable to IL-4-switched IgE and IL-5-induced eosinophilia, and against pathogens which are removed primarily through humoral mechanisms.

Infections with **Mycobacterium tuberculosis,** the etiologic agent of tuberculosis, demonstrate well the clinical significance of these T-helper cell subsets. Successful control of infection is dependent upon an adequate TH1 response. These cells, by promoting IFNγ production will activate macrophages to reduce bacterial load and to release TNF, which is essential for granuloma production.

Infections with *Leishmania* organisms are also influenced by the pattern of cytokines produced by TH1 and TH2 cells. In the localized cutaneous form of the disease, IL-2 and IFNγ mRNA predominate in the lesions indicating that TH1 cells are limiting the infection. In the more severe chronic muco-cutaneous disease, however, the lesions have an abundance of IL-4 mRNA suggesting a predominantly TH2 response with inadequate cellular control. In the most severe visceral form of the disease, circulating lymphocytes are unable to produce IFNγ or IL-12 in response to the etiologic agent, *Leishmania donovani*, but addition of anti-IL-10 antibody results in an augmented IFNγ response. These findings may have significant therapeutic possibilities as therapies that increase activity of TH1 cytokines or decrease TH2 cytokines may enhance resolution of leishmania lesions. IFNγ in particular, since it enhances macrophage killing of parasites, has been shown to have some beneficial effect in treating severely ill patients and those with refractory disease.

ACTIVATED T-CELLS PROLIFERATE IN RESPONSE TO CYTOKINES

Amplification of T-cells following activation is critically dependent upon IL-2 (figure 8.5). This lymphokine acts only on cells which express high-affinity IL-2 receptors. These receptors are not present on resting cells, but are synthesized within a few hours after activation (figure 8.1). The number of these receptors on the cell increases under the action of antigen and of IL-2, and as antigen is cleared, so the receptor numbers decline and, with that, the responsiveness to IL-2.

The T-cell blasts also produce an impressive array of other cytokines and the proliferative effect of IL-2 is reinforced by the action of IL-4 and, to some extent, IL-6, which react with corresponding receptors on the dividing T-cells. We must not lose sight of the importance of control mechanisms such as transforming growth factor-β (TGFβ), which

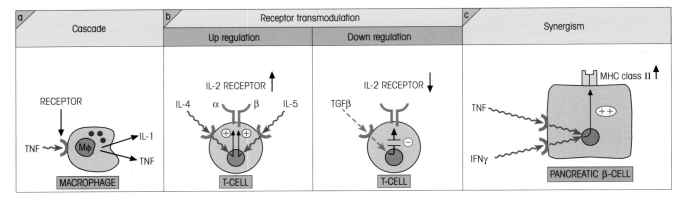

Figure 8.3 Network interactions of cytokines. (a) Cascade: in this example TNF induces secretion of IL-1 and of itself (autocrine) in the macrophage (note all diagrams in this figure are simplified in that the effects on the nucleus are due to messengers resulting from combination of cytokine with its surface receptor). (b) Receptor transmodula-tion showing upregulation of each chain forming the high-affinity IL-2 receptor in an activated T-cell by individual lymphokines and downregulation by TGFβ. (c) Synergy of TNF and IFNγ in upregulation of surface MHC class II molecules on cultured pancreatic insulin-secreting cells.

blocks IL-2-induced proliferation (figure 8.3b) and the cytokines IFNγ, IL-4 and IL-10, which mediate the mutual antagonism of TH1 and TH2 subsets.

T-CELL EFFECTORS IN CELL-MEDIATED IMMUNITY

Cytokines mediate chronic inflammatory responses

In addition to their role in the adaptive response, the T-cell lymphokines are responsible for generating antigen-specific chronic inflammatory reactions which deal with intracellular microorganisms (figure 8.6).

Early events

The initiating event is probably a local inflammatory response to tissue injury caused by the infectious agent which would upregulate the synthesis of adhesion molecules such as vascular cell adhesion molecule (VCAM-1) and intercellular adhesion molecule (ICAM-1) on adjacent vascular endothelial cells. These would permit entry of memory T-cells to the infected site through their VLA-4 and LFA-1 homing receptors. Contact with processed antigen derived from the intracellular organism will activate the specific T-cell and induce the release of secreted cytokines. TNF will further enhance the expression of endothelial accessory molecules and increase the chances of other memory cells in the circulation homing in to meet the antigen provoking inflammation.

Chemotaxis

The recruitment of T-cells and macrophages to the inflammatory site is greatly enhanced by the action of chemotactic cytokines termed **chemokines** (chemoattractant cytokine). The main stimuli to the production of chemokines are the proinflammatory cytokines such as IL-1 and TNFα, but bacterial and viral products may also do this. Chemokines, of which nearly 40 have now been identified, are divided into two families: the α-chemokines, of which IL-8 is an example, attract neutrophils but not monocytes; and the β-chemokines, including MCP, MIP and RANTES (cf. Table 11.1, p. 96), attract monocytes, eosinophils, T-cells and NK-cells (figure 8.6). Chemokines activate specific receptors on target cells, and a growing family of chemokine receptors have been identified. Receptor activation leads to a cascade of cellular events that ultimately results in activation of the cellular machinery necessary to propel the cell in a particular direction. Although these receptors are specific for chemokines, some are now known to act as co-receptors for the HIV virus, allowing the virus which has attached to the CD4 molecule to gain entrance to the T-cell or the monocyte.

Macrophage activation

Macrophages with intracellular organisms are activated by agents such as IFNγ, GM-CSF, IL-2 and TNF (figure 8.6) and become endowed with microbicidal powers. During this process, some macrophages may die (helped along by cytotoxic T-cells?) and release living organisms, but these will be dealt with by fresh macrophages brought to the site by

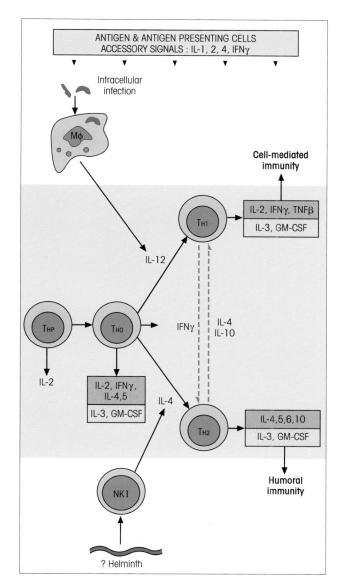

Figure 8.4 The generation of Tн1 and Tн2 CD4 subsets. Following initial stimulation of T-cells, a range of cells producing a spectrum of cytokine patterns emerges. Under different conditions, the resulting population can be biased towards two extremes. IL-12, possibly produced through an 'innate' type effect of an intracellular infection on macrophages, encourages the development of Tн1 cells which produce the cytokines characteristic of *cell-mediated immunity*. IL-4, possibly produced by interaction of microorganisms with NK cells, skews the development to production of Tн2 cells whose cytokines assist the progression of B-cells to antibody secretion and the provision of *humoral immunity*. Cytokines produced by polarized Tн1 and Tн2 subpopulations are mutually inhibitory. Tнp = T-helper precursor; Tн0 = early helper cell producing a spectrum of cytokines; other abbreviations as in table 8.1.

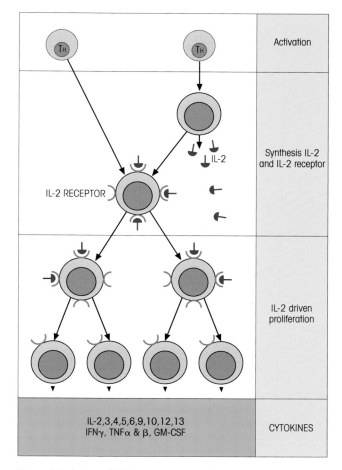

Figure 8.5 Activated T-blasts expressing surface receptors for IL-2 proliferate in response to IL-2 produced by itself or by another T-cell subset. The expanded population secretes a wide variety of biologically active lymphokines of which IL-4 also enhances T-cell proliferation.

chemotaxis and activated by local cytokines, so that they have passed the stage of differentiation at which the intracellular organisms can subvert their killing mechanisms.

Combating viral infection

Virally infected cells require a different strategy, and one strand of that strategy exploits the innate interferon mechanism to deny the virus access to the cell's replicative machinery. TNF has cytotoxic potential against virally infected cells, which is particularly useful since death of an infected cell before viral replication has occurred is obviously beneficial to the host. The cytotoxic potential of TNF was first recognized using tumor cells as targets (hence the name), and recent work with cloned products reveals a synergism

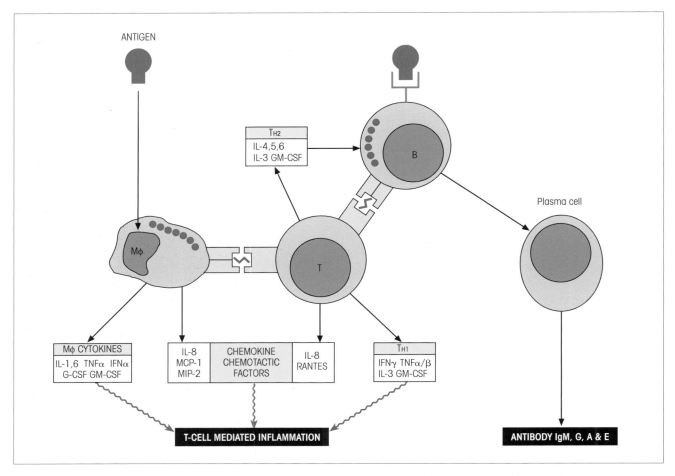

Figure 8.6 Cytokines controlling the antibody and T-cell-mediated inflammatory responses. Abbreviations as in tables 8.1 and 11.1.

between IFNγ and lymphotoxin α (TNFβ) in which IFNγ sets up the cell for destruction by inducing the formation of TNF receptors.

Killer T-cells

The generation of cytotoxic T-cells

Cytotoxic T-cells (Tc) represent the other major arm of the cell-mediated immune response and are generally thought to be of strategic importance in the killing of virally infected cells and possibly in contributing to the postulated surveillance mechanisms against cancer cells.

The cytotoxic cell precursors recognize antigen on the surface of cells in association with class I major histocompatibility complex (MHC) molecules, and like B-cells they require help from T-cells. The mechanism by which help is proffered may, however, be quite different. Effective T–B collaboration involves capture of the native antigen by the surface Ig receptors on the B-cells, which process it internally and present it to the TH as a peptide in association with MHC class II. With TH and cytotoxic cell precursor (TCP) interactions, it seems most likely that both cells bind to the same APC which has processed viral antigen and displays processed viral peptides in association with both class II (for the TH cell) and class I (for the TCP) on its surface; one cannot exclude the possibility that the APC could be the virally infected cell itself. Cytokines from the triggered TH will be released in close proximity to the TCP which is engaging the antigen–MHC signal and will be stimulated to proliferate and differentiate into a Tc under the influence of IL-2 and other cytokines.

The lethal process

Cytotoxic T-cells (Tc) are usually of the CD8 subset and their binding to the target cell through T-receptor recognition of antigen plus class I MHC is assisted by association between

CD8 and class I and by other accessory molecules such as LFA-1 and CD2 (see figure 7.2). MHC recognition is important for this binding as is the intimate signaling to the T-receptor or the CD3 transducer. In some circumstances CD4+ T-cells may also mediate cytotoxicity through the Fas-FasL pathway.

Tc are **unusual secretory cells** which use a modified lysosome to secrete their lytic proteins. Following delivery of the TCR/CD3 signal, the **lytic granules** are driven along the microtubule system and delivered to the point of contact between the Tc and its target (figure 8.7). This guarantees the specificity of killing dictated by TCR recognition of the target and limits any damage to bystander cells. As argued earlier when we discussed cytotoxicity by NK cells which have comparable granules, there is evidence for exocytosis of the granule contents, including perforins, granzymes and TNF, which cause lesions in the target cell membrane and death by inducing apoptosis. Tc are endowed with a second killing mechanism involving Fas and its ligand (cf. pp. 12 and 153)

Videomicroscopy shows that Tc are serial killers. After the 'kiss of death', the T-cell can disengage and seek a further victim, there being rapid synthesis of new granules. One should also not lose sight of the fact that CD8 cells synthesize other cytokines such as IFNγ which also have antiviral potential.

Inflammation must be regulated

Once the inflammatory process has cleared the inciting agent, the body needs to switch off the immune response to that antigen. A variety of anti-inflammatory cytokines are produced during humoral and cell-mediated immune responses. IL-10 has profound anti-inflammatory and immunoregulatory effects, acting on macrophages and TH1 cells to inhibit release of proinflammatory factors such as IL-1/IFNγ and TNFα. It induces the release of soluble TNF receptors which are endogenous inhibitors of TNF, and downregulates surface TNF receptor. IL-1, a potent proinflammatory cytokine, can be regulated by soluble IL-1 receptors released during inflammation which act to decoy IL-1, and by the IL-1 receptor antagonist (IL-1Ra). This latter cytokine, which is structurally similar to IL-1, is produced by monocytes and macrophages during inflammation and competes with IL-1 for IL-1 receptors thereby antagonizing IL-1 activity. Production of IL-1Ra is stimulated by IL-4, which also inhibits IL-1 production and, as we have indicated previously, also acts to constrain TH1 cells. The role of TGFβ is more difficult to tease out because it has some pro- and other anti-inflammatory effects, although it

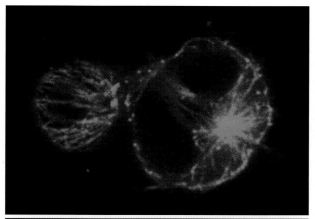

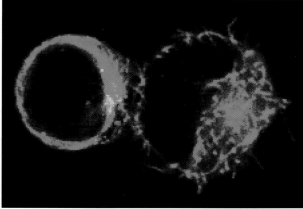

Figure 8.7 Conjugation of a cytotoxic T-cell (on left) to its target, here a mouse mastocytoma, showing polarization of the granules towards the target at the point of contact. The cytoskeletons of both cells are revealed by immunofluorescent staining with an antibody to tubulin (green) and the lytic granules with an antibody to granzyme A (red). Twenty minutes after conjugation the target cell cytoskeleton may still be intact (*above*), but this rapidly becomes disrupted (*below*). (Photographs kindly provided by Dr Gillian Griffiths.)

undoubtedly promotes tissue repair after resolution of the inflammation.

These anti-inflammatory cytokines have considerable potential for the treatment of those human diseases where proinflammatory cytokines are responsible for clinical manifestations. Such a situation exists in septic shock, where many of the clinical features are due to the massive production of IL-1, TNFα and IL-6. Studies in rabbits showed that pre-treatment with IL-1Ra blocked endotoxin-induced septic shock and death. In studies in humans, however, treatment with IL-1Ra has not been shown to reduce mortality in patients with sepsis, and further trials on this and other anti-inflammatory cytokines are in progress.

PROLIFERATION AND MATURATION OF B-CELL RESPONSES ARE MEDIATED BY CYTOKINES

The activation of B-cells by TH through the TCR recognition of MHC-linked antigenic peptide plus the costimulatory **CD40L/CD40 interaction**, leads to upregulation of the surface receptors for interleukins. Copious local release of cytokines such as IL-2, IL-4 and IL-13 from the TH then drives powerful clonal proliferation and expansion of the activated B-cell population (figure 8.8).

Under the influence of IL-4 alone, the expanded clones can differentiate and mature into IgE-synthesizing cells. TGFβ encourages cells to switch their Ig class to IgA, and IL-5 can then stimulate them to become IgA producers. IgM plasma cells emerge under the tutelage of IL-4 plus IL-5, and IgG producers result from the combined influence of IL-4, 5 and 6 with a probable contribution from IFNγ (figure 8.8).

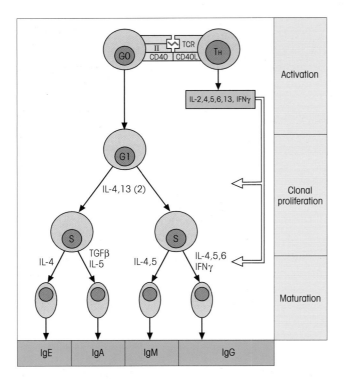

Figure 8.8 B-cell response to thymus-dependent antigen: clonal expansion and maturation of activated B-cells under the influence of T-cell-derived soluble factors. Costimulation through the CD40L/CD40 interaction is essential for primary and secondary immune responses to TD antigens and for the formation of germinal centers and memory.

Thymus-independent antigens can activate B-cells directly but nonetheless still need cytokines for efficient proliferation and Ig production.

WHAT IS GOING ON IN THE GERMINAL CENTER?

Secondary challenge with antigen or immune complexes induces enlargement of germinal centers, formation of new ones, appearance of B-memory cells and development of Ig-producing cells of higher affinity. B-cells entering the germinal center become **centroblasts**, which divide with a very short cycle time of 6 h, and then become nondividing **centrocytes** in the basal light zone, many of which die from apoptosis (figure 8.9). As the surviving centrocytes mature, they differentiate either into **immunoblast plasma cell precursors**, which secrete Ig in the absence of antigen, or **memory B-cells**.

What then is the underlying scenario? Following secondary antigen challenge, primed B-cells may be activated by paracortical TH cells in association with interdigitating dendritic cells or macrophages, and migrate to the germinal center. There they divide in response to powerful stimuli from complexes on follicular dendritic cells, and **somatic mutation** of B-cell Ig genes occurs with high frequency. Mutated cells with surface antibody of higher affinity will be positively selected so leading to maturation of antibody affinity during the immune response. The cells also undergo **Ig class-switching** and further differentiation will now occur. The cells either migrate to the sites of plasma cell activity (e.g. lymph node medulla) or go to expand the memory B-cell pool.

IMMUNOGLOBULIN CLASS-SWITCHING OCCURS IN INDIVIDUAL B-CELLS

The synthesis of antibodies belonging to the various immunoglobulin classes proceeds at different rates. Usually there is an early IgM response which tends to fall off rapidly. IgG antibody synthesis builds up to its maximum over a longer time period. On secondary challenge with antigen, the synthesis of IgG antibodies rapidly accelerates to a much higher titer and there is a relatively slow fall-off in serum antibody levels (figure 8.10). The same probably holds for IgA, and in a sense both these immunoglobulin classes provide the main immediate defense against future penetration by foreign antigens.

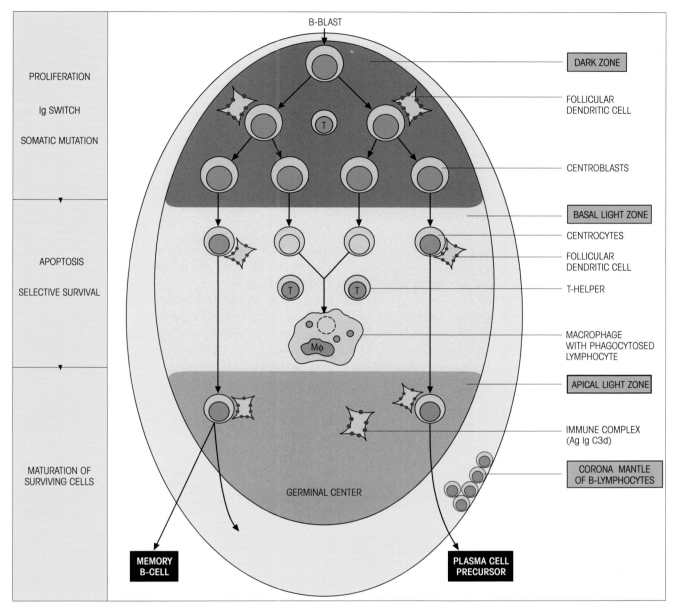

Figure 8.9 The events occurring in lymphoid germinal centers. Germinal center B-cells show numerous mutations in antibody genes. Expression of LFA-1 and ICAM-1 on B-cells and follicular dendritic cells (FDC) in the germinal center makes them 'sticky'. Through their surface receptors, FDC bind immune complexes containing antigen and C3 which, in turn, are very effective B-cell stimulators since coligation of the surface receptors for antigen and C3 lowers their threshold for activation. The costimulatory molecules CD40 and B7 play pivotal roles, and antibodies to CD40 or B7 prevent formation of germinal centers.

Antibody synthesis in most classes shows considerable dependence upon T-cooperation in that the responses in T-deprived animals are strikingly deficient. Similarly, the switch from IgM to IgG and other classes appears to be largely under T-cell control critically mediated by CD40 and presumably also by cytokines as described earlier. In addi-

tion to being brisker the secondary responses tend to be of higher affinity because once the primary response gets under way and the antigen concentration declines to low levels, only successively higher-affinity cells will bind sufficient antigen to maintain proliferation.

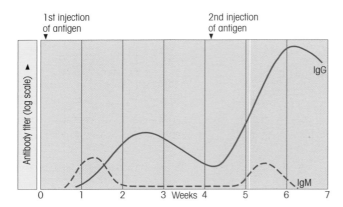

Figure 8.10 Synthesis of IgM and IgG antibody classes in the primary and secondary responses to antigen.

MEMORY CELLS

Memory of early infections such as measles is long-lived and the question arises as to whether the memory cells are long-lived or are subject to repeated antigen stimulation from persisting antigen or subclinical reinfection. Fanum in 1847 described a measles epidemic on the Faroe Islands in the previous year in which almost the entire population suffered from infection except for a few old people who had been infected 65 years earlier. While this evidence favors the long half-life hypothesis it is envisaged that B-cell memory is a dynamic state in which survival of the memory cells is maintained by recurrent signals from follicular dendritic cells in the germinal centers, the only long-term repository of antigen.

T-cell memory exists for both CD4 and CD8 cells and is also probably dependent upon repeated stimulation by antigen. If we accept the proposition that antigen usually only persists as complexes on follicular dendritic cells, one must further assume that these cells are driven by germinal center memory B-cells which capture and process this complexed antigen before presenting it to the T-cells.

The memory population is not simply an expansion of corresponding naive cells

In general, memory cells are more readily stimulated by a given dose of antigen because they have a higher affinity. In the case of B-cells we have been satisfied by the evidence linking mutation and antigen selection to the creation of high-affinity memory cells within the germinal center of secondary lymph node follicles. Virgin B-cells lose their surface IgM and IgD and switch receptor isotype on becoming memory cells. The costimulatory molecules B7.1 and B7.2 are rapidly upregulated on memory B-cells and their potent antigen-presenting capacity for T-cells could well account for the brisk and robust nature of secondary responses.

REVISION

See the accompanying website (www.roitt.com) for multiple choice questions.

A succession of genes are upregulated by T-cell activation
• Within 15–30 minutes genes for transcription factors concerned in the progression G0 to G1 and control of IL-2 are expressed.
• Up to 14 hours cytokines and their receptors are expressed.
• Later, a variety of genes related to cell division and adhesion are upregulated.

Cytokines act as intercellular messengers
• Cytokines act transiently and usually at short range, although circulating IL-1 and IL-6 can mediate release of acute-phase proteins from the liver.
• They act through high-affinity cell surface receptors.
• Cytokines are pleiotropic, i.e. have multiple effects in the general areas of (i) control of lymphocyte growth, (ii) activation of innate immune mechanisms (including inflammation), and (iii) control of bone marrow hematopoiesis
• Cytokines may act sequentially, through one cytokine inducing production of another or by transmodulation of the receptor for another cytokine; they can also act synergistically or antagonistically.

Different CD4 T-cell subsets can make different cytokines
• As immunization proceeds, TH tend to develop into two subsets: TH1 cells concerned in inflammatory processes, macrophage activation and delayed sensitivity make IL-2 and 3, IFNγ, TNFβ and GM-CSF; TH2 cells help B-cells to synthesize antibody and secrete IL-3, 4, 5, 6 and 10, TNFα and GM-CSF.

- Early interaction of antigen with macrophages producing IL-12 or with a T-cell subset secreting IL-4 will skew the responses to TH1 or TH2 respectively.

  Different patterns of cytokine production influence the severity and clinical manifestations of various infectious diseases.

Activated T-cells proliferate in response to cytokines

- IL-2 acts as an autocrine growth factor for TH1 and paracrine for TH2 cells which have upregulated their IL-2 receptors.
- Cytokines act on cells which express receptors.

T-cell effectors in cell-mediated immunity

- Cytokines mediate chronic inflammatory responses.
- α-Chemokines are cytokines which chemoattract neutrophils, and β-chemokines attract T-cells, macrophages and other inflammatory cells.

  Some chemokine receptors act as co-receptors for the HIV virus.
- TNF synergizes with IFNγ in killing cells.

Killer T-cells

- Cytotoxic T-cells are generated against cells (e.g. virally infected) which have intracellularly derived peptide associated with surface MHC class I.
- Tc proliferate under the influence of IL-2 released by helper T-cells in close proximity.
- Tc are CD8 cells which secrete lytic proteins to the point of contact between the Tc and its target.
- The granules contain perforins and TNF, which produce lesions in the target cell membrane, and granzymes, which also cause death by apoptosis.

Control of inflammation

- Various anti-inflammatory cytokines are produced during the immune response;

- T-cell-mediated inflammation is strongly downregulated by IL-10.
- IL-1 is inhibited by the IL-1 receptor antagonist and by IL-4.

Proliferation of B-cell responses is mediated by cytokines

- Early proliferation is mediated by IL-4, which also aids IgE synthesis.
- IgA producers are driven by TGFβ and IL-5.
- IL-4 plus IL-5 promotes IgM, and IL-4, 5 and 6 plus IFNγ stimulate IgG synthesis.

Events in the germinal center

- There is clonal expansion, isotype switch and mutation in the centroblasts.
- The B-cell centroblasts become nondividing centrocytes which differentiate into plasma cell precursors or into memory cells.

Ig class-switching occurs in individual B-cells

- IgM produced early in the response switches to IgG, particularly with thymus-dependent antigens. The switch is under T-cell control.
- IgG, but not IgM, responses improve on secondary challenge.

  Secondary responses show increased affinity for antigen.

Memory cells

- It has been suggested that activated memory cells are sustained by recurrent stimulation with antigen.
- This must occur largely in the germinal centers since the complexes on the surface of follicular dendritic cells are the only long-term source of antigen.
- Memory cells have higher affinity than naive cells.

FURTHER READING

Capra J.D. (1996) Germinal centers: a new lease of life for B-cells and 'B-cell-ologists'. *The Immunologist* **4** (3), 84.

Kelsoe G. (1999) VDJ hypermutation and receptor revision. *Current Opinion in Immunology* **11** (1), 70.

Linsley P.S. & Reth M. (eds) (1999) Section on Lymphocyte Activation and Effector Functions. *Current Opinion in Immunology* **11** (3).

Raynaud C.-A. & Weill J.-C. (eds) (1996) Somatic mutation: mechanisms and signals. *Seminars in Immunology* **8**, 125.

Sallusto F., Lanzavecchia A. & Mackay C.R. (1998) Chemokines and chemokine receptors in T-cell priming and TH1/TH2-mediated responses. *Immunology Today* **19** (12), 568.

Stout R.D. & Suttles J. (1996) The many roles of CD40 in cell-mediated inflammatory responses. *Immunology Today* **17**, 487–492.

Swain S.L. & Cambier J.C. (eds) (1996) Lymphocyte activation and effector functions. *Current Opinion in Immunology* **8**, 309–418.

Vicari A.P. & Zlotnik A. (1996) Mouse NK1.1+ T-cells: a new family of T-cells. *Immunology Today* **17**, 71.

CHAPTER 9

Control mechanisms

ANTIGEN IS A MAJOR FACTOR IN CONTROL

The acquired immune response evolved so that it would come into play when contact with an infectious agent was first made. The appropriate antigen-specific cells expand, the effectors eliminate the antigen and then the response quietens down and leaves room for reaction to other infections. Feedback mechanisms must operate to limit antibody production, otherwise, after antigenic stimulation, we would become overwhelmed by the responding clones of antibody-forming cells and their products. There is abundant evidence to support the view that antigen is a major regulatory factor and that antibody production is driven by the presence of antigen, falling off in intensity as the antigen concentration drops (figure 9.1). Furthermore, clearance of antigen by injection of excess antibody during the course of an immune response leads to a dramatic decrease in antibody synthesis and in the number of antibody- secreting cells.

ANTIBODY EXERTS FEEDBACK CONTROL

A useful control mechanism is to arrange for the product of a reaction to be an inhibitor, and this type of negative feedback is seen with antibody. Thus removal of circulating antibody by plasmapheresis during an on-going response leads to an increase in synthesis, whereas injection of preformed IgG antibody markedly hastens the fall in the number of antibody-forming cells consistent with feedback control on overall synthesis.

T-CELL REGULATION

T-helper cells

We have deliberated at length on the role of T-helper (TH) cells in the facilitation of cytotoxic T-cell (Tc) and B-cell responses, and in the production of class-switching and memory responses. We should perhaps note that the TH cells do not expand B-cell and Tc clone sizes indefinitely since the maturation factors inhibit the action of the proliferative lymphokines.

As one might anticipate, there is a built-in braking system on T-cell expansion in the form of Fas-mediated apoptosis of activated mature cells. Both Fas and Fas-ligand are expressed and this can lead to suicide or mutual homicide, particularly between the daughter cells of mitotic division.

T-cell suppression

We raised the question of suppression as distinct from help and perhaps it is inevitable that Nature, having evolved a functional set of T-cells which promote immune responses, should also develop a regulatory set whose job is to modulate the helpers. Over the years, T-cell suppression has been shown to modulate a variety of humoral and cellular responses, the latter including delayed-type hypersensitivity, cytotoxic T-cells and antigen-specific T-cell proliferation. Mutual inhibition between TH1 and TH2 cells may appear as suppression. Anergic T-cells produced by defective, incomplete or abortive antigen-specific stimulation, can suppress other T-cells reacting with the same antigen-presenting cells by so-called 'infectious tolerance'. There is also evidence for a phenotypically distinct population of T-cells which regulate the activity of potentially autoreactive lymphocytes.

IDIOTYPE NETWORKS

Jerne's network hypothesis

The hypervariable loops on the immunoglobulin molecule which go to form the antigen-combining site have individual characteristic shapes which can be recognized by the appropriate antibodies as idiotypic determinants. There are hun-

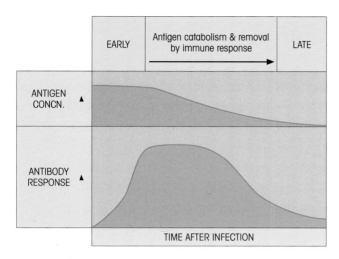

Figure 9.1 Antigen drives the immune response. As the antigen concentration falls due to catabolism and elimination by antibody, the intensity of the immune response declines but is maintained for some time at a lower level by antigen trapped on the follicular dendritic cells of the germinal centers.

dreds of thousands, if not more, of different idiotypes in one individual.

Jerne reasoned brilliantly that the great diversity of idiotypes would to a considerable extent mirror the diversity of antigenic shapes in the external world. Thus, he said, if lymphocytes can recognize a whole range of foreign antigenic determinants, they should be able to recognize the idiotypes on other lymphocytes. They would therefore form a large network or series of networks depending upon idiotype–anti-idiotype recognition between lymphocytes of the various T- and B-subsets (figure 9.2), and the response to an external antigen perturbing this network would be conditioned by the state of the idiotypic interactions. There is no doubt that the elements which can form an idiotypic network are present in the body. Individuals can be immunized against idiotypes on their own antibodies, and such autoanti-idiotypes have been identified during the course of responses induced by antigens. It seems likely that similar interactions will be established for early T-cells, possibly linking with the B-cell network. Certainly, anti-idiotypic reactivity can be demonstrated in T-cell populations,

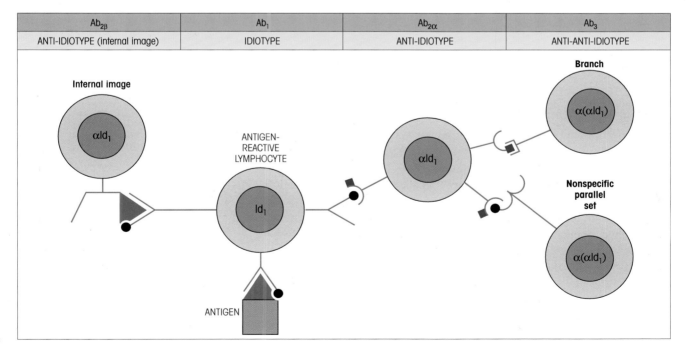

Figure 9.2 Elements in an idiotypic network in which the antigen receptors on one lymphocyte reciprocally recognize an idiotype on the receptors of another. T–T interactions could occur through direct recognition of one T-cell receptor (TCR) by the other, or more usually

by recognition of a processed TCR peptide associated with MHC. One of the anti-idiotype sets, $Ab_2\beta$, may bear an idiotype of similar shape to (i.e. provides an **internal image** of) the antigen.

and it is likely that relatively closed Id–anti-Id circuits contribute to a regulatory system.

THE INFLUENCE OF GENETIC FACTORS

Some genes affect general responsiveness

Mice can be selectively bred for high or low antibody responses through several generations to yield two lines, one of which consistently produces high-titer antibodies to a variety of antigens, and the other antibodies of relatively low titer. Out of the ten or so different genetic loci involved, some gave rise to a higher rate of B-cell proliferation and differentiation, while one or more affect macrophage behavior. The two lines are comparable in their ability to clear carbon particles or sheep erythrocytes from the blood by phagocytosis, but macrophages from the high responders present antigen more efficiently. On the other hand, the low responders survive infection by *Salmonella typhimurium* better and their macrophages support much slower replication of *Listeria*, indicative of an inherently more aggressive microbicidal ability.

ARE THERE REGULATORY IMMUNONEUROENDOCRINE NETWORKS?

There is a danger, as one focuses more and more on the antics of the immune system, of looking at the body as a collection of myeloid and lymphoid cells roaming around in a big sack and of having no regard to the integrated physiology of the organism. Within the wider physiological context, attention has been drawn increasingly to interactions between immunologic and neuroendocrine systems, which is generating a whole new subject of 'psychoimmunology'.

Immunologic cells have the receptors which enable them to receive signals from a whole range of hormones: corticosteroids, insulin, growth hormone, estradiol, testosterone, β-adrenergic agents, acetylcholine, endorphins and enkephalins. There is an extensive literature concerning their influence on immune function, but by and large, glucocorticoids and androgens depress immune responses, whereas estrogens, growth hormone, thyroxine and insulin do the opposite.

A neuroendocrine feedback loop affecting immune responses

The secretion of glucocorticoids is a major response to stresses induced by a wide range of stimuli such as extreme changes of temperature, fear, hunger and physical injury. They are also released as a consequence of immune responses and limit those responses in a neuroendocrine feedback loop. Thus, IL-1, IL-6 and tumor necrosis factor α (TNFα) are capable of stimulating glucocorticoid synthesis and do so through the hypothalamic–pituitary–adrenal axis. This, in turn, leads to downregulation of TH1 and macrophage activity so completing the negative feedback circuit (figure 9.3).

Sex hormones come into the picture

Estrogen is said to be the major factor influencing the more active immune responses in females relative to males. They have higher serum Ig and secreted IgA levels, a higher antibody response to T-independent antigens, relative resistance

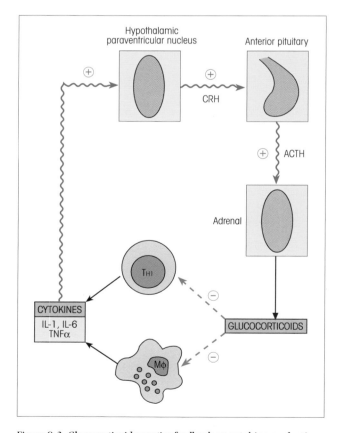

Figure 9.3 Glucocorticoid negative feedback on cytokine production. CRH = corticotropin-releasing hormone; ACTH = adrenocorticotropic hormone. Cells of the immune system in both primary and secondary lymphoid organs can produce hormones and neuropeptides, while classical endocrine glands as well as neurones and glial cells can synthesize cytokines and appropriate receptors.

to T-cell tolerance and greater resistance to infections. Females are also far more susceptible to autoimmune disease, an issue that will be discussed in greater depth in Chapter 17, but here let us note that oral contraceptives can induce flares of the autoimmune disorder systemic lupus erythematosus (SLE).

Malnutrition diminishes the effectiveness of the immune response

The greatly increased susceptibility of undernourished individuals to infection can be attributed to many factors: poor sanitation and personal hygiene, overcrowding and inadequate health education. But in addition there are gross effects of protein calorie malnutrition on immunocompetence. The widespread atrophy of lymphoid tissues and the 50% reduction in circulating CD4 T-cells underlies serious impairment of cell-mediated immunity. Antibody responses may be intact but they are of lower affinity; phagocytosis of bacteria is relatively normal but the subsequent intracellular destruction is defective.

Deficiencies in pyridoxine, folic acid and vitamins A, C and E result in generally impaired immune responses. Vitamin D is an important regulator. It is produced not only by the UV-irradiated dermis but also by activated macrophages, the hypercalcemia associated with sarcoidosis being attributable to production of the vitamin by macrophages in the active granulomas. The vitamin is a potent inhibitor of T-cell proliferation and of cytokine production by TH1 cells. This generates a neat feedback loop at sites of inflammation where macrophages activated by IFNγ produce vitamin D which suppresses the T-cells making the interferon. It also downregulates antigen presentation by macrophages and promotes multinucleated giant cell formation in granulomatous lesions. Nonetheless, in further emphasis of the potential duality of the CD4 helper subsets, it promotes TH2 activity, especially at mucosal surfaces. Zinc deficiency is rather interesting; this greatly affects the biological activity of thymus hormones and has a major effect on cell-mediated immunity.

Of course there is another side to all this in that moderate restriction of total calorie intake and/or marked reduction in fat intake, ameliorate age-related diseases such as autoimmunity.

REVISION

See the accompanying website (www.roitt.com) for multiple choice questions.

Control by antigen
• Immune responses are largely antigen driven and as the level of exogenous antigen falls, so does the intensity of the response.

Feedback control by antibody
• IgG antibodies inhibit responses via the Fcγ receptor on B-cells.

T-cell regulation
• TH cells may use their surface receptors for Ig isotypes to augment the expansion of B-cells expressing the related isotype.
• Activated T-cells express Fas and FasL which can restrain unlimited clonal expansion (p. 12).
• At high levels of antigen, T-cells which suppress T-helpers emerge, presumably as feedback control of excessive TH expansion.

Idiotype networks
• Antigen-specific receptors on lymphocytes can interact with the idiotypes on the receptors of other lymphocytes to form a network (Jerne).

Genetic factors influence the immune response
• Approximately ten genes control the overall antibody response to complex antigens: some affect macrophage antigen processing and microbicidal activity and some the rate of proliferation of differentiating B-cells.

Immunoneuroendocrine networks
• Immunologic, neurologic and endocrinologic systems can all interact.
• Regulatory interdependent circuits are being described, of which the feedback by cytokines augmenting the production of corticosteroids is important because this shuts down TH1 and macrophage activity.

• Estrogens may be largely responsible for the more active immune responses in females relative to males.

Effects of diet and other factors on immunity
• Protein-calorie malnutrition grossly impairs cell-mediated immunity and phagocyte microbicidal potency.

• Exercise, trauma, age and environmental pollution can all act to impair immune mechanisms. The pattern of cytokines produced by peripheral blood cells changes with age, IL-2 decreasing and TNFα, IL-1 and IL-6 increasing.

FURTHER READING

Chandra R.K. (1992) Nutrition and the immune system. In: *Encyclopedia of Immunology* (eds I.M. Roitt & P.J. Delves), p. 1369. Academic Press, London. [See also other relevant articles in the *Encyclopedia*: 'Aging and the immune system', p. 45; 'Behavioural regulation of immunity', p. 228; 'Vitamin D', p. 1567.]

Cohen I.R. & Young D.B. (1991) Autoimmunity, microbial immunity and the immunological homunculus. *Immunology Today* **12**, 105.

Goetz H. (1994) Exercise and the immune system: a model of the stress response. *Immunology Today* **15**, 382.

Linsley P.S. & Reth M. (eds) (1999) Section on Lymphocyte Activation and Effector Functions. *Current Opinion in Immunology* **11** (3).

Swain S.L. & Cambier J.C. (eds) (1996) Lymphocyte activation and effector functions. *Current Opinion in Immunology* **8**, 309–418.

Talal N. (1992) Sex hormones and immunity. In: *Encyclopedia of Immunology* (eds I.M. Roitt & P.J. Delves), p. 1369. Academic Press, London.

van Eden W. *et al.* (1998) Do heat shock proteins control the balance of T-cell regulation in inflammatory diseases? *Immunology Today* **19** (7), 303.

CHAPTER 10

Ontogeny

THE MULTIPOTENTIAL HEMATOPOIETIC STEM CELL GIVES RISE TO THE FORMED ELEMENTS OF THE BLOOD

Hematopoiesis originates in the early yolk sac and as embryogenesis proceeds, this function is taken over by the fetal liver and finally by the bone marrow where it continues throughout life. The hematopoietic stem cell which gives rise to the formed elements of the blood (figure 10.1) can be shown to be multipotent, to seed other organs and to have a relatively unlimited capacity to renew itself through the creation of further stem cells. Thus an animal can be completely protected against the lethal effects of high doses of radiation by injection of bone marrow cells which will repopulate its lymphoid and myeloid systems. This forms the basis of human bone marrow transplantation.

We have come a long way towards the goal of isolating highly purified populations of hematopoietic stem cells, although not all agree that we have yet achieved it. CD34 is a marker of an extremely early cell but there is some debate as to whether this identifies the holy pluripotent stem cell itself.

THE THYMUS PROVIDES THE ENVIRONMENT FOR T-CELL DIFFERENTIATION

The thymus is organized into a series of lobules based upon meshworks of epithelial cells which form well-defined cortical and medullary zones (figure 10.2). This framework of cells provides the microenvironment for T-cell differentiation. There are subtle interactions between the extracellular matrix proteins and a variety of integrins on different lymphocyte subpopulations which play a role in the homing of progenitors to the thymus and their subsequent migration within the gland. In addition, the epithelial cells produce a series of peptide hormones including thymulin, α_1- and β_4-

thymosin, and thymopoietin which seem capable of promoting the appearance of T-cell differentiation markers.

The specialized large epithelial cells in the outer cortex are known as 'nurse' cells because they can each be associated with large numbers of lymphocytes which appear to be lying within their cytoplasm. The epithelial cells of the deep cortex have branched dendritic processes rich in class II MHC. They connect through desmosomes to form a network through which cortical lymphocytes must pass on their way to the medulla (figure 10.2). The cortical lymphocytes are densely packed compared with those in the medulla, many are in division and a surprising number are undergoing apoptosis as a result of positive and negative selection (see later). A number of bone marrow-derived interdigitating dendritic cells are present in the medulla and the epithelial cells have broader processes than their cortical counterparts and express high levels of both class I and class II MHC.

In the human, thymic involution commences within the first 12 months of life, reducing by around 3% a year to middle age and by 1% thereafter. The size of the organ gives no clue to these changes because there is replacement by adipose tissue. In a sense, the thymus is progressively disposable because, as we shall see, it establishes a long-lasting peripheral T-cell pool which enables the host to withstand loss of the gland without catastrophic failure of immunologic function, witness the minimal effects of thymectomy in the adult compared with the **dramatic influence in the neonate**.

T-CELL ONTOGENY

Differentiation is accompanied by changes in surface markers

T-lymphocytes originate from hematopoietic stem cells which are attracted to the thymus by some chemotactic factor. The T-cell precursors stain positively for CD34 and for

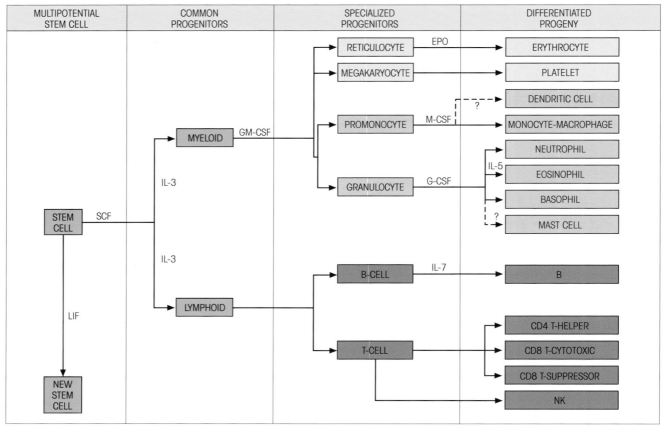

Figure 10.1 The multipotential hematopoietic stem cell and its progeny which differentiate under the influence of a series of growth factors within the microenvironment of the bone marrow. SCF = stem cell factor; LIF = leukemia inhibitory factor; IL-3 = interleukin-3, often termed the multi-CSF because it stimulates progenitors of platelets, mast cells and all the other types of myeloid and erythroid cells; GM-

CSF = granulocyte–macrophage colony-stimulating factor, so called because it promotes the formation of mixed colonies of these two cell types from bone marrow progenitors either in tissue culture or on transfer to an irradiated recipient where they appear in the spleen; G-CSF = granulocyte colony-stimulating factor; M-CSF = monocyte colony-stimulating factor; EPO = erythropoietin.

the enzyme terminal deoxynucleotidyl transferase (TdT), which is thought to be involved in the insertion of nucleotide sequences at the N-terminal region of D and J variable region segments to increase diversity of the T-cell receptors (TCRs). Under the influence of interleukin-1 (IL-1) and tumor necrosis factor (TNF) they differentiate into prothymocytes, committed to the T-lineage. At this stage the cells begin to express various TCR chains and are then expanded, ultimately expressing CD3, the invariant signal-transducing complex of the TCR, and becoming **double-positive** for CD4+, CD8+. Finally the cells traverse the cortico-medullary junction to the medulla where they appear as separate immunocompetent populations of **single-positive CD4+ T-helpers** and **CD8+ cytotoxic T-cell precursors**. The γδ cells remain double-negative, i.e. CD4−8−, except for a small subset which express CD8. The rearrangement of V, D and J region genes

required to generate the TCR has not yet taken place at the prothymocyte stage.

Receptor rearrangement

The development of T-cell receptors

The earliest T-cell precursors have TCR genes in the germline configuration, and the first rearrangements to occur involve the γ and δ loci. The αβ receptors are only detected a few days later. The V_β is first rearranged in the double-negative CD4−8− cells and associates with a conserved pre-α-chain and a CD3 molecule to form a single 'pre-TCR'. Expression of this complex leads the pre-T-cells to proliferate and become double-positive CD4+8+ cells. Further development now requires rearrangement of the V_α

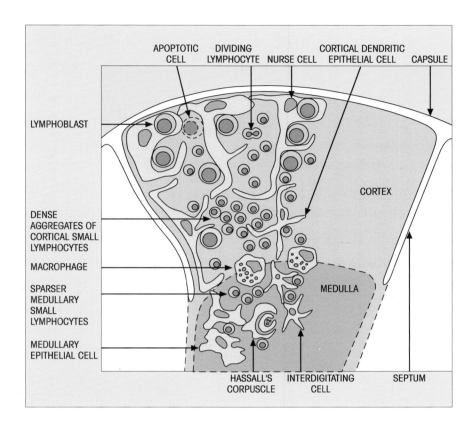

Figure 10.2 Cellular features of a thymus lobule. See text for description. (Adapted from Hood L.E., Weissman I.L., Wood W.B. & Wilson J.H. (1984) *Immunology*, 2nd edn. p. 261. Benjamin Cummings, California.)

gene segments so allowing formation of the mature αβ TCR, and the cells are now ready for subsequent bouts of positive and negative receptor editing as will be discussed shortly. Rearrangement of the V_β genes on the sister chromatid is suppressed by a process called **allelic exclusion**.

Cells are positively selected for self MHC restriction in the thymus

The ability of T-cells to recognize antigenic peptides in association with self MHC is developed in the thymus gland. A small proportion of the double-positive (CD4+8+) T-cells bearing their T-cell receptors, will bind to thymic cortical epithelial cells with low avidity and will be positively selected to complete their progress to mature T-cells. The rest of the cells which do not recognize their own MHC are eliminated and will die in 3 or 4 days. Another feature of this selection phase of T-cell development is that CD4+8+ cells bearing receptors which recognize self MHC on the epithelial cells are positively selected for differentiation to CD4+8− or CD4−8+ single-positive cells. A cell coming into contact with self MHC class I molecules will mature as a CD8+ cell, whereas if contact is made with MHC class II molecules the

cells will develop as CD4+ T-cells. In the rare immunodeficiency disorder called the bare lymphocyte syndrome, MHC molecules do not appear on the surface of cells. As a result CD8+ cells will not develop in those cases which lack class I MHC, while CD4+ cells fail to appear in those cases without class II MHC molecules.

Self-reactive cells are removed in the thymus by negative selection

Many of the cells which survive positive selection have receptors for self antigen and if allowed to mature would produce immune responses to autoantigens. These thymocytes therefore undergo negative selection, which is crucial for maintaining tolerance to self antigens. In this process self antigens are presented to the maturing thymocytes by dendritic cells or macrophages and any cell responding with high avidity is eliminated. The result of positive and negative selection is that all mature T-cells moving out of the thymic cortex into the medulla will either be CD4 or CD8 positive, will recognize foreign peptide only in the context of self MHC, and will not have the potential to mount immune responses against self antigens.

T-CELL TOLERANCE

The induction of immunologic tolerance is necessary to avoid self-reactivity

In essence, lymphocytes recognize foreign antigens through complementariness in shape mediated by the intermolecular forces we have described previously. To a large extent the building blocks used to form microbial and host molecules are the same, so it is the assembled shapes of *self* and *nonself* molecules which must be discriminated by the immune system if potentially disastrous autoreactivity is to be avoided. Many self-reacting T-cells are eliminated by negative selection in the thymus and others are tolerized in the periphery by contact with self antigens in a 'nonstimulatory' context. The restriction of each lymphocyte to a single specificity makes the job of establishing self-tolerance that much easier, simply because it just requires a mechanism which functionally deletes self-reacting cells and leaves the remainder of the repertoire unscathed. The most radical difference between self and nonself molecules lies in the fact that, in early life, the developing lymphocytes are surrounded by self and normally only meet nonself antigens at a later stage and then usually associated with the danger signals induced by the adjuvanticity and cytokine release characteristic of infection. With its customary efficiency, the blind force of evolution has exploited these differences to establish the mechanisms of **immunologic tolerance to host constituents**.

DEVELOPMENT OF B-CELL SPECIFICITY

The sequence of immunoglobulin gene rearrangements

Stage 1. Initially, the *D-J* segments on both heavy chain coding regions (one from each parent) rearrange (figure 10.3).

Stage 2. A *V–DJ* recombinational event now occurs on one heavy chain. If this proves to be a *nonproductive* rearrangement (i.e. adjacent segments are joined in an incorrect reading frame or in such a way as to generate a termination codon downstream from the splice point), then a second *V–DJ* rearrangement will occur on the sister heavy chain region. If a productive rearrangement is not achieved, we can wave the pre-B-cell a fond farewell.

Stage 3. Assuming a productive rearrangement is made, the pre-B-cell can now synthesize μ chains. At around the same time, two genes, V_{preB} and λ_5, with homology for the V_L and C_L segments of λ-light chains respectively, are temporarily transcribed to form a 'pseudo light chain' which associates with the μ chains to generate a surface surrogate 'IgM' receptor together with the Ig-α and Ig-β chains conventionally required to form a functional B-cell receptor. This surrogate receptor closely parallels the pre-Tα/β receptor on pre-T-cell precursors of native TCR-bearing cells.

Stage 4. The surface receptor is signaled, perhaps by a stromal cell, to suppress any further rearrangement of heavy chain genes on a sister chromatid. This is termed **allelic exclusion**.

Stage 5. It is presumed that the surface receptor now initiates the next set of gene rearrangements which occur on the κ light chain gene loci. These involve V–J recombinations on first one and then the other κ allele until a productive V_κ–J rearrangement is accomplished. Were that to fail, an attempt would be made to achieve productive rearrangement of the λ alleles. Synthesis of conventional sIgM now proceeds.

Stage 6. The sIgM molecule now prohibits any further gene shuffling by allelic exclusion of any unrearranged light chain genes. B-cells bearing self-reactive receptors of moderately high affinity are eliminated by a negative selection process akin to that operating on autoreactive T-cells in the thymus.

At the next stage of differentiation, the cell develops a commitment to producing a particular antibody class and either bears surface IgM alone or in combination with IgA or IgG. The further addition of surface IgD now marks the readiness of the virgin B-cell for priming by antigen. Some cells, therefore, bear surface Ig of three different classes: M, G and D or M, A and D, but all Ig molecules on a single cell have the same idiotype and therefore are derived from the same V_H and V_L genes, presumably by splicing of a long RNA transcript. IgD is lost on antigenic stimulation so that memory cells lack this Ig. At the terminal stages in the life of a fully mature plasma cell, virtually all surface Ig is shed.

The importance of allelic exclusion

Since each cell has chromosome complements derived from each parent, the differentiating B-cell has four light- and two heavy-chain gene clusters to choose from. We have described how once the *VDJ* DNA rearrangement has occurred within one light- and one heavy-chain cluster, the *V* genes on the other four chromosomes are held in the embryonic state by an allelic exclusion mechanism so that the cell is able to express only one light and one heavy chain.

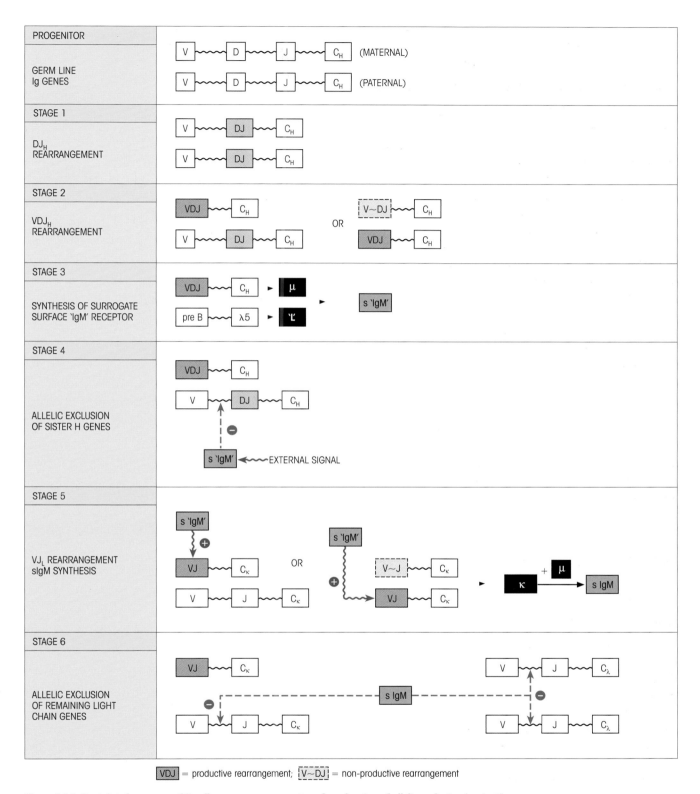

VDJ = productive rearrangement; V~DJ = non-productive rearrangement

Figure 10.3 Postulated sequence of B-cell gene rearrangements and mechanism of allelic exclusion (see text).

This is essential for clonal selection to work since the cell is then programmed only to make the one antibody it uses as a cell surface receptor to recognize antigen.

THE OVERALL RESPONSE IN THE NEONATE

Lymph node and spleen remain relatively underdeveloped in the fetus except where there has been intrauterine exposure to antigens, as in congenital infections with rubella or other organisms. The ability to reject grafts and to mount an antibody response is reasonably well developed by birth but the immunoglobulin levels, with one exception, are low, particularly in the absence of intrauterine infection. The exception is IgG, which is acquired by placental transfer from the mother, a process dependent upon Fc structures specific to this Ig class. Maternal IgG is catabolized with a half-life of approximately 30 days so that serum levels fall over the first 3 months, accentuated by the increase in blood volume of the growing infant. Thereafter the rate of synthesis overtakes the rate of breakdown of maternal IgG and the overall concentration increases steadily. The other immunoglobulins do not cross the placenta and the low but significant levels of IgM in cord blood are synthesized by the baby (figure 10.4). IgM reaches adult levels by 9 months of age. Only trace levels of IgA, IgD and IgE are present in the circulation of the newborn.

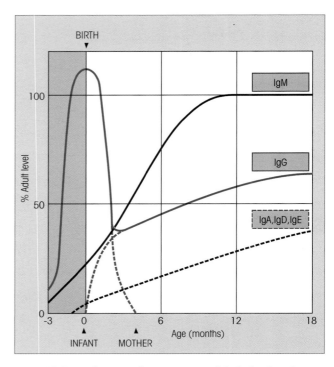

Figure 10.4 Development of serum immunoglobulin levels in the human. (After Hobbs J.R. (1969) In: *Immunology and Development* (ed. M. Adinolfi), p. 118. Heinemann, London.)

REVISION

See the accompanying website (www.roitt.com) for multiple choice questions.

Multipotential stem cells from the bone marrow give rise to all the formed elements of the blood
• Expansion and differentiation are driven by soluble growth (colony-stimulating) factors and contact with reticular stromal cells.

The differentiation of T-cells occurs within the microenvironment of the thymus
• Bone marrow stem cells become immunocompetent T-cells in the thymus. Numerous cortical lymphocytes undergo apoptosis due to positive and negative selection.
• Thymic involution commences within the first 12 months of life.

T-cell ontogeny
• Differentiation to immunocompetent T-cell subsets is accompanied by changes in the surface phenotype which can be recognized with monoclonal antibodies.
• CD34 positive stem cells differentiate into prothymocytes and begin expressing various TCR chains and CD3.
• Double-negative CD4-8- pre-T-cells are driven and expanded by the pre-receptor to become double-positive CD4+8+.
• As the cells traverse the cortico-medullary junction, they become either CD4+ or CD8+.

Receptor rearrangement
• The first TCR rearrangement involves the γ and δ loci.

- Rearrangements of first the $V\beta$ locus and later the $V\alpha$ locus form the mature $\alpha\beta$ TCR 2.

T-cells are positively and negatively selected in the thymus

- The thymus epithelial cells **positively select** CD4+8+ T-cells with avidity for their MHC haplotype so that single-positive CD4+ or CD8+ T-cells develop that are restricted to the recognition of antigen in the context of the epithelial cell haplotype.
- The rest of the cells which do not recognize their own MHC are eliminated.
- Cells which have receptors for self antigen undergo negative selection and are also eliminated.

Development of B-cell specificity

- The sequence of Ig variable gene rearrangements is *DJ* and then *VDJ*.
- *VDJ* transcription produces μ chains which associate with $V_{preB} \cdot \lambda_5$ chains to form a surrogate surface IgM-like receptor.
- This receptor signals allelic exclusion of unrearranged heavy chains.
- If the rearrangement at any stage is unproductive, i.e. does not lead to an acceptable gene reading frame, the allele on the sister chromosome is rearranged.
- The next set of gene rearrangements occur on the k light gene, or if this fails, on the λ light chain gene.
- The cell now develops a commitment to producing a particular class of antibody.
- The mechanisms of allelic exclusion ensure that each lymphocyte is programmed for only one antibody (figure 10.3).

The overall response in the neonate

- Maternal IgG crosses the placenta and provides a high level of passive immunity at birth.

FURTHER READING

Arnold B., Schönrich G. & Hammerling G.J. (1993) Multiple levels of peripheral (T-cell) tolerance. *Immunology Today* **14**, 12.

Camacho S.A., Kosco-Vilbois M.H. & Berek C. (1998) The dynamic structure of the germinal center. *Immunology Today* **19** (11), 511.

Chothia C. (1992) One thousand families for the molecular biologist. *Nature* **357**, 543.

Horton J. & Ratcliffe N. (1996) Evolution of immunity. In: *Immunology*, 4th edn (eds I.M. Roitt, J. Brostoff & M.K. Male), p. 15.1. Mosby, London.

Kruisbeek A.M. & Storb U. (eds) (1996) Lymphocyte development. *Current Opinion in Immunology* **8**, 257.

Liu Y-J. & Banchereau J. (1996) The paths and molecular controls of peripheral B-cell development. *The Immunologist* **4** (2), 55.

Miller J.F.A.P. (1994) The thymus: maestro of the immune system. *Bioessays* **16**, 509. [An intriguing historical account of the unravelling of the role of the thymus.]

Nemazee D. & Fowlkes B.J. (eds) (1999) Lymphocyte Development. *Current Opinion in Immunology* **11** (2).

Turner R.J. (ed.) (1994) *Immunology: A Comparative Approach*. John Wiley, Chichester.

Youinou P., Jamin C. & Lydyard P.M. (1999) CD5 expression in human B-cell populations. *Immunology Today* **20** (7), 312.

CHAPTER 11

Adversarial strategies during infection

We are engaged in constant warfare with the microbes which surround us, and the processes of mutation and evolution have tried to select microorganisms with the means of evading our defense mechanisms. In this chapter, we look at the varied, often ingenious, adversarial strategies which we and our enemies have developed over very long periods of time.

INFLAMMATION REVISITED

The acute inflammatory process involves a protective influx of white cells, complement, antibody and other plasma proteins into a site of infection or injury and was discussed in broad outline in the introductory chapters.

Mediators of inflammation

A complex variety of mediators is involved in acute inflammatory responses. Some act directly on the smooth muscle wall surrounding the arterioles to alter blood flow. Others act on the venules to cause contraction of the endothelial cells with transient opening of the interendothelial junctions and consequent transudation of plasma. The migration of leukocytes from the bloodstream is facilitated by cytokines, which upregulate the expression of adherence molecules on both endothelial and white cells, and chemokines, which lead the leukocytes to the inflamed site.

Leukocytes bind to endothelial cells through paired adhesion molecules

The adherence of leukocytes to the endothelial vessel wall through the interaction of complementary binding of cell surface molecules is an absolutely crucial step in inflammation. Several classes of molecule subserve this function, some acting as lectins to bind a carbohydrate ligand on the complementary partner.

Initiation of the acute inflammatory response

A very early event is the upregulation of P-selectin and platelet activating factor (PAF) on the endothelial cells lining the venules by histamine or thrombin released by the original inflammatory stimulus. Engagement of P-selectin molecule with ligands on polymorphonuclear neutrophils (PMN)) causes the neutrophil to **roll** along the endothelial wall and helps PAF to dock onto its corresponding receptor. This, in turn, increases surface expression of the integrin, lymphocyte function associated molecule-1 (LFA-1), which now binds the neutrophil very firmly to the endothelial surface (figure 11.1).

Activation of the neutrophils also makes them more responsive to chemotactic agents and, under the influence of C5a and leukotriene-B4, the PMNs exit from the circulation by moving purposefully through the gap between endothelial cells, across the basement membrane (**diapedesis**) and up the chemotactic gradient to the inflammation site.

The ongoing inflammatory process

Tissue macrophages under the stimulus of local infection or injury secrete an imposing array of mediators. These include the cytokines interleukin-1 (IL-1) and tumor necrosis factor α (TNFα), which stimulate the endothelial cells to upregulate the adhesion molecule E-selectin, and a group of **chemokines** (*chemo*tactic cyto*kines*; table 11.1) such as IL-8, which are highly effective PMN chemotaxins. In general, chemokines of the C-X-C subfamily (defined in table 11.1) such as IL-8 are specific for neutrophils and, to varying extents, lymphocytes, whereas chemokines with the C-C motif are chemotactic for monocytes and variably for natural killer (NK) cells, basophils and eosinophils. Eotaxin is highly specific for eosinophils and the presence of significant concentrations of this mediator together with RANTES

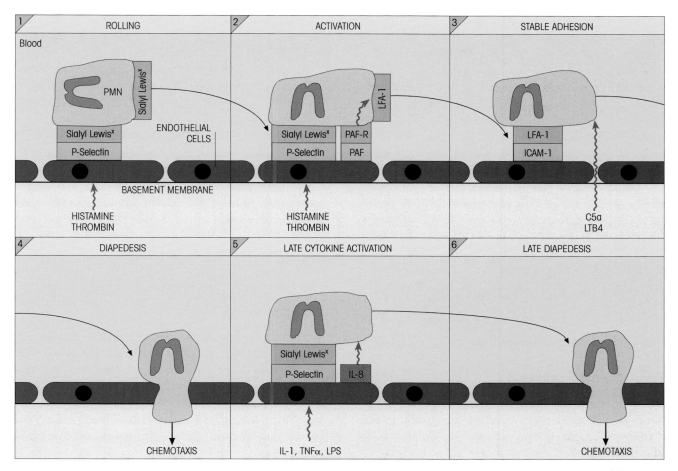

Figure 11.1 Early events in inflammation affecting neutrophil margination and diapedesis. Recognition of extracellular gradients of the chemotactic mediators by receptors on the polymorphonuclear neutrophil (PMN) surface triggers intracellular signals which generate motion. Sialyl Lewis^x is a carbohydrate ligand on the PMN. The neutrophils crawl rather than swim, and migration along the extracellular matrix vitronectin is dependent upon very rapid cycles of integrin-dependent adhesion and detachment regulated by calcineurin.

(*r*egulated upon *a*ctivation *n*ormal *T*-cell *e*xpressed and *s*ecreted) in mucosal surfaces could account for the enhanced population of eosinophils in those tissues.

Clearly this whole operation serves to focus the immune defenses around the invading microorganisms. These become coated with antibody, C3b and certain acute phase proteins and are ripe for phagocytosis by the activated granulocytes and macrophages.

Of course it is beneficial to recruit lymphocytes to sites of infection and we should remember that endothelial cells in these areas express VCAM-1, which acts as a homing receptor for VLA-4-positive activated memory T-cells. In addition, the endothelial cells themselves, when activated, release the chemokines IL-8 and lymphotactin, which will attract lymphocytes to the site of the inflammatory response.

Regulation and resolution of inflammation

With its customary prudence, evolution has established regulatory mechanisms to prevent inflammation from getting out of hand. At the humoral level we have a series of complement regulatory proteins such as C1 inhibitor, the C3 control proteins factors H and I, complement receptor CR1, and decay accelerating factor (DAF).

At the cellular level, PGE$_2$, transforming growth factor β (TGFβ) and glucocorticoids are powerful regulators. PGE$_2$ is a potent inhibitor of lymphocyte proliferation and cytokine production by T-cells and macrophages. TGFβ deactivates macrophages by inhibiting the production of reactive oxygen intermediates and downregulating MHC class II expression, and it inhibits cytotoxic activity of γ-interferon (IFNγ)-activated NK cells.

Chronic inflammation

If an inflammatory agent persists, either because of its resistance to metabolic breakdown or through the inability of a deficient immune system to clear an infectious microbe, the character of the cellular response changes. The site becomes dominated by macrophages with varying morphology: many have an activated appearance, some form arrays of what are termed 'epithelioid' cells and others fuse to form giant cells. If an adaptive immune response is involved, lymphocytes in various guises will also be present. This characteristic **granuloma** walls off the persisting agent from the remainder of the body (see section on type IV hypersensitivity in Chapter 14, p. 135, and figure 14.13).

EXTRACELLULAR BACTERIA SUSCEPTIBLE TO KILLING BY PHAGOCYTOSIS AND COMPLEMENT

Bacterial survival strategies

The variety and ingenuity of escape mechanisms demonstrated by bacteria are most intriguing and, as with virtually all infectious agents, if you can think of a possible avoidance strategy, some microbe will already have used it.

A common mechanism by which virulent forms escape phagocytosis is by synthesis of an outer **capsule**, which does not adhere readily to phagocytic cells and covers carbohydrate molecules on the bacterial surface which could otherwise be recognized by phagocyte receptors. Other organisms have actively **antiphagocytic** cell surface molecules, and some go as far as to secrete **exotoxins**, which actually poison the leukocytes. Many organisms have developed mechanisms to resist complement activation and lysis. For example, Gram-positive organisms have evolved thick peptidoglycan layers which prevent the insertion of the lytic C5b–9 membrane attack complex into the bacterial cell membrane.

The host counter-attack

The defense mechanisms exploit the specificity and variability of the antibody molecule. Antibodies can defeat these devious attempts to avoid engulfment by neutralizing the antiphagocytic molecules and by binding to the surface of the organisms to focus the site for fixation of complement, so 'opsonizing' the organisms for ingestion by polymorphs and

Chemokine	Type	Chemoattractant specificity					
		Neutrophils	Basophils	Eosinophils	NK cells	Monocytes	Lymphocytes
IL-8	CXC	+++					+++
ENA-78	CXC	+++					
NAP-2	CXC	++					
IP-10	CXC						+++
Eotaxin	CC			+++			
RANTES	CC		+++	++	+	+++	
MCP-1	CC		++		+++	++	+
MCP-2	CC					+	
MCP-3	CC		++	++		++	
MIP-1α	CC			++	+++	+++	
MIP-1β	CC				+++	+++	
Lymphotactin	C						+++

Table 11.1 Chemokines: leukocyte chemoattractant specificities.

CXC=chemokine with any amino acid X intervening between the first + second conserved cysteines of the four which characterize the chemokine structural motif; CC=no intervening residue; C=lacks first and third cysteines of the motif; except for IP-10, the CXC motif is preceded by the amino acids E-L-R; ENA-78=epithelial derived neutrophil attractant-78; NAP-2=neutrophil activating protein-2; IP-10=interferon-inducible protein-10; RANTES=regulated upon activation normal T-cell expressed and secreted; MCP=monocyte chemotactic proteins; MIP=macrophage inflammatory protein.
(Data summarized from Schall T.J. & Bacon K.B. (1994) *Current Opinion in Immunology* **6**, 865.)

macrophages or preparing them for the terminal membrane attack complex.

Toxin neutralization

Circulating antibodies act to neutralize the soluble antiphagocytic molecules and other exotoxins released by bacteria. In its complex with antibody, the toxin may be unable to diffuse away rapidly and will be susceptible to phagocytosis.

Opsonization of bacteria

Mannose-binding protein is a molecule with a similar ultra-structure to C1q which can bind to terminal mannose on the bacterial surface and can lead to the antibody-independent activation of the classical complement pathway. Encapsulated bacteria which resist phagocytosis become extremely attractive to polymorphs and macrophages when coated with antibody and C3b, and their rate of clearance from the bloodstream is strikingly enhanced (figures 11.2 & 11.3). Furthermore, complexes containing C3b may show immune adherence to the CR1 complement receptors on red cells to provide aggregates which are transported to the liver for phagocytosis.

Some elaboration on **complement receptors** may be pertinent at this stage. The CR1 receptors for C3b are also present on neutrophils, macrophages, B-cells and follicular dendritic cells in lymph nodes. Together with the CR3 receptor, they have the main responsibility for clearance of complexes containing C3.

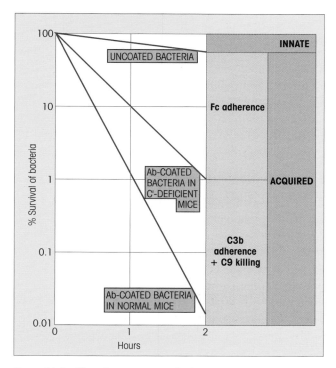

Figure 11.2 Effect of opsonizing antibody and complement on rate of clearance of virulent bacteria from the blood. The uncoated bacteria are phagocytosed rather slowly (*innate immunity*) but, on coating with antibody, adherence to phagocytes is increased many-fold (*acquired immunity*). The adherence is less effective in animals temporarily depleted of complement. This is a hypothetical but realistic situation; the natural proliferation of the bacteria has been ignored.

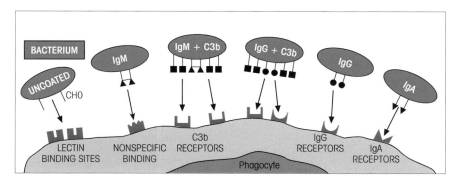

Figure 11.3 Immunoglobulin and complement coats greatly increase the adherence of bacteria (and other antigens) to macrophages and polymorphs. Uncoated bacteria adhere to lectin-like sites, including the mannose-binding receptor. There are no specific binding sites for IgM (▲▲) but there are high-affinity receptors for IgG (Fc) (●) and iC3b (■: CR1 and CR3 types) on the macrophage surface which considerably enhance the strength of binding. The augmenting effect of complement is due to the fact that two adjacent IgG molecules can fix many C3b molecules, thereby increasing the number of links to the macrophage. Although IgM does not bind specifically to the macrophage, it promotes adherence through complement fixation. Specific receptors for the Fcα domains of IgA have also been defined.

CR2 receptors, which bind to various breakdown products of C3 such as C3dg and iC3b, are present on B-cells and follicular dendritic cells and transduce accessory signals for B-cell activation especially in the germinal centers (cf. pp. 52,78). Their affinity for the Epstein–Barr virus (EBV) provides the means for entry of the virus into the B-cell.

CR3 receptors on polymorphs, macrophages and NK cells all bind the inactivated form C3bi.

The secretory immune system protects the external mucosal surfaces

We have earlier emphasized the critical nature of the mucosal barriers, particularly in the gut where there is a potentially hostile interface with the microbial hordes. With an area of around 400 square meters, give or take a tennis court or two, the epithelium of the adult mucosae represents the most frequent portal of entry for common infectious agents, allergens and carcinogens. The need for well-marshalled, highly effective mucosal immunity is glaringly obvious.

The mucosal surfaces are mainly defended by secretory IgA and IgM, with IgA1 predominating in the upper areas and IgA2 in the large bowel. The size of the task is high-lighted by the fact that 80% of the Ig-producing B-cells in the body are present in the secretory mucosae and exocrine glands. IgA antibodies afford protection in the external body fluids, tears, saliva, nasal secretions and those bathing the surfaces of the intestine (so-called 'coproantibodies') and lung, by coating bacteria and viruses and preventing their adherence to the epithelial cells of the mucous membranes. In addition high-affinity Fc receptors for this Ig class have been identified on macrophages and polymorphs and can mediate phagocytosis (figure 11.4).

Where the opsonized organism is too large for phagocytosis, it can be killed by antibody-dependent cell-mediated cytotoxicity (ADCC), discussed earlier (p. 19). This is particularly important in controlling parasitic infections.

BACTERIA WHICH GROW IN AN INTRACELLULAR HABITAT

Cell-mediated immunity is crucial for the control of intracellular organisms

Some strains of bacteria, such as the tubercle and leprosy bacilli and *Listeria* and *Brucella* organisms, escape the wrath of the immune system by cheekily fashioning an intracellular life within one of its strongholds, the macrophage no less

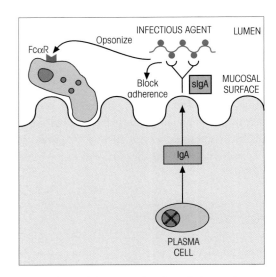

Figure 11.4 Defense of the mucosal surfaces. IgA opsonizes organisms and prevents adherence to the mucosa.

(figure 11.5). Mononuclear phagocytes are a good target for such organisms in the sense that they are very mobile and allow wide dissemination throughout the body. Entry of opsonized bacteria is facilitated by phagocytic uptake after attachment to Fcγ and C3b receptors but once inside many of them defy the mighty macrophage by subverting the innate killing mechanisms.

In an elegant series of experiments, Mackaness demonstrated the importance of cell-mediated immune (CMI) reactions for the killing of these intracellular parasites and the establishment of an immune state. Animals infected with moderate doses of *Mycobacterium tuberculosis* overcome the infection and are immune to subsequent challenge with the bacillus. The immunity can be transferred to a normal recipient by means of T-lymphocytes but not macrophages or serum from an immune animal. Supporting this view, that specific immunity is mediated by T-cells, is the greater susceptibility of patients with T-cell defects such as HIV infection, to infection with mycobacteria or other intracellular organisms.

Activated macrophages kill intracellular parasites

Resting macrophages can be activated in several stages, but the ability to kill obligate intracellular microbes only comes after stimulation by macrophage activating factor(s) such as IFNγ released from stimulated lymphokine-producing T-cells. Foremost amongst the killing mechanisms which are upregulated are those mediated by reactive oxygen intermediates and NO. The activated macrophage is undeniably a

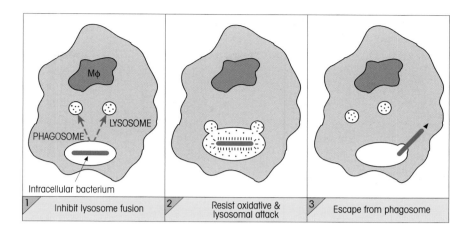

Figure 11.5 Evasion of phagocytic death by intracellular bacteria.

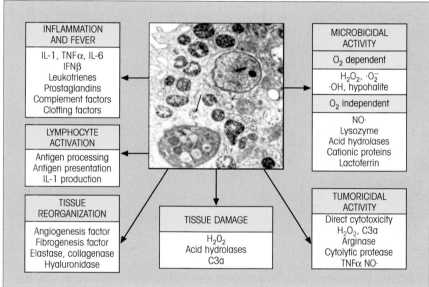

Figure 11.6 The role of the activated macrophage in the initiation and mediation of chronic inflammation with concomitant tissue repair, and in the killing of microbes and tumor cells. It is possible that macrophages differentiate along distinct pathways to subserve these different functions. The electron micrograph shows a highly activated macrophage with many lysosomal structures, which have been highlighted by the uptake of thorotrast; one (arrowed) is seen fusing with a phagosome containing the protozoan *Toxoplasma gondii*. (Photograph kindly supplied by Professor C. Jones.)

remarkable and formidable cell, capable of secreting 60 or more substances which are concerned in chronic inflammatory reactions (figure 11.6).

The mechanism of T-cell-mediated immunity now becomes clear. Specifically primed T-cells react with processed antigen derived from the intracellular bacteria present on the surface of the infected macrophage in association with MHC II; the subsequent release of lymphokines activates the macrophage and endows it with the ability to kill the organisms it has phagocytosed (figure 11.7). Where the host has difficulty in effectively eliminating these organisms, the chronic CMI response to local antigen leads to the accumulation of densely packed macrophages, which release angiogenic and fibrogenic factors and stimulate the formation of granulation tissue and ultimately fibrosis. The activated macrophages, perhaps under the stimulus of IL-4,

transform to epithelioid cells and fuse to become giant cells. As suggested earlier, the resulting granuloma represents an attempt by the body to isolate a site of persistent infection.

IMMUNITY TO VIRAL INFECTION

Protection by serum antibody

The antibody molecule can neutralize viruses by a variety of means. It may stereochemically inhibit combination with the receptor site on cells, thereby preventing penetration and subsequent intracellular multiplication — the protective effect of antibodies to influenza viral hemagglutinin providing a good example. Antibody may destroy a free virus

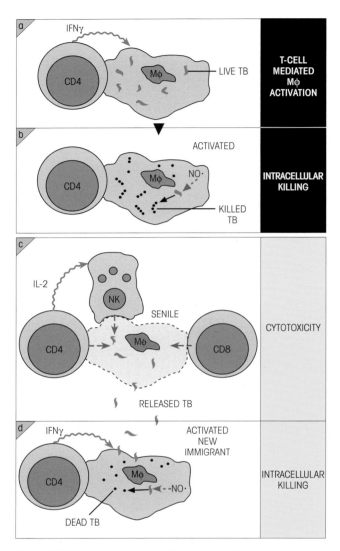

Figure 11.7 The 'cytokine connection': nonspecific murine macrophage killing of intracellular bacteria triggered by a specific T-cell mediated immunity reaction. (a) Specific CD4 Th1 cell recognizes mycobacterial peptide associated with MHC class II and releases Mφ-activating IFNγ. (b) The activated Mφ kills the intracellular tubercle bacilli (TB), mainly through generation of toxic NO. (c) A 'senile' Mφ, unable to destroy the intracellular bacteria, is killed by CD8 and CD4 cytotoxic cells and possibly by IL-2-activated NK cells. The Mφ then releases live TB which are taken up and killed by newly recruited Mφ susceptible to IFNγ activation. Human monocytes require activation by both IFNγ and IL-4 plus a CD23-mediated signal for induction of iNO synthase and production of NO.

particle directly through activation of the classical complement pathway or produce aggregation, enhanced phagocytosis and intracellular death by mechanisms already discussed.

Local factors

With some viral diseases, such as influenza and the common cold, there is a short incubation time as the final target organ for the virus is the same as the portal of entry. There is little time for a primary antibody response to be mounted and in all likelihood the **rapid production of interferon** is the most significant mechanism used to counter the viral infection. Antibody, as assessed by the serum titer, seems to arrive on the scene much too late to be of value in aiding recovery. However, recent investigations have shown that antibody levels may be elevated in the local fluids bathing the infected surfaces, for example nasal mucosa and lung, despite low serum titers, and it is the production of **antiviral antibody** (most prominently IgA) by locally deployed immunologically primed cells which is of major importance for the **prevention of subsequent infection**. Unfortunately, in so far as the common cold is concerned, a subsequent infection is likely to involve an antigenically unrelated virus so that general immunity to colds is difficult to achieve.

Cell-mediated immunity gets to the intracellular virus

In Chapter 2 we emphasized the general point that antibody dealt with extracellular infective agents and CMI with intracellular ones. The same holds true for viruses which try to shelter from antibody in an intracellular habitat. Local or systemic antibodies can block the spread of cytolytic viruses which are released from the host cell they have just killed. Antibodies alone, however, are usually inadequate in controlling those viruses which bud off from the surface as infectious particles because they spread to adjacent cells without becoming exposed to antibody (figure 11.8). The importance of CMI for recovery from infection with these agents is underlined by the inability of children with primary T-cell immunodeficiency to cope with such viruses, whereas patients with Ig deficiency but intact CMI are not troubled in this way.

NK cells can kill virally infected targets

In earlier chapters we have explained how early recognition and killing of a virally infected cell before replication occurs is of obvious benefit to the host. The surface of a virally infected cell undergoes modification, probably in its surface carbohydrate structures, making it an attractive target for NK cells. The NK cell possesses two families of surface receptors. One binds to the novel structures expressed by the infected cell, the other recognizes specificities common

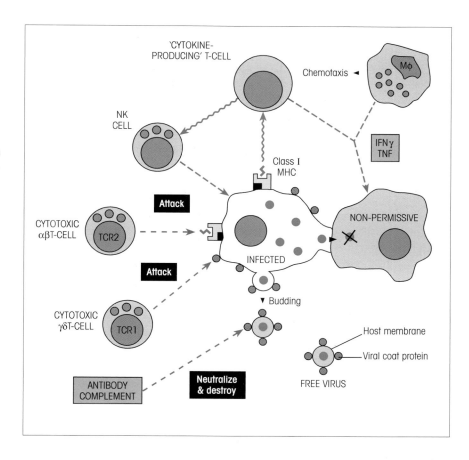

Figure 11.8 Control of infection by 'budding' viruses. Free virus released by budding from the cell surface is neutralized by antibody. Specific cytotoxic T-cells kill virally infected targets directly. Interaction with a (separate?) subpopulation of T-cells releases lymphokines, which attract macrophages, prime contiguous cells with IFNγ and TNF to make them resistant to viral infection, and activate cytotoxic NK cells. NK cells are large granular lymphocytes, powerful producers of IFNγ and GM-CSF. Possibly they recognize neocarbohydrates on the infected cell membrane and antibody coating viral envelope protein (by ADCC). Included in this group of budding viruses are: oncorna (= oncogenic RNA virus, e.g. murine leukemogenic); orthomyxo (influenza); paramyxo (mumps, measles); toga (dengue); rhabdo (rabies); arena (lymphocytic choriomeningitis); adeno, herpes (simplex, varicella zoster, cytomegalo, Epstein–Barr, Marek's disease); pox (vaccinia); papova (SV40, polyoma) and rubella viruses.

to several MHC class I alleles. The first activates killing but the recognition of class I delivers an inhibitory signal. Thus, the sensitivity of the target cell is closely related to self MHC class I expression; sensitive targets have low class I but transfection with the self MHC molecule will generally protect them. It has been suggested that whereas T-cells search for the presence of foreign shapes, NK cells survey tissues for the absence of self as indicated by aberrant or absent expression of MHC class I, which might occur in tumorigenesis or certain viral infections. The production of IFNα during viral infection not only protects surrounding cells but also activates NK cells and upregulates MHC expression on the adjacent cells, making them more resistant to cytotoxicity.

Cytotoxic T-cells (Tc) are crucial elements in immunity to infection by budding viruses

T-lymphocytes from a sensitized host are directly cytotoxic to cells infected with viruses, the new MHC-associated peptide antigens on the target cell surface being recognized by specific αβ receptors on the aggressor lymphocytes. Downregulation of MHC class I poses no problems for γδ T-cells, which

recognize native viral coat protein (e.g. herpes simplex virus glycoprotein) on the cell surface (figure 11.8).

Tc cells can usually be detected in the peripheral blood lymphocytes of individuals who have recovered from infection with influenza, cytomegalovirus (CMV) or EBV by re-exposure *in vitro* to appropriately infected cells. Studies on volunteers, showing that high levels of cytotoxic activity before challenge with live influenza correlated with low or absent shedding of virus, speak in favour of the importance of Tc in human viral infection.

After a natural infection, both antibody and Tc cells are generated; subsequent protection is long lived without reinfection. By contrast, injection of killed influenza produces antibodies but no Tc and protection is only short term.

Cytokines recruit effectors and provide a 'cordon sanitaire'

A number of studies on transfer of protection to influenza and other viral infections focus on CD8 rather than CD4 T-cells as the major defensive force. The knee-jerk response would be to implicate cytotoxicity but it is becoming increasingly clear that CD8 cells also produce cytokines. This may well be crucial when viruses escape the cytotoxic mechanism and manage to sidle laterally into an adjacent cell. CMI can now play some new cards: if T-cells (CD8?) stimulated by viral antigen release lymphokines such as IFNγ and macrophage or monocyte chemotaxin, the mononuclear phagocytes attracted to the site will be activated to secrete TNF, which will synergize with the IFNγ to render the contiguous cells nonpermissive for the replication of any virus acquired by intercellular transfer (figure 11.8). In this way the site of infection can be surrounded by a cordon of resistant cells. Like IFNα, IFNγ may also increase the nonspecific cytotoxicity of NK cells for infected cells. This generation of 'immune interferon' (IFNγ) and TNF in response to nonnucleic acid viral components provides a valuable back-up mechanism when dealing with viruses which are intrinsically poor stimulators of interferon synthesis.

IMMUNITY TO FUNGI

Many fungal infections become established in immunocompromised hosts or when the normal commensal flora are upset by prolonged administration of broad-spectrum antibiotics. T-cells are important in defense and can interact directly with the surface of organisms such as *Cryptococcus neoformans* and *Candida albicans*, killing them by the granzyme system. NK cells can also lyse *C. neoformans*.

IMMUNITY TO PARASITIC INFECTIONS

The consequences of infection with the major parasitic organisms could be at one extreme a lack of immune response leading to overwhelming superinfection, and at the other an exaggerated life-threatening immunopathologic response. To be successful, a parasite must steer a course *between* these extremes, avoiding wholesale killing of the human host and yet at the same time escaping destruction by the immune system. In practice, each type of parasite is virtually a world unto itself in the complexity of the mechanisms by which this is achieved.

The host responses

A wide variety of defensive mechanisms are deployed by the host but the rough generalization may be made that a humoral response develops when the organisms invade the bloodstream (e.g. malaria, trypanosomiasis), whereas parasites which grow within the tissues (e.g. cutaneous leishmaniasis) usually elicit CMI.

Humoral immunity

Antibodies of the right specificity present in adequate concentrations and affinity are reasonably effective in providing protection against blood-borne parasites such as *Trypanosoma brucei* and the sporozoite and merozoite stages of malaria. Thus individuals receiving IgG from solidly immune adults in malaria endemic areas are themselves temporarily protected against infection, the effector mechanisms being opsonization and phagocytosis, and complement-dependent lysis.

A marked feature of the immune reaction to helminthic infections such as *Trichinella spiralis* is the eosinophilia and the high level of IgE antibody produced. Serum levels of IgE can rise from normal values of around 100 ng/ml to as high as 10 000 ng/ml. These changes have all the hallmarks of response to TH2-type lymphokines, and it is notable that in animals infected with helminths, injection of anti-IL-4 greatly reduces IgE production and anti-IL-5 suppresses the eosinophilia. It is relevant to note that schistosomules, the early immature form of the schistosome, can be killed in cultures containing both specific IgG and eosinophils by the ADCC mechanism.

Cell-mediated immunity

Just like mycobacteria, many parasites have adapted to life within the macrophage despite the possession by that cell of potent microbicidal mechanisms including NO·. Intracellular organisms such as *Toxoplasma gondii*, *Trypanosoma cruzi* and *Leishmania* spp. use a variety of ploys to subvert the macrophage killing systems but again, as with mycobacterial infections, cytokine-producing T-cells are crucially important for the stimulation of macrophages to release their killing power and dispose of the unwanted intruders.

In vivo, the balance of cytokines produced may be of the utmost importance. Infection of mice with *Leishmania major* is instructive in this respect: the organism produces fatal disease in susceptible mice but other strains are resistant. In susceptible mice there is excessive stimulation of TH2-like cells producing IL-4, whereas resistant strains are characterized by the expansion of TH1-type cells which secrete IFNγ in response to antigen presented by macrophages harboring *living* protozoa.

Organisms such as malarial plasmodia, and incidentally rickettsiae and chlamydiae, that live in cells which are not professional phagocytes, may be eliminated through activation of intracellular defense mechanisms by IFNγ released from CD8-positive T-cells or even by direct cytotoxicity.

REVISION

See the accompanying website (www.roitt.com) for multiple choice questions.

Immunity to infection involves a constant battle between the host defenses and the mutant microbes trying to evolve evasive strategies. Specific acquired responses amplify and enhance innate immune mechanisms.

Inflammation revisited

• Inflammation is a major defensive reaction initiated by infection or tissue injury.
• The mediators released upregulate adhesion molecules on endothelial cells and leukocytes, which pair together causing first rolling of leukocytes along the vessel wall and then passage across the blood vessel up the chemotactic gradient to the site of inflammation.
• IL-1, TNFα and chemokines such as IL-8 are involved in maintaining the inflammatory process.
• Inflammation is controlled by complement regulatory proteins, PGE$_2$, TGFβ and glucocorticoids.
• Inability to eliminate the initiating agent leads to a chronic inflammatory response dominated by macrophages and often forming granulomas.

Extracellular bacteria susceptible to killing by phagocytosis and complement

• Bacteria try to avoid phagocytosis by surrounding themselves with capsules, secreting exotoxins which kill phagocytes or impede inflammatory reactions, diverting complement to inoffensive sites, or by colonizing relatively inaccessible locations.
• Antibody combats these tricks by neutralizing the toxins, making complement deposition more even on the bacterial surface, overcoming the antiphagocytic nature of the capsules by opsonizing them with Ig and C3b.
• The secretory immune system protects the external mucosal surfaces. IgA inhibits adherence of bacteria and can opsonize them. IgE bound to mast cells can initiate the influx of protective IgG, complement and polymorphs to the site by a miniature acute inflammatory response.

Bacteria which grow in an intracellular habitat

• Intracellular bacteria such as tubercle and leprosy bacilli grow within macrophages.

• They are killed by CMI: specifically sensitized T-helpers release lymphokines on contact with infected macrophages, which powerfully activate the formation of nitric oxide (NO·), reactive oxygen intermediates (ROI) and other microbicidal mechanisms.

Immunity to viral infection

• Antibody neutralizes free virus and is particularly effective when the virus has to travel through the bloodstream before reaching its final target.
• Where the target is the same as the portal of entry, e.g. the lungs, interferon is dominant in recovery from infection.
• Antibody is important in preventing reinfection.
• 'Budding' viruses which can invade lateral cells without becoming exposed to antibody are combated by CMI. Infected cells express a processed viral antigen peptide on their surface in association with MHC class I a short time after entry of the virus, and rapid killing of the cell by cytotoxic αβ-T-cells prevents viral multiplication. γδ-Tc recognize native viral coat protein on the target cell surface. NK cells are also cytotoxic.

Immunity to fungi

• T-cells can kill by direct contact.

Immunity to parasitic infections

• Diseases involving *protozoal parasites* and *helminths* affect hundreds of millions of people. Antibodies are usually effective against the blood-borne forms. IgE production is notoriously increased in worm infestations; schistosomes coated with IgG or IgE are killed by adherent eosinophils through extracellular mechanisms involving release of cationic proteins and peroxidase.
• Organisms such as *Leishmania* spp., *Trypanosoma cruzi* and *Toxoplasma gondii* hide from antibodies inside macrophages and use the same strategies as intracellular parasitic bacteria to survive. Like them they are killed when the macrophages are activated by TH1 cytokines produced during cell-mediated immune responses. NO· is an important killing agent.
• CD8 cells also have a protective role.

FURTHER READING

Bloom B. & Zinkernagel R. (eds) (1996) Immunity to infection. *Current Opinion in Immunology* **8**, 465.

Brandtzaeg P. (1995) Basic mechanisms of mucosal immunity: a major adaptive defense system. *The Immunologist* **3**, 89–96.

Cotran R.S., Kumar V. & Robbins S.L. (1989) *Pathologic Basis of Disease*, chs 1 & 2. W.B. Saunders, Philadelphia.

Mims C.A., Playfair J.H.L., Roitt I.M., Wakelin D. & Williams R. (1993) *Medical Microbiology*. C.V. Mosby, London. [Based on conflict of host vs microbe; systems treatment of infections; reference tables of organisms.]

Ogra P.E. *et al.* (eds) (1994) *Handbook of Mucosal Immunology*. Academic Press, Orlando.

Price D.A., Klennerman P., Booth B.L., Phillips R.E. & Sewell A.K. (1999) Cytotoxic T lymphocytes, chemokines and antiviral immunity. *Immunology Today* **20** (5), 212.

Rappuoli R., Pizza M., Douce G. & Dougan G. (1999) Structure and mucosal adjuvanticity of cholera and *Escherichia coli* heat-labile enterotoxins. *Immunology Today* **20** (11), 493.

Spriggs M.K. & Sher A. (eds) (1999) Section on Immunity to Infection. *Current Opinion in Immunology* **11** (4).

CHAPTER 12

Prophylaxis

Immunization against infectious disease represents one of science's greatest triumphs. Many of the epidemic diseases of the past are now controlled and all but eliminated in developed countries, and new vaccines promise protection against a variety of more recently recognized infectious diseases including the various forms of hepatitis, Lyme disease and hopefully HIV infection. Modern vaccine biology is now targeting not only infectious diseases but also autoimmune and malignant disease. This chapter will review various procedures for stimulating antibody production or activating T-cell responses against defined prophylactically administered antigens.

PASSIVELY ACQUIRED IMMUNITY

Temporary protection against infection can be established by giving preformed antibody from another individual of the same or a different species (table 12.1). As the acquired antibodies are utilized by combination with antigen or catabolized in the normal way, this protection is gradually lost.

Horse globulins containing antitetanus and antidiphtheria toxins have been extensively employed prophylactically, but with the advent of antibiotics the requirement for such antisera has diminished. One complication of this form of therapy is serum sickness developing in response to the foreign protein. This is more likely to occur in subjects already sensitized by previous contact with horse globulin; thus individuals who have been given horse antitetanus (e.g. for immediate protection after receiving a wound) are later advised to undergo a course of active immunization to obviate the need for further injections of horse protein in any subsequent emergency.

Maternally acquired antibody

In the first few months of life, protection is afforded by maternally derived antibodies acquired by placental transfer and by intestinal absorption of colostral immunoglobulins. The major immunoglobulin in milk is secretory IgA, which is not absorbed by the baby but remains in the intestine to protect the mucosal surfaces. The sIgA antibodies are directed against bacterial and viral antigens often present in the intestine, and it is presumed that IgA-producing cells, responding to gut antigens, migrate and colonize breast tissue where the antibodies they produce appear in the milk.

Pooled human γ-globulin

Regular injection of pooled human adult γ-globulin collected from the plasma of normal donors is an essential treatment for patients with long-standing humoral immunodeficiency. Preparations containing high titers of antibodies to specific antigens may be used to modify the effects of chickenpox or measles in patients with defective immune responses due to prematurity, protein malnutrition, steroid treatment or patients with immune deficiency due to leukemia. Contacts with cases of infectious hepatitis may also be afforded protection by γ-globulin, especially when in the latter case the material is derived from the serum of individuals vaccinated some weeks previously. Cytomegalovirus human immune globulin is now administered to recipients of organ transplants taken from CMV-positive donors, and rabies immune globulin may be given together with active immunization to patients bitten by a potentially rabid animal. Curiously, pooled γ-globulin is being increasingly used as a treatment for autoimmune diseases such as idiopathic thrombocytopenic purpura. The effect is presumed to be due to the presence of anti-idiotype antibodies in the pooled globulin. The bioengineering of custom-designed antibodies is of increasing importance (see Chapter 3).

Table 12.1 Passive immunotherapy with antibody.

INFECTION	SOURCE OF ANTIBODY		USE
	HORSE	HUMAN	
Tetanus Diphtheria	√	√	Prophylaxis Treatment
Botulism Gas gangrene Snake or scorpion bite	√	–	Treatment
Varicella zoster	–	√	Treatment immunodeficiency
Rabies	–	√	Post-exposure to vaccine
Hepatitis B	–	√	Treatment
Hepatitis A Measles	–	Pooled Ig	Prophylaxis (Travel) Treatment

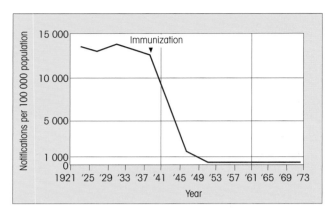

Figure 12.1 Notification of diphtheria in England and Wales per 100 000 population showing dramatic fall after immunization. (Reproduced from Dick G. (1978) *Immunisation*. Update Books, with kind permission of the author and publishers.)

VACCINATION

Herd immunity

In the case of tetanus, active immunization is of benefit to the individual but not to the community since it will not eliminate the organism, which persists in the soil as highly resistant spores. Where a disease depends on human transmission, immunity in just a proportion of the population can help the whole community if it leads to a fall in the reproduction rate (i.e. the number of further cases produced by each infected individual) to less than one; under these circumstances the disease will die out, witness for example the disappearance of diphtheria from communities in which around 75% of the children have been immunized (figure 12.1). But this figure must be maintained; there is no room for complacency. In contrast, focal outbreaks of poliomyelitis have occurred in communities which object to immunization on religious grounds, raising an important point for parents in general.

Strategic considerations

The objective of vaccination is to provide effective immunity by establishing adequate levels of antibody and a primed population of memory cells which can rapidly expand on renewed contact with antigen and so provide protection against infection. Sometimes, as with polio infection, a high blood titer of antibody is required; in mycobacterial diseases such as tuberculosis (TB), a macrophage-activating cell-mediated immunity (CMI) is most effective, whereas with influenza virus infection, antibodies and cytotoxic T-cells play a significant role. The site of the immune response

Table 12.2 Factors required for a successful vaccine.

FACTOR	REQUIREMENTS
Effectiveness	Must evoke protective levels of immunity: at the appropriate site of relevant nature (Ab, T_c, T_{H1}, T_{H2}) of adequate duration
Availability	Readily cultured in bulk or accessible source of subunit
Stability	Stable under extreme climatic conditions, preferably not requiring refrigeration
Cheapness	What is cheap in the West may be expensive in developing countries but WHO tries to help
Safety	Eliminate any pathogenicity

evoked by vaccination may also be most important. For example in cholera, antibodies need to be in the gut lumen to inhibit adherence to and colonization of the intestinal wall.

In addition to an ability to engender effective immunity, a number of mundane but nonetheless crucial conditions must be satisfied for a vaccine to be considered successful (table 12.2). The antigens must be readily available, the preparation should be stable on storage, and it should be cheap, easy to administer and, certainly, safe.

KILLED ORGANISMS AS VACCINES

The simplest way to destroy the ability of microbes to cause disease yet maintain their antigenic constitution is to prevent their replication by killing in an appropriate manner. Parasitic worms and, to a lesser extent, protozoa are extremely difficult to grow up in bulk to manufacture killed vaccines. This problem does not arise for many bacteria and viruses and, in these cases, the inactivated microorganisms have generally provided safe antigens for immunization. Examples are typhoid, cholera and killed poliomyelitis (Salk) vaccines. Care has to be taken to ensure that important protective antigens are not destroyed in the inactivation process.

LIVE ATTENUATED ORGANISMS HAVE MANY ADVANTAGES AS VACCINES

The objective of attenuation is to produce a modified organism which mimics the natural behavior of the original microbe without causing significant disease. In many instances the immunity conferred by killed vaccines, even when given with adjuvant (see below), is often inferior to that resulting from infection with live organisms. This must be partly because the replication of the living microbes confronts the host with a **larger and more sustained dose of antigen** and that, with budding viruses, infected cells are required for the establishment of good **cytotoxic T-cell memory**. Another significant advantage of using live organisms is that the immune **response takes place largely at the site of the natural infection**. This is well illustrated by the nasopharyngeal IgA response to immunization with polio vaccine. In contrast with the ineffectiveness of parenteral injection of killed vaccine, intranasal administration evoked a good local antibody response which declined over a period of 2 months. Oral immunization with *live attenuated* virus produced an even better response with a persistently high IgA antibody level (figure 12.2).

Classical methods of attenuation

The objective of attenuation, that of producing an organism which causes only a very mild form of the natural disease, can be equally well attained by employing heterologous strains which are virulent for another species, but avirulent in man. The best example of this was Jenner's seminal demonstration that cowpox infection would protect against smallpox. Since then, a truly remarkable global effort by the World Health Organization, combining extensive vaccination and selective epidemiological control methods, **has completely eradicated the human disease**—a wonderful achievement.

Attenuation itself can be achieved by modifying the conditions under which an organism grows. Pasteur first achieved the production of live but nonvirulent forms of chicken cholera bacillus and anthrax by culturing at higher temperatures and under anaerobic conditions. A virulent

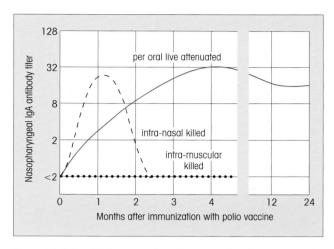

Figure 12.2 Local IgA response to polio vaccine. Local secretory antibody synthesis is confined to the specific anatomical sites which have been directly stimulated by contact with antigen. (Data from Ogra P.L. *et al.* (1975) In: *Viral Immunology and Immunopathology* (ed. A.L. Notkins), p. 67. Academic Press, New York.)

strain of *Mycobacterium tuberculosis* became attenuated by chance in 1908 when Calmette and Guérin at the Institut Pasteur, Lille, added bile to the culture medium in an attempt to achieve dispersed growth. After 13 years of culture in bile-containing medium, the strain remained attenuated and was used successfully to vaccinate children against tuberculosis. The same organism, BCG (bacille Calmette–Guérin), is widely used today for immunization of tuberculin-negative individuals in many countries. It should be stressed that an individual receiving BCG immunization will convert from being tuberculin skin test-negative to the positive state. Although the immunization often confers protection, the feeling in the USA is that a negative skin test is important in excluding a diagnosis of TB, and BCG negates the use of the skin test. For this reason therefore, BCG is not employed in the USA.

Attenuation of viruses usually requires cultivation in nonhuman cells where after many rounds of culture they develop multiple random genetic mutations, some of which lead to a loss of ability to infect human cells. Unfortunately on very rare occasions pathogenicity may return by further mutations of the organism, as was seen with the polio virus vaccine where reversions to the wild type resulted in clinical cases of the disease occurring in vaccinated children.

Attenuation by recombinant DNA technology

Instead of the random mutations achieved by classic attenuation procedures, genetic recombination is now being used to develop various attenuated strains of viruses.

Microbial vectors for other genes

An ingenious trick is to use a virus as a 'piggyback' for genes from another virus, particularly one that cannot be grown successfully, or which is inherently dangerous. Large DNA viruses, such as vaccinia, can act as carriers for one or many foreign genes while retaining infectivity for animals and cultured cells. The proteins encoded by these genes are appropriately expressed *in vivo*, and are processed for major histocompatibility complex (MHC) presentation by the infected cells, thus effectively endowing the host with both humoral and CMI.

A wide variety of genes have been expressed by vaccinia virus vectors including hepatitis surface antigen (HBsAg), which has protected chimpanzees against the clinical effects of hepatitis B virus. Spectacular neutralizing antibody titers were produced by a construct with the gene encoding rabies virus glycoprotein, which also protected animals against intracerebral challenge. It is even possible to make a vector with two inserts.

Another approach is to employ attenuated bacteria such as BCG, as vehicles for antigens required to evoke CD4-mediated T-cell immunity. The organism is avirulent, has a low frequency of serious complications, can be administered any time after birth, has strong adjuvant properties, gives long-lasting CMI after a single injection and is a bargain at around US$ 0.05 a shot. Since *Salmonella* can elicit **mucosal responses by oral immunization**, organisms made to express proteins from other pathogens could be useful potential oral vaccines.

SUBUNIT VACCINES CONTAINING INDIVIDUAL PROTECTIVE ANTIGENS

A whole parasite or bacterium usually contains many antigens which are not concerned in the protective response of the host but may provoke hypersensitivity. Vaccination with the isolated protective antigens may avoid these complications, and identification of these antigens then opens up the possibility of producing them synthetically.

Bacterial exotoxins such as those produced by diphtheria and tetanus bacilli have long been used as immunogens. First, they must of course be detoxified and this is achieved by formaldehyde treatment, which fortunately does not destroy the major immunogenic determinants (figure 12.3). Immunization with the resulting **toxoid** will therefore provoke the formation of protective antibodies, which neutralize the toxin by stereochemically blocking the active site. The toxoid is generally given after adsorption to aluminum

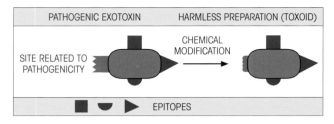

Figure 12.3 Modification of toxin to harmless toxoid without losing many of the antigenic determinants. Thus antibodies to the toxoid will react well with the original toxin.

hydroxide, which acts as an adjuvant and produces higher antibody titers.

Antigens can be synthesized through gene cloning

The emphasis now is to move towards gene cloning of individual proteins once they have been identified immunologically and biochemically. Recombinant DNA technology enables us to make genes encoding part or the whole of a protein peptide chain almost at will, and express them in an appropriate vector. This approach has been used to produce a commercial hepatitis vaccine employing the product secreted by yeast cells expressing the HBsAg gene. The potential of gene cloning is clearly vast and, in principle, economical, but there are sometimes difficulties in identifying a good expression vector and in obtaining correct folding of the peptide chain to produce an active protein.

One restriction to gene cloning is that carbohydrate antigens cannot be synthesized directly by recombinant DNA technology, although preliminary attempts to clone the cohort of genes which encode the cascade of synthetic enzymes needed to produce complex carbohydrates are underway.

The naked gene itself acts as a vaccine

It has recently been appreciated that injected DNA functions as a source of immunogen and can induce strong immune responses both humoral and cell-mediated. The gene is stitched in place in a DNA plasmid with appropriate promoters and enhancers and injected into muscle where it can give prolonged expression of protein. Broad immune responses are observed including induction of Tc cells, presumably reflecting the cytosolic expression of the protein and its processing with MHC class I.

DNA for this procedure can be obtained directly from current clinical material without having to select specific mutant strains. Altogether, the speed and simplicity mean that the two years previously needed to make a recombinant vaccine can be reduced to months. DNA vaccines do not need the cumbersome and costly protein synthesis and purification procedures that subunit formulations require; they can be prepared in a highly stable powder and, above all, they are incredibly cheap. Before there is widespread use in humans, however, a number of safety considerations, such as the possibility of permanent incorporation of a plasmid into the host genome, need to be addressed.

CURRENT VACCINES

The established vaccines in current use and the schedules for their administration are set out in table 12.3.

ADJUVANTS

For practical and economic reasons, prophylactic immunization should involve the minimum number of injections and the least amount of antigen. We have referred to the undoubted advantages of replicating attenuated organisms in this respect but nonliving organisms, and especially purified products, frequently require an adjuvant, which by definition is a substance incorporated into or injected simultaneously with antigen which potentiates the immune response (Latin *adjuvare* to help). The mode of action of adjuvants involves a number of mechanisms, one of which is to counteract the dispersion of free antigen and localize it, either at an extracellular location or within macrophages. The most common adjuvants of this type used in man are **aluminum compounds** (phosphate and hydroxide). Virtually all adjuvants stimulate antigen-presenting cells and improve their immunogenicity by the provision of accessory costimulatory signals to direct lymphocytes towards an immune response rather than tolerance, and by the secretion of soluble stimulatory factors (e.g. interleukin (IL-1)), which influence the proliferation of lymphocytes.

Table 12.3 Current vaccination practice.

VACCINE		ADMINISTRATION		
		UK	USA	OTHER COUNTRIES
CHILDREN				
Triple (DTP) vaccine: diphtheria, tetanus, pertussis	Primary	2–6 mo (3x/4 weekly)		Japan: 2 yr
	Boost	3–5yr	15 mo/4 yr DT every 10 yr	
Polio: live	Primary	Concomitant with DTP		
	Boost	4/6 yr	15 mo, 4 yr high-risk adult	
killed		Immunocompromised		
MMR vaccine: measles, mumps rubella	Primary	12–18		Africa: 6 mo
	Boost	3–5yr 10–14 yr seronegative girls selectively with rubella		
BCG (TB, leprosy)		10–14 yr	high risk only	Tropics: at birth
Haemophilus		18 mo		
Varicella		Neonates at risk, immunocompromised		
ELDERLY				
Pneumococcal polysaccharide serotypes		Aged & high risk		
Influenza		Aged & high risk		
SPECIAL GROUPS				
Hepatitis B		Travellers, high risk groups		
Hepatitis A Meningitis (A+C)		Travellers to endemic areas		
Yellow fever Typhoid Cholera		Travellers to endemic areas		Tropics: infants Yellow fever: boost residents and frequent visitors every 10 yr
Rabies		Prophylactically in high risk groups Post-exposure to contacts in endemic areas		

REVISION

See the accompanying website (www.roitt.com) for multiple choice questions.

Passively acquired immunity
• Horse antisera have been extensively used in the past but their use is now more restricted because of the danger of serum sickness.

• Passive immunity can be acquired by maternal antibodies or from homologous pooled γ-globulin.
• Sera containing high-titer antibodies against a specific pathogen are useful in treating or preventing various

viral diseases such as severe chickenpox, CMV infection or rabies.

Vaccination

• Active immunization provides a protective state through contact with a harmless form of the organism.
• A good vaccine should be based on antigens which are easily available, cheap, stable under extreme climatic conditions and nonpathogenic.

Killed organisms as vaccines

• Killed bacteria and viruses have been widely used.

Live attenuated organisms

• The advantages are: replication gives a bigger dose, and the immune response is produced at the site of the natural infection.
• Attenuated vaccines are produced by altering the conditions under which organisms are cultivated.
• Attenuated vaccinia can provide a 'piggyback' carrier for genes from other organisms which are difficult to attenuate.
• BCG is a good vehicle for antigens requiring CD4 T-cell immunity, and salmonella constructs may give oral and systemic immunity. Intranasal immunization is fast gaining popularity.
• Risks are reversion to the virulent form and danger to immunocompromised individuals.

Subunit vaccines

• Whole organisms have a multiplicity of antigens, some of which are not protective, may induce hypersensitivity or might even be frankly immunosuppressive.

• It makes sense in these cases to use purified components.
• Toxoids are exotoxins treated with formaldehyde which destroys the pathogenicity of the organism but leaves antigenicity intact.
• There is greatly increased use of recombinant DNA technology to produce these antigens. Expression in bananas provides a very cheap way of achieving oral immunization in the developing world.
• Naked DNA encoding the vaccine subunit can be injected directly into muscle, where it expresses the protein and produces immune responses. The advantages are stability, ease of production and cheapness.

Current vaccines

• Children in the USA and UK are routinely immunized with diphtheria and tetanus toxoids and pertussis (DTP triple vaccine) and attenuated strains of measles, mumps and rubella (MMR) and polio. BCG is given at 10–14 years in the UK.
• Subunit forms of pertussis lacking side-effects are being introduced.
• The capsular polysaccharide of *H. influenzae* has to be linked to a carrier.
• The elderly receive vaccines of influenza and *Pneumococcus* polysaccharides.
• Vaccines for hepatitis A and B, meningitis, yellow fever, typhoid, cholera and rabies are available for travellers and high-risk groups.

Adjuvants

• Adjuvants work by producing depots of antigen, and by activating antigen-presenting cells; they sometimes have direct effects on lymphocytes.

FURTHER READING

Dietrich G., Gentschev I., Hess J., Ulmer J.B., Kaufmann S.H. & Goebel W. (1999) Delivery of DNA vaccines by attenuated intracellular bacteria. *Immunology Today* **20** (6), 251.

Kumar V. & Sercarz E. (1996) Genetic vaccination: The advantages of going naked. *Nature Medicine* **2** (8), 857–859.

Lambert P.H. (1993) New vaccines for the world—needs and prospects. *The Immunologist* **1**, 50–55.

Mims C.A., Playfair J.H.L., Roitt I.M., Wakelin D. & Williams R. (1993) *Medical Microbiology*. Mosby, London.

Peter G. (1992) Current concepts: childhood immunizations. *New England Journal of Medicine* **327**, 1794–1800.

Sherwood J.K. *et al.* (1996) Controlled release of antibodies for long-term topical passive immunoprotection of female mice against genital herpes. *Nature Biotechnology* **14** (4), 468.

CHAPTER 13

Immunodeficiency

PRIMARY IMMUNODEFICIENCY STATES IN THE HUMAN

In accord with the dictum that 'most things that can go wrong, do so', a multiplicity of immunodeficiency states in man which are **not secondary** to environmental factors, have been recognized. We have earlier stressed the manner in which the interplay of complement, antibody and phagocytic cells constitutes the basis of a tripartite defense mechanism against pyogenic (pus-forming) infections with bacteria which require prior opsonization before phagocytosis. Hence it is not surprising that deficiency in any one of these factors may predispose the individual to repeated infections of this type. Patients with T-cell deficiency of course present a markedly different pattern of infection, being susceptible to those viruses, intracellular bacteria, fungi and parasites which are normally eradicated by cell-mediated immunity (CMI).

The following sections examine various forms of these primary immunodeficiencies.

DEFICIENCIES OF INNATE IMMUNE MECHANISMS

Phagocytic cell defects

Quantitative neutrophil disorders will clearly lead to recurrent infections, usually with endogenous organisms. Primary defects in neutrophil number are rare as most cases are due to treatment with cytotoxic drugs usually associated with malignant disease. As would be expected these patients are prone to pyogenic infections but not to parasitic, viral or fungal disease.

Chronic granulomatous disease (CGD) is a rare disease in which the monocytes and polymorphs fail to produce reactive oxygen intermediates (figure 13.1) required for the intracellular killing of phagocytosed organisms. This results

in severe recurrent bacterial and fungal infections which when unresolved may lead to granulomas that may obstruct the gastrointestinal and urogenital systems. Curiously, the range of infectious pathogens which trouble these patients is relatively restricted. The most common pathogen is *Staphylococcus aureus* but certain Gram-negative bacilli and fungi such as *Aspergillus fumigatus* and *Candida albicans* are frequently involved.

The disease is due to mutations in cytochrome $b558$ which is crucial for the production of NADPH oxidase, an enzyme important in the generation of superoxide in phagocytes.

The treatment of CGD is aimed primarily at aggressive treatment of infections with antibiotics. γ-Interferon (IFNγ) has been shown to stimulate the production of superoxide by CGD neutrophils resulting in considerably fewer infectious episodes, and this is now a commonly used therapy. Because CGD results from a single gene defect in phagocytic cells, the ideal treatment of the disease would be the transfer of the correct gene into the bone marrow stem cells. Initial work in this area is encouraging. Some patients have been effectively treated by bone marrow transplantation from a normal MHC-matched sibling, but the significant mortality of this procedure needs to be weighed against the much improved quality of life that patients can now expect from conservative treatments with antibiotics and IFNγ.

Chediak–Higashi disease is a rare autosomal recessive disease due to various mutations in a gene called the CHS gene. In this condition neutrophils, monocytes and lymphocytes contain giant lysosomal granules which result from increased granule fusion. This gives rise to phagocytic cells which are defective in chemotaxis, phagocytosis and microbicidal activity, and NK cells which lack cytotoxic activity. In addition to increasing susceptibility to pyogenic infections, these lysosomal defects affect melanocytes causing albinism and platelets giving rise to bleeding disorders.

Leukocyte adhesion deficiency results from lack of the CD18 β-subunit of the β_2-integrins, which include LFA-1. Children with this defect suffer from repeated pyogenic infections because phagocytic cells which would normally

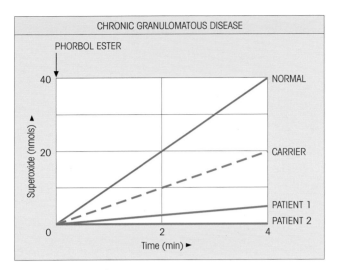

Figure 13.1 Defective respiratory burst in neutrophils of patients with chronic granulomatous disease. The activation of the NADP/cytochrome oxidase is measured by superoxide anion ($\cdot O_2^-$; cf. figure 1.9) production following stimulation with phorbol myristate acetate. Patient 2 has a p92*phox* mutation which prevents expression of the protein, whilst patient 1 has the variant p92*phox* mutation producing very low but measurable levels. Many carriers of the X-linked disease express intermediate levels, as in the individual shown who is the mother of patient 2. (Data from Smith R.M. & Curnutte J.T. (1991) *Blood* 77, 673–686.)

be recruited to a site of infection cannot emigrate through the vessel walls to the infected tissue. They also have problems with wound healing and delayed separation of the umbilical cord is the earliest manifestation of this defect. Fortunately bone marrow transplantation has resulted in restoration of neutrophil function and is now the treatment of choice.

Complement system deficiencies

As we have seen previously, activation of the complement system plays an important role in host defense against bacterial infections and is also crucial for the clearance of immune complexes from the circulation. Genetic deficiencies in almost all the complement proteins have now been described and as would be expected these result in either recurrent infections or failure to clear immune complexes.

Deficiency of early classical pathway proteins results in increased susceptibility to immune-complex disease

This has been observed in patients with deficiency of the C1 proteins, C2 or C4 who have some increase in susceptibility

to infection but also have an unusually high incidence of an SLE (systemic lupus erythematosus)-like disease. Although the reason for this is unclear it could be due to a decreased ability to mount an adequate host response to infection with a putative etiologic agent or, more probably, to eliminate antigen–antibody complexes effectively.

Deficiency of C3 or the control proteins factor H or factor I, results in severe recurrent infections

Although deficiency of C3 is rare, the clinical picture seen in these patients is instructive in emphasizing the crucial role of C3 in both the classical and alternative pathways. Complete absence of this component causes a block in both pathways resulting in defective opsonizing and chemotactic activities. Factor H or factor I deficiency produce a similar clinical picture, because there is inability to destroy C3b. This results in continuous activation of the alternative pathway through the feedback loop, leading to consumption of C3, the levels of which may fall to zero.

Permanent deficiencies in C5, C6, C7 and C8 result in susceptibility to neisserial infection

Many of the individuals with these rare disorders are quite healthy and not particularly prone to infection apart from an increased susceptibility to disseminated *Neisseria gonorrhoeae* and *N. meningitidis* infection. Presumably the host requires a complete and intact complement pathway with its resulting cytolytic activity, to destroy these particular organisms.

Deficiency of C9 does not result in any clinical disorder

A number of individuals, particularly in Japan, have been described as being deficient in the C9 protein, yet show no ill effects. Thus full operation of the terminal complement system does not appear to be essential for survival, and adequate protection must be largely afforded by opsonizing antibodies and the immune adherence mechanism.

Deficiency of the C1 inhibitor causes hereditary angioedema

C1INH acts on the classical complement system by inhibiting the binding of C1r and C1s to C1q and also inhibits factor XII of the clotting system (figure 13.2). Absence of C1INH leads to recurring episodes of acute circumscribed noninflammatory edema mediated by the unrestricted pro-

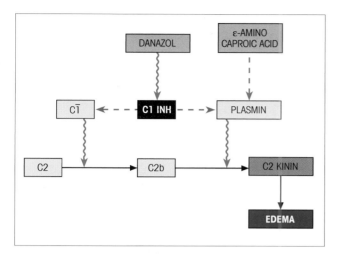

Figure 13.2 C1 inhibitor deficiency and angioedema. C1 inhibitor stoichiometrically inhibits C1, plasmin, kallikrein and activated Hageman factor and deficiency leads to formation of the vasoactive C2 kinin by the mechanism shown. The synthesis of C1 inhibitor can be boosted by methyltestosterone or preferably the less masculinizing synthetic steroid, danazol; alternatively, attacks can be controlled by giving ε-aminocaproic acid to inhibit the plasmin.

duction of the vasoactive C2a fragment. Lack of C1INH also leads to an increase in generation of bradykinin, which adds to the increased permeability of small vessels causing the edema associated with this disease. These patients therefore present with recurrent episodes of swelling of the skin, acute abdominal pain due to swellings of the intestine, and obstruction of the larynx which may rapidly cause complete laryngeal obstruction. Attacks are precipitated by trauma or excessive exercise and can be controlled by anabolic steroids such as danazol, which for unknown reasons suppress the symptoms of hereditary angioedema.

PRIMARY B-CELL DEFICIENCY

Bruton's X-linked agammaglobulinemia (XLA) is one of several immunodeficient syndromes which have been mapped to the X-chromosome (figure 13.3). The defect is due to mutations in the Bruton's tyrosine kinase (*Btk*) gene, which is expressed early in B-cell development and which is crucial for maturation of the B-cell series. Over 100 different *Btk* mutations are now recorded in the XLA mutation registry. Early B-cells are generated in the bone marrow but fail to mature and the production of immunoglobulin in affected males is grossly depressed. B-cells are reduced or absent in the peripheral blood and there are few lymphoid follicles or plasma cells in the lymph nodes.

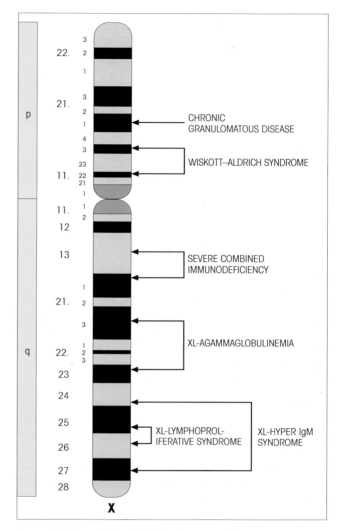

Figure 13.3 Loci of the X-linked (XL) immunodeficiency syndromes.

Affected boys are usually well for the first few months of life as they are protected by transplacentally acquired maternal antibody. They are then subject to repeated infection by pyogenic bacteria—*Staphylococcus aureus, Streptococcus pyogenes* and *pneumoniae, Neisseria meningitidis, Haemophilus influenzae*—and by *Giardia lamblia* which chronically infects the gastrointestinal tract. Resistance to viruses and fungi, which depends on T-lymphocytes, is normal, with the exception of hepatitis and enteroviruses. Therapy involves the repeated administration of human γ-globulin to maintain adequate concentrations of circulating immunoglobulin.

IgA deficiency due to a failure of IgA-bearing lymphocytes to differentiate into plasma cells, is encountered with relative frequency. Antibodies to IgA are often detectable but it is uncertain whether these antibodies prevented development of the IgA system or whether lack of tolerance resulting from an absent IgA system allowed the body to make antibodies to exogenous determinants immunologically related to IgA.

Common variable immunodeficiency is the most common form of primary immunodeficiency, but the least well characterized. It is a heterogeneous disease usually appearing in adult life and is associated with a high incidence of autoimmune diseases and malignant disease, particularly of the lymphoid system. It probably results from inadequate T-cell signal transduction which causes imperfect interactions between T- and B-cells. In the absence of suitable T-cell interactions there is defective terminal differentiation of B-lymphocytes into plasma cells in some cases or defective ability to secrete antibody in others. The genetic basis of this disease is as yet unknown but a large proportion of the cases possess the same HLA haplotypes as patients with IgA deficiency, suggesting a common underlying disorder.

X-linked **hyper-IgM syndrome** is a rare disorder characterized by recurrent bacterial infections, very low levels or absence of IgG, A and E, and normal to raised concentrations of serum IgM and IgD. The disease is due to point mutations, usually single amino acid substitutions in the CD40L expressed by CD4⁺ T-cells. Such defects will interfere with the normal interaction between CD40L and its counter-receptor CD40 on B-cells, a reaction which is crucial for the generation of memory B-cells and for immunoglobulin class-switching. Furthermore, it has been shown that interaction between CD40L on activated T-cells and CD40 on macrophages will stimulate IL-12 secretion, which is important in eliciting an adequate immune response against intracellular pathogens. This may explain why these patients are also unduly susceptible to the intracellular organism *Pneumocystis carinii*.

Transient hypo-γ-globulinemia of infancy, characterized by recurrent respiratory infections, is associated with low IgG levels which often return somewhat abruptly to normal by 4 years of age. There is a deficiency in the number of circulating lymphocytes and in their ability to generate help for Ig production by B-cells but this returns to normal as the disease resolves spontaneously.

PRIMARY T-CELL DEFICIENCY

The **DiGeorge** and **Nezelof syndromes** are characterized by a failure of the thymus to develop normally from the third and fourth pharyngeal pouches during embryogenesis (DiGe-orge children also lack parathyroids and have severe cardiovascular abnormalities). Consequently, stem cells cannot differentiate to become T-lymphocytes and the 'thymus-dependent' areas in lymphoid tissue are sparsely populated; in contrast lymphoid follicles are seen but even these are poorly developed (figure 13.4). Cell-mediated immune responses are undetectable and although the infants can deal with common bacterial infections, they may be overwhelmed by vaccinia (figure 13.5) or measles, or by bacille Calmette–Guérin (BCG) if given by mistake. Humoral antibodies can be elicited but the response is subnormal, presumably reflecting the need for the cooperative involvement of T-cells. Treatment by fetal thymus transplantation or bone marrow transplantation from an HLA-identical donor leads to restoration of immunocompetence. Complete absence of the thymus is, however, pretty rare and more often one is dealing with a 'partial DiGeorge'. These patients tend to improve with time and T-cell function and numbers may become normal even without treatment.

PRIMARY T-CELL DYSFUNCTION

A number of syndromes due to abnormal T-cell function have been described. These differ from severe combined immunodeficiency (SCID; see below) by having T-cells in the peripheral blood. They include patients who lack the γ-chain of the CD3 molecule resulting in T-cells with defective function. Another group have a defective form of ZAP-70, a tyrosine kinase crucial for T-cell signal transduction, and a further subset of patients have abnormal IL-2 production resulting from an IL-2 gene transcription failure. The clinical picture produced by these defects is similar to that seen in patients with SCID, and bone marrow transplantation offers the only hope of long-term cure.

An interesting group of patients who are selectively susceptible to poorly pathogenic mycobacterial species and other intracellular bacteria have defects in the type-1 cytokine pathway. These patients have mutations in the IFN-γ receptor or the IL-12 receptor, resulting in defective activation of macrophages and inability to control intracellular infections.

SEVERE COMBINED IMMUNODEFICIENCY (SCID)

SCID is a heterogeneous group of diseases involving T-cell immunodeficiency with or without B-cell immunodeficiency, resulting from any one of several genetic defects. The

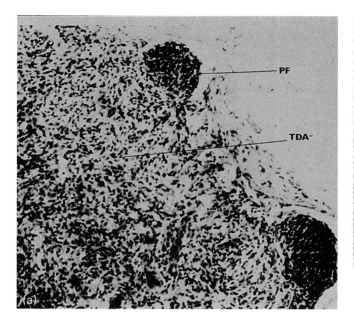

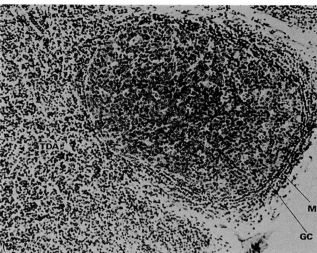

Figure 13.4 Lymph node cortex. (a) From patient with DiGeorge syndrome showing depleted thymus-dependent area (TDA) and small primary follicles (PF). (b) From normal subject: the populated T-cell area and the well-developed secondary follicle with its mantle of small lymphocytes (M) and pale-staining germinal center (GC) provide a marked contrast. (DiGeorge material kindly supplied by Dr D. Webster; photograph by Mr C.J. Sym.)

cases are characterized by severe lymphopenia with deficient cellular and humoral immunity. These children suffer recurrent infections early in life. Prolonged diarrhea resulting from gastrointestinal infections and pneumonia due to *Pneumocystis carinii* are common; *Candida albicans* grows vigorously in the mouth or on the skin. If vaccinated with attenuated organisms (cf. figure 13.5) these children usually die of progressive infection and most will not survive the first year of life unless their immune systems are reconstituted by bone marrow transplantation.

Mutation in the common cytokine receptor γ_c chain is the commonest cause of SCID

SCID occurs in both an X-linked recessive and an autosomal form, but over half of the cases are X-linked (X-SCID) and derive from mutations in the common γ chain of the IL-2 receptor. This γ_c chain is also found in the receptors for interleukins 4, 7, 9 and 15. A number of mutations of this gene have been described and each results in a complex associa-tion of defects in the five affected cytokine/cytokine receptor systems. Isolated cases of human SCID involving mutations in the *RAG* genes which catalyse the introduction of the double-strand breaks (p. 24) have been reported.

SCID can be due to mutations in purine salvage pathway enzymes

Many SCID patients with the autosomal recessive form of the disease have a genetic deficiency of the purine degradation enzymes, especially adenosine deaminase (ADA) and less commonly purine nucleoside phosphorylase (PNP). This results in the accumulation of metabolites (dATP and dGTP respectively) that are toxic to lymphoid stem cells. Half the ADA-deficient SCID patients do reasonably well on transfusions of normal red cells containing the enzyme, whereas others with a longer-standing, more severe deficiency also require treatment with the enzyme modified by polyethylene glycol, which extends its half-life. These patients are excellent candidates for gene therapy. Children have been treated with periodic infusion of their own T-cells corrected by transfection with the *ADA* gene linked to a retroviral vector. Significant reconstitution of antibody responses and delayed-type skin tests to environmental antigens have been achieved without apparent complications. Hematopoietic stem cells from umbilical cord blood transfected with the *ADA* gene could be detected up to 18 months of age but the level of expression was very low and until the technology is improved, such patients must be maintained on enzyme replacement therapy.

the class II MHC genes themselves. MHC class I deficiency has also been described in rare families who present with recurrent infections. Interaction between MHC class I molecules on thymic cells is essential for CD8+ cell maturation and therefore these patients have very low or absent CD8+ cells but normal numbers of functioning CD4+ cells. The rapidly fatal variant of severe combined immunodeficiency associated with lack of myeloid cell precursors is termed **reticular dysgenesis**. The molecular basis of this disease is unknown but the defect presumably affects the bone marrow stem cells.

OTHER COMBINED IMMUNODEFICIENCY DISORDERS

Wiskott–Aldrich syndrome (WAS) is an X-linked disease characterized by thrombocytopenia, eczema and immunodeficiency especially associated with inability to produce antibodies to thymic-independent antigens. This results in bleeding and recurrent infections. The abnormal gene encodes the so-called WAS protein, which is important in the organization of the cytoskeleton of both lymphocytes and platelets. This accounts for the disorganization of the cytoskeleton and loss of microvilli seen in T-cells from these patients, a feature that can be used to diagnose these cases prenatally.

Ataxia telangiectasia is an autosomal recessive disorder of childhood characterized by progressive cerebellar ataxia due to degeneration of Purkinje cells, associated with vascular malformations (telangiectasia), increased incidence of malignancy and defects of both T- and B-cells. These patients also display a hypersensitivity to X-rays, which, together with the unduly high incidence of cancer, has been laid at the door of a defect in DNA repair mechanisms.

An attempt has been made to summarize the cellular basis of the various deficiency states in figure 13.6.

RECOGNITION OF IMMUNODEFICIENCIES

Defects in immunoglobulins can be assessed by quantitative immunoglobulin estimations and then by attempting to induce active immunization with diphtheria, tetanus, pertussis and killed poliomyelitis—but not with live vaccines. B-cells can be enumerated by flow cytometry using CD19, CD20 and CD22.

Enumeration of T-cells is most readily achieved by flow cytometry using CD3 monoclonal antibody or other anti-

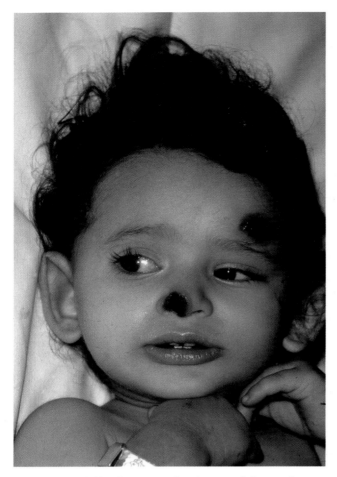

Figure 13.5 A child with severe combined immunodeficiency showing skin lesions due to infection with vaccinia gangrenosum resulting from smallpox immunization. Lesions were widespread over the whole body. (Reproduced by kind permission of Professor R.J. Levinsky and the Medical Illustration Department of the Hospital for Sick Children, Great Ormond Street, London.)

Other SCID variants

A variety of other rare defects have been identified in individual SCID patients. These include mutations in the gene encoding Jak-3 kinase, which is crucial for transducing the signal when IL-2 and other cytokines bind their receptors. The '**bare lymphocyte syndrome**' is a rare form of immunodeficiency due to defective expression of class II MHC molecules. Since the expression of class II MHC is crucial for the selection of CD4+ cells in the thymus, few of these cells develop and those that do are inadequately stimulated by antigen-presenting cells lacking class II molecules. Because MHC class I molecules are normal, CD8+ cells are present. The condition is due to mutations in one of a number of genes that regulate class II MHC expression rather than in

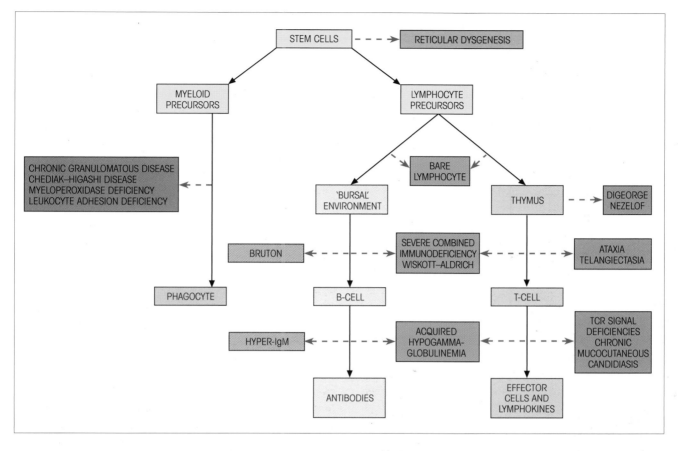

Figure 13.6 The cellular basis of immunodeficiency states. The red arrows indicate the cell type or differentiation process which is defective. Complement deficiencies have not been included.

bodies directed against T-cells such as CD2, CD5, CD7 or CD4 and CD8. Patients with T-cell deficiency will be hypore-active or unreactive in skin tests to such antigens as tuber-culin, *Candida*, tricophytin, streptokinase/streptodornase and mumps, and the reactivity of their peripheral blood mononuclear cells to phytohemagglutinin (PHA) or other nonspecific mitogens will be depressed or absent.

In vitro tests for complement and for the bactericidal and other functions of polymorphs are available, while the reduction of Nitroblue Tetrazolium (NBT) or the stimulation of superoxide production provides a measure of the oxida-tive enzymes associated with active phagocytosis.

SECONDARY IMMUNODEFICIENCY

Immune responsiveness can be depressed nonspecifically by many factors. CMI in particular may be impaired in a state of malnutrition, even of the degree which may be encountered in urban areas of the more affluent regions of the world.

Viral infections are not infrequently immunosuppressive, and in the case of measles in man, Newcastle disease in chickens and rinderpest in cattle, this has been attributed to a direct cytotoxic effect of virus on the lymphoid cells. The most notorious immunosuppressive virus, human immuno-deficiency virus (HIV), is elaborated upon below.

Many therapeutic agents such as X-rays, cytotoxic drugs and corticosteroids, although often used in a nonimmuno-logic context, can nonetheless have dire effects on the immune system (see p. 144). **B-lymphoproliferative disor-ders** like chronic lymphocytic leukemia, myeloma and Waldenström's macroglobulinemia are associated with varying degrees of hypo-γ-globulinemia and impaired anti-body responses. Their common infections with pyogenic bacteria contrast with the situation in Hodgkin's disease where the patients display all the hallmarks of defective CMI — susceptibility to tubercle bacillus, *Brucella*, *Cryptococ-cus* and herpes zoster virus.

ACQUIRED IMMUNODEFICIENCY SYNDROME (AIDS)

AIDS is due to the human immunodeficiency virus (HIV) of which there are two main variants called HIV-1 and HIV-2. The virus is transmitted inside infected CD4 cells and macrophages and the disease is therefore spread sexually or through blood or blood products such as encountered by intravenous drug users. Virus may also be transmitted from an infected mother to her infant, in which case babies born with a high viral load progress more rapidly than those with lower viral loads. The disease causes widespread immune dysfunction leading eventually to very low CD4 cell numbers and depressed cell-mediated immunity. Death is usually due to pulmonary infection, but serious complications involving the nervous system are appearing in about 30% of cases. In essence, there is a sudden onset of immunodeficiency associated with opportunistic infections involving, most commonly, *Pneumocystis carinii*, but also cytomegalovirus, Epstein–Barr (EB) and herpes simplex viruses, fungi such as *Candida*, *Aspergillus* and *Cryptococcus*, and the protozoan *Toxoplasma*; additionally, there is exceptional susceptibility for Kaposi's sarcoma induced by a herpes virus (HHV8).

AIDS results from infection by a human immunodeficiency virus (HIV)

Transmission of the disease is usually through infection with blood or semen containing the HIV-1 virus or the related HIV-2. HIV-1/2 are members of the lentivirus group, which produce disease with a long latency and are adept at evading the immune system. They are budding viruses whose genome is relatively complex and tightly compressed (figure 13.7b). The many virion proteins (figure 13.7a) are generated by RNA splicing and cleavage by the viral protease.

The infection of cells by HIV

The envelope glycoprotein gp120 of HIV **binds avidly to cell-surface CD4** molecules (figure 13.7c). Helper T-cells with their abundant CD4 are a major target for infection but the presence of even relatively low densities of CD4 on macrophages and microglia makes them susceptible to infection, and in the latter case is suspected of being a major factor in the cerebral complications of the disease. After binding to CD4, gp41 on the viral membrane fuses with the cell membrane and enters the cell. For complete fusion to occur various co-receptors present on the CD4 cell are required. CXCR4 (fusin) was the first of a series of membrane glycoproteins to be discovered. Similar chemokine receptors (e.g. CCR5) act as cofusion factors for macrophages. As would be expected individuals who lack such a receptor are more resistant to infection, and mutation or complete absence of the receptor has been described in 1% of Caucasians, but not in people of African descent.

HIV is an RNA retrovirus which utilizes a **reverse transcriptase** to convert its genetic RNA into the corresponding DNA. This is integrated into the host genome where it can remain latent for long periods (figure 13.7c). Stimulation of latently infected T-cells or macrophages activates HIV replication through an increase in the intracellular concentration of NFκB dimers, which bind to consensus sequences in the HIV enhancer region. This initiation of HIV gene transcription occurs when the host cells are activated by cytokines or by specific antigen. It is significant that tumor necrosis factor α (TNFα), which upregulates HIV replication through this NFκB pathway, is present in elevated concentrations in the plasma of HIV-infected individuals, particularly in the advanced stage when they are infected with multiple organisms. Perhaps also, the more rapid progression of HIV infection in Africa may be linked to activation of the immune system through continual microbial insult.

The AIDS infection depletes helper T-cells

Natural history of the disease

The sequence of events following HIV-1 infection is charted in figure 13.8. The virus normally enters the body by infecting Langerhans cells in the rectal or vaginal mucosa and then moves to local lymph nodes where it replicates. The virus is then disseminated by a viremia which is associated with an acute early syndrome of fever, myalgia and arthralgia. A dominant nucleocapsid viral antigen, p24, can be detected in the blood during this phase. An immune response to the virus identifiable by circulating antibodies to p24 and the envelope proteins gp120 and gp41, and by the production of gp120-specific cytotoxic T-cells, curtails the viremia and leads to **sequestration of HIV in lymphoid tissue**. Trapping of viral particles complexed with antibody and complement stimulates follicular hyperplasia and infection of the follicular dendritic cells (FDC). In effect the follicles become the principal site for viral replication and infection of other cells of the immune system. Eventually, follicular involution leads to a gradual degeneration of the FDC network with an increase in viral burden and replication in peripheral blood mononuclear cells. Crucially, **circulating CD4 T-cell numbers fall progressively** but it may take

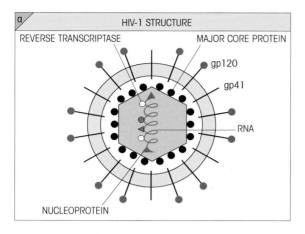

a HIV-1 STRUCTURE

REVERSE TRANSCRIPTASE MAJOR CORE PROTEIN

gp120

gp41

RNA

NUCLEOPROTEIN

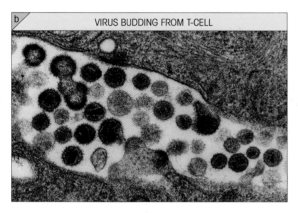

b VIRUS BUDDING FROM T-CELL

Figure 13.7 Characteristics of the HIV-1 AIDS virus. (a) HIV-1 structure. (b) Electron micrograph of mature and budding HIV-1 particles at the surface of human PHA blasts. (c) Intracellular life cycle of HIV. (Photograph kindly supplied by Drs Carol Upton and S. Martin.)

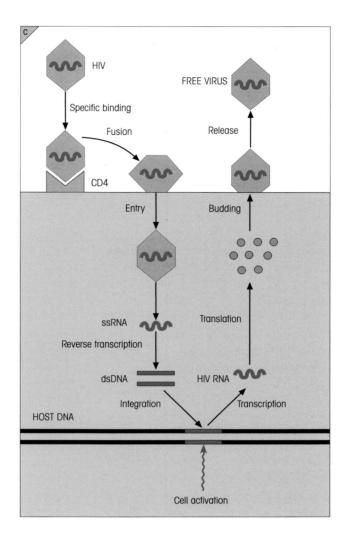

c

HIV

Specific binding

FREE VIRUS

Fusion

Release

CD4

Entry

Budding

ssRNA

Translation

Reverse transcription

dsDNA

HIV RNA

Integration

Transcription

HOST DNA

Cell activation

many years before they are profoundly depleted with levels below, say, 50 mm^{-3}. The patient is now wide open to life-threatening infections caused by normally nonpathogenic (i.e. opportunistic) agents such as *Pneumocystis carinii* and cytomegalovirus characteristic of AIDS.

Mechanisms of depletion

The major immunologic feature of AIDS is the elimination of CD4 cells, a phenomenon which cannot be solely explained by the direct cytopathic effect of HIV. There is certainly no shortage of hypotheses to account for CD4 depletion with the corresponding change in the CD4:CD8 ratio. These include:

1 A direct cytopathic effect by the virus either on single cells or through the formation of multinucleate syncytia between infected and noninfected CD4 cells.

2 Behavior of HIV as a superantigen combining with and deleting certain TCR families.

3 Susceptibility to programmed cell death (apoptosis). Stimulation of CD4 T-cells in asymptomatic HIV-infected individuals leads to apoptosis. There is some evidence that HIV-infected cells are particularly sensitive to Fas-induced apoptosis, and this may relate to the expression of Fas on infected or uninfected T-cells induced by gp120 and tat proteins produced by HIV.

4 Antibodies against HIV proteins may bind to infected cells which may then be destroyed by antibody-dependent cellular cytotoxicity.

5 Cytotoxic CD8 cells are crucial in reducing viral load early in the HIV infection. They expand rapidly in infected patients and may play an important role in lysing infected CD4-positive cells.

6 There is now good evidence that not only are T-cells destroyed during HIV infection, but that production of new T-cells from the thymus or bone marrow is inhibited.

It is likely that a combination of several of these mecha-

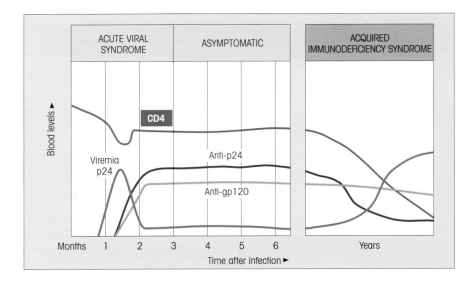

Figure 13.8 **The natural history of HIV-1 infection.** The changes in p24 antigen and antibody shown late in the disease are seen in some but not all patients.

nisms will ultimately act to tip the balance in favor of the virus.

Laboratory diagnosis of AIDS

Patients with HIV infection will demonstrate the presence of viral antibodies within a few weeks of infection. CD4 levels decrease rapidly after infection as is shown by a reversal of the normal CD4 : CD8 ratio. Quantitative HIV-RNA plasma viral load measurement is now routinely employed to evaluate and monitor patients with HIV infection. This includes measuring the baseline of viral load prior to initiation of antiretroviral therapy and assessing the efficacy of antiviral drug treatment. Quantitative HIV-RNA measurements are also thought to be the best indicator of the development of AIDS-defining opportunistic infections and subsequent progression of the disease. Associated with the decline in CD4 cells many tests of cell-mediated immunity will show defects, including the delayed hypersensitivity skin response to recall antigens.

Treatment of HIV disease

Although a major focus of managing HIV disease is reducing viral load and preventing infectious complications, it is important that emotional, social, psychological and financial aspects of this disease be understood and dealt with by the physician. Prolonged survival depends on the use of antiretroviral agents, immunization and chemoprophylaxis and aggressive treatment of infectious and malignant complications when they occur. An increasing number of antiretroviral agents have been developed and these include both non-nucleoside and nucleoside reverse transcriptase inhibitors and protease inhibitors. Although the optimal time to initiate these therapies is controversial, they should always be used in symptomatic patients and in any infected person with a CD4 count below $500\,mm^{-3}$ or with a viral load greater than 50000 copies per milliliter. The major drawback of these drugs is their enormous expense, which limits their use in those communities of the world where they are most needed.

REVISION

See the accompanying website (www.roitt.com) for multiple choice questions.

Primary immunodeficiency states
• These occur in the human, albeit somewhat rarely, as a result of a defect in almost any stage of differentiation in the whole immune system.
• Rare X-linked mutations produce disease in males.
• Defects in phagocytic cells, the complement pathways or the B-cell system lead in particular to infection with bacte-

ria, which are disposed of by opsonization and phagocytosis.
• Patients with T-cell deficiencies are susceptible to viruses and molds, which are normally eradicated by CMI.

Deficiencies of innate immune mechanisms
• Chronic granulomatous disease results from mutations in the NADPH oxidase of phagocytic cells.

• Chediak–Higashi leukocytes contain giant lysosomal granules which interfere with their function.

• Leukocyte adhesion deficiency involves mutations in the CD18 subunit of β_2-integrins.

• Deficiency of one of the early components of the classical complement may result in immune complex disease.

• Deficiency of C3 results in severe recurrent pyogenic infections.

• Deficiency of the late complement components results in increased susceptibility to recurrent neisserial infections.

• Lack of C1 inhibitor leads to hereditary angioedema.

• Deficiencies in C1, 4 or 2 are associated with SLE–like syndromes.

Primary B-cell deficiency

• Congenital X-linked agammaglobulinemia (Bruton), involving differentiation arrest at the pre-B stage, is caused by mutations in a novel tyrosine kinase gene.

• Patients with IgA deficiency are susceptible to infections of the respiratory and gastrointestinal tract.

• In common variable immunodeficiency the B-cells fail to secrete antibody, probably due to abnormal interactions with T-cells.

• Deletions in the T-cell CD40L gene provide the basis for hyper-IgM syndrome.

Primary T-cell deficiency

• DiGeorge syndrome results from failure of thymic development.

Primary T-cell dysfunction

• This group of patients have circulating T-cells, but their function is abnormal due a variety of genetic defects.

Severe combined immunodeficiency (SCID)

• Half the patients with SCID have mutations in the gene for the γ-chain common to receptors for IL-2, 4, 7, 9 and 15.

• Many SCID patients have a genetic deficiency of the purine degradation enzymes PNP and ADA, which leads to accumulation of toxic products. Patients with ADA deficiency are being corrected by transfection of autologous T-cells with the normal gene.

• The bare lymphocyte syndrome is due to defective expression of MHC class II molecules.

Other combined immunodeficiency disorders

• Wiskott–Aldrich males have a syndrome characterized by thrombocytopenia, eczema and immunodeficiency.

• Defective DNA repair mechanisms are found in patients with ataxia telangiectasia.

Recognition of immunodeficiencies

• Humoral immunodeficiency can be assessed initially by quantitating immunoglobulins in the blood.

• B- and T-cell numbers can be enumerated by flow cytometric analysis.

Secondary immunodeficiency

• Immunodeficiency may arise as a secondary consequence of malnutrition, lymphoproliferative disorders, agents such as X-rays and cytotoxic drugs, and viral infections.

Acquired immunodeficiency syndrome (AIDS)

• AIDS results from infection by the RNA retroviruses HIV-1 and HIV-2.

• HIV infects T-helper cells through binding of its envelope gp120 to CD4 with the help of a cofactor molecule, CXCR4 and other similar cytokine receptors. It also infects macrophages, microglia, T-cell-stimulating dendritic cells and FDCs, the latter through a CD4-independent pathway.

• Within the cell, the RNA is converted by the reverse transcriptase to DNA which can be incorporated into the host's genome where it lies dormant until the cell is activated by stimulators such as TNFα which increase NFκB levels.

• There is usually a long asymptomatic phase after the early acute viral infection has been curtailed by an immune response, and the virus is sequestered to the FDC in the lymphoid follicles where it progressively destroys the dendritic cell meshwork.

• A disastrous fall in CD4 cells destroys cell-mediated defenses and leaves the patient open to life-threatening infections through opportunist organisms such as Pneumocystis carinii and cytomegalovirus.

• There is a tremendous battle between the immune system and the virus, with extremely high rates of viral destruction and CD4 T-cell replacement.

• CD4 T-cell depletion may eventually occur as a result of direct pathogenicity, apoptosis, ADCC, direct cytotoxicity by CD8 cells or disruption of normal T-cell production.

• AIDS is diagnosed in an individual with opportunistic infections, by low CD4 but normal CD8 T-cells in blood, poor delayed-type skin tests, positive tests for viral antibodies and p24 antigen, lymph node biopsy and isolation of live virus or demonstration of HIV genome by the polymerase chain reaction (PCR).

FURTHER READING

Bolognesi D.P. & Cooper M.D. (eds) (1995) Immunodeficiency. *Current Opinion in Immunology* **7**, 433–470.

Brostoff J., Scadding G.K., Male D. & Roitt I.M. (eds) (1991) *Clinical Immunology*, chs 23–25. Gower Medical Publishing, London.

Chapel H. & Haeney M. (1993) *Essentials of Clinical Immunology*, 3rd edn. Blackwell Scientific Publications, Oxford.

Conley M.E. (ed) (1999) Section on Genetic Effects on Immunity. *Current Opinion in Immunology* **11** (4).

Fischer A. (ed.) (1996) Genetic effects on immunity. *Current Opinion in Immunology* **8**, 510.

Heeney J.L. *et al.* (1999) Immune correlates of protection from HIV and AIDS – more answers but yet more questions. *Immunology Today* **20** (6), 247.

Landau N.R. (ed) (1999) Section on HIV. *Current Opinion in Immunology* **11** (4).

Lokki M.-L. & Colten H.R. (1995) Genetic deficiencies of complement. *Annals of Medicine* **27**, 451.

Stiehm E.R. (ed.) (1989) *Immunological Disorders in Infants and Children*, 3rd edn. W.B. Saunders, Philadelphia.

CHAPTER 14

Hypersensitivity

INAPPROPRIATE IMMUNE RESPONSES CAN LEAD TO TISSUE DAMAGE

When an individual has been immunologically primed, further contact with antigen leads to secondary boosting of the immune response. However, the reaction may be excessive and lead to tissue damage (hypersensitivity). It should be emphasized that the mechanisms underlying these inappropriate reactions are those normally employed by the body in combating infection, as discussed in Chapter 11. We speak of **hypersensitivity reactions** and a state of **hypersensitivity**. Coombs and Gell defined four types of hypersensitivity. Types I, II and III depend on the interaction of antigen with humoral antibody, whereas Type IV involves T-cell recognition. Because of the longer time course this has in the past been referred to as 'delayed-type hypersensitivity'.

TYPE I: ANAPHYLACTIC HYPERSENSITIVITY

The phenomenon of anaphylaxis

The earliest accounts of inappropriate responses to foreign antigens relate to **anaphylaxis**. The phenomenon can be readily reproduced in guinea-pigs which, like man, are a highly susceptible species. A single injection of 1 mg of an antigen such as egg albumin into a guinea-pig has no obvious effect. However, if the injection is repeated 2–3 weeks later, the sensitized animal reacts very dramatically with the symptoms of generalized anaphylaxis; almost immediately the guinea-pig begins to wheeze and within a few minutes dies from asphyxia. Examination shows intense constriction of the bronchioles and bronchi and generally there is: (i) contraction of smooth muscle and (ii) dilatation of capillaries. Similar reactions can occur in human subjects and have been observed following wasp and bee stings or injections of penicillin in appropriately sensitive individuals. In many instances only a timely injection of epinephrine to counter the smooth muscle contraction and capillary dilatation can prevent death.

Type I allergic reactions are due to the overproduction of IgE antibodies

The reasons why some individuals will produce an IgE response to certain antigens (allergens) while others will produce an IgG response are not clear. Allergic reactions are caused by a limited number of allergens which are deposited on mucosal epithelium or skin from where they are ingested and processed by Langerhans cells or other antigen-presenting cells. As with any other antigen they are proteolytically cleaved into small peptides and presented to uncommitted TH0 cells. In the case of allergy, however, these cells now differentiate into TH2 lymphocytes which release various cytokines important in the allergic reaction. These include IL-3, IL-4, IL-5, IL-10 and a variety of other cytokines which inhibit TH1 cell activation (IL-4, IL-13). These cytokines together with signals delivered by the B-cell surface molecule CD40, induce isotype switching in newly generated IgM-bearing B-cells from μ to ε resulting in subsequent production of IgE. It has been shown that allergic individuals not only have larger numbers of allergen-specific TH2 cells in their blood, but these cells produce greater amounts of IL-4 per cell than TH2 cells from normal people.

There is a strong genetic component to allergic diseases

Genetic susceptibility to allergic reactions has not been clearly defined but high levels of IgE are noted in certain allergic (atopic) families. HLA linkage is associated with allergic responses to a number of allergens including ragweed and house dust mite. A further major genetic locus which regulates serum IgE levels has been identified on chromosome 5q in the region containing the genes for IL-4, IL-5 and IL-9, cytokines that are important in regulating IgE synthesis.

Anaphylaxis is triggered by clustering of IgE receptors on mast cells through cross-linking

Mast cells display a high-affinity receptor (FcεR1) for the Cε2:Cε3 junction region of IgE Fc, a property shared with their circulating counterpart, the basophil.

Cross-linking of IgE antibodies bound to a mast cell by a multivalent hapten will trigger the release of inflammatory mediators which are responsible for the acute allergic reaction. The critical event is aggregation of the receptors by cross-linking, as clearly shown by the ability of antibodies reacting directly with the receptor to trigger the mast cell (figure 14.1). Activation is rapidly followed by the breakdown of phosphatidylinositol to inositol triphosphate (IP3), the generation of diacylglycerol (DAG) and an increase in intracytoplasmic free calcium. The biochemical cascade allows the granules to fuse with the plasma membrane and release their preformed mediators into the surrounding tissue. It also results in synthesis of lipid mediators including a series of arachidonic acid metabolites formed by the cyclo-oxygenase and lipoxygenase pathways, and a variety of cytokines which are responsible for the late phase of the acute allergic reaction.

Mast cell and basophil mediators

Mast cell degranulation is the major initiating event of the acute allergic reaction. The preformed mediators released from the granules include histamine, heparin, neutral protease and various eosinophil and neutrophil chemotactic factors. Histamine itself is responsible for many of the immediate symptoms of allergic reactions including bronchoconstriction, vasodilatation, mucus secretion and edema caused by leakage of plasma proteins from small

vessels. These effects can all be visualized in the immediate skin test where allergen injected into the skin gives rise to a characteristic wheal and flare reaction with redness, edema and pruritus (itchiness).

Activation of the mast cells also results in the liberation of newly formed lipid mediators which include the leukotrienes LTB4, LTC4 and LTD4, the prostaglandin PGD_2 and platelet activating factor (PAF). PGD_2, the leukotrienes and PAF are highly potent bronchoconstrictors which also increase vascular permeability and are chemotactic for inflammatory cells.

The late phase of the allergic reaction is mediated by cytokines

Mast cells and basophils are responsible for significant production of proinflammatory cytokines including TNF, IL-1, IL-4 and IL-5. Within 12 hours of an acute allergic reaction a late-phase reaction occurs which is characterized by a cellular infiltrate of CD4+ cells, monocytes and eosinophils. These cells will themselves release a variety of TH2-type cytokines, especially IL-4 and IL-5, which are responsible for further inflammation at the site of the allergen. This late reaction, therefore, resembles a delayed hypersensitivity reaction because of the infiltration of T-cells and the effects of the cytokines. A differentiating feature, however, is the presence of eosinophils and TH2 cells in the late phase of the allergic response and their absence from delayed hypersensitivity reactions.

The sudden degranulation of mast cells, therefore, leads to release of a complex cascade of mediators which generally results in the symptoms of acute allergic reactions. Under normal circumstances, these mediators help to orchestrate the development of a defensive acute inflamma-

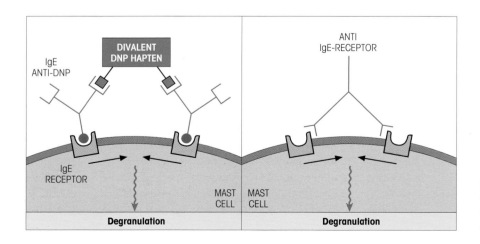

Figure 14.1 Clustering of IgE receptors either by multivalent hapten or antibody to the receptors themselves leads to mast cell degranulation.

tory reaction. When there is a massive release of these mediators under abnormal conditions, as in atopic disease, their bronchoconstrictive and vasodilatory effects predominate and become distinctly threatening.

Eosinophils are prominent in the allergic reaction

The preferential accumulation of eosinophils is a characteristic feature of allergic diseases and is due to the eosinophil chemoattractants RANTES, eotaxin and IL-5. The source of the IL-5 which is such a major player in the eosinophil infiltration could come partly from local mast cells but also from TH2-type cells. Activation of the eosinophils is mediated by the actions of eotaxin, IL-3, IL-5 and GM-CSF; IL-5 also inhibits the natural apoptosis of eosinophils which regulates their normal lifespan, and increases eosinophil adhesion to vascular endothelium via β_2 integrins. The eosinophil granules release very basic, highly charged polypeptides including major basic protein and eosinophil peroxidase which may themselves cause tissue damage including destruction of the respiratory epithelium in asthmatics. Eosinophils are also an important source of leukotrienes, PAF, cytokines including IL-3 and IL-5, and a variety of eosinophil chemoattractants which further amplify the eosinophil response.

Atopic allergy

Examples of clinical responses to inhaled allergens

Allergic rhinitis

Nearly 10% of the population suffer to a greater or lesser degree from allergies involving localized IgE-mediated anaphylactic reactions to extrinsic allergens such as grass pollens, animal danders, the feces from mites in house dust (figure 14.2) and so on. The most common manifestation is allergic rhinitis, often known as hay fever, where the target organs are the mucus membranes of the nose and eyes (figure 14.3) resulting in congestion, itchiness and sneezing which is so characteristic of this condition. An increasing number of causative allergens have now been cloned and expressed including **Der p1** from house dust mites and **Lol pI–V** from ryegrass pollen. Exposure to these and other allergens produces the typical symptoms within minutes. Many atopic patients, however, develop long-lasting symptoms after exposure to allergen due to the late-acting mediators.

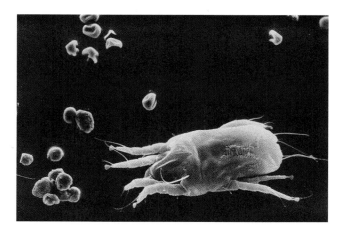

Figure 14.2 House dust mite—a major cause of allergic disease. The electron micrograph shows the rather nasty looking mite, graced by the name *Dermatophagoides pteronyssinus*, and fecal pellets on the bottom left which are the major source of allergen. The biconcave pollen grains (top left), shown for comparison, indicate the size of particles which can become airborne and reach the lungs. The mite itself is much too large for that. (Reproduced courtesy of Dr E. Tovey.)

Asthma

Asthma is a chronic disease characterized by increased responsiveness of the tracheobronchial tree to a variety of stimuli resulting in reversible airflow limitation and inflammation of the airways. It is thought that exposure to indoor allergens early in infancy predisposes to the disease regardless of a family history, but the development of asthma is influenced by multiple genetic and environmental factors. Bronchial biopsy and lavage of asthmatic patients reveals involvement of **mast cells and eosinophils** as the major mediator-secreting effector cells, while T-cells provide the microenvironment required to sustain the inflammatory response which is an essential feature of the histopathology (figure 14.4). Cytokines released by all these infiltrating cells give rise to allergic inflammation resulting in variable airflow obstruction and bronchial hyper-responsiveness which are the cardinal clinical and physiological features of the disease.

Latex allergy

This is a hypersensitivity reaction to proteins contained in latex, the name given to the sap of the rubber tree. It is becoming increasingly recognized in health-care workers and others who have significant exposure to rubber gloves or other rubber-containing materials. The acute allergic reaction may present with skin rashes, itching or redness of the

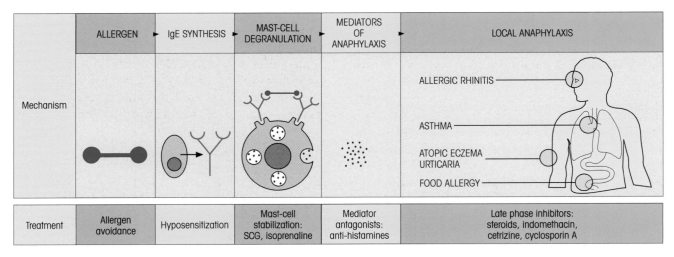

	ALLERGEN	IgE SYNTHESIS	MAST-CELL DEGRANULATION	MEDIATORS OF ANAPHYLAXIS	LOCAL ANAPHYLAXIS
Mechanism					ALLERGIC RHINITIS ASTHMA ATOPIC ECZEMA URTICARIA FOOD ALLERGY
Treatment	Allergen avoidance	Hyposensitization	Mast-cell stabilization: SCG, isoprenaline	Mediator antagonists: anti-histamines	Late phase inhibitors: steroids, indomethacin, cetrizine, cyclosporin A

Figure 14.3 Atopic allergies: sites of local responses and possible therapies. SCG = sodium cromoglycate.

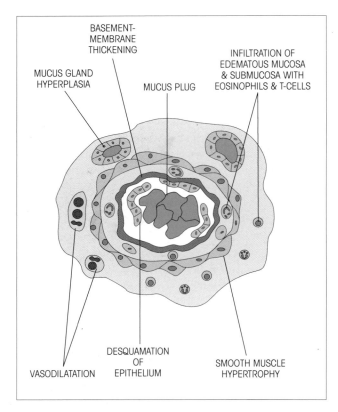

BASEMENT-MEMBRANE THICKENING

MUCUS GLAND HYPERPLASIA

MUCUS PLUG

INFILTRATION OF EDEMATOUS MUCOSA & SUBMUCOSA WITH EOSINOPHILS & T-CELLS

VASODILATATION

DESQUAMATION OF EPITHELIUM

SMOOTH MUSCLE HYPERTROPHY

Figure 14.4 Pathologic changes in asthma. Diagram of cross-section of an airway in severe asthma.

powder and cause acute respiratory symptoms in allergic individuals. As with other allergies, avoidance of the allergen is crucial. In the case of hospital workers this may entail avoiding all contact with airway masks and straps, catheters, anesthesia bags, chest tubes, catheter bags and many other rubber-containing products at home. There is some evidence that latex-allergic individuals may develop symptoms from various fruits, especially avocado and banana, which contain proteins that cross-react with latex.

Food allergy

Awareness of the importance of IgE sensitization to food allergens in the gut has increased dramatically so that allergy to peanuts or peanut butter is necessitating major changes in school lunch programs. Many foods have been incriminated, especially nuts, shellfish, milk and eggs, and food additives such as sulfiting agents can also cause adverse reactions. Sensitization to egg white and cows' milk may even occur in early infancy through breast-feeding, with antigen passing into the mother's milk. Contact of the food with specific IgE on mast cells in the gastrointestinal tract may produce local reactions such as diarrhea and vomiting, or may allow the allergen to enter the body by causing a change in gut permeability through mediator release resulting in systemic reactions including skin eruptions (urticaria), bronchospasm and anaphylactic shock.

Clinical tests for allergy

Sensitivity is normally assessed by the response to intradermal challenge with antigen. The release of histamine and

eyes, nasal symptoms or coughing, wheezing and shortness of breath. In severe cases anaphylactic shock may occur. Aerosols of latex may occur when rubber gloves containing powders are removed because the latex can bind to the

other mediators rapidly produces a **wheal and flare reaction** at the site (figure 14.5a), maximal within 30 minutes and then subsiding. This immediate reaction may be followed by the late-phase reaction, which sometimes lasts for 24 hours and is characterized by dense infiltration with eosinophils and T-cells and is more edematous than the early reaction. The similarity to the histopathology of the inflammatory

infiltrate in chronic asthma is obvious, and these late-phase reactions can also be seen following challenge of the bronchi and nasal mucosa of allergic subjects.

Allergen-specific serum IgE can also be measured by a **radioallergosorbent test (RAST)**, the results of which correlate well with skin test results. In some instances, intranasal challenge with allergen may provoke a response even when

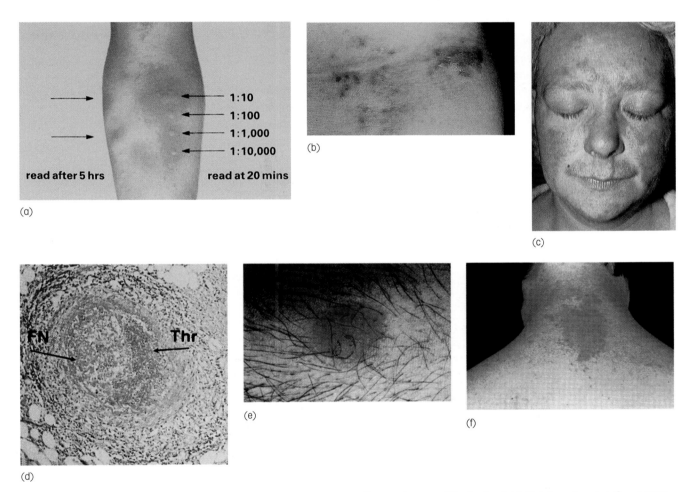

(a) read after 5 hrs / read at 20 mins / 1:10 / 1:100 / 1:1,000 / 1:10,000

(b)

(c)

(d) FN / Thr

(e)

(f)

Figure 14.5 Hypersensitivity reactions.

Type I (a) Skin prick tests with grass pollen allergen in a patient with typical summer hay fever. Skin tests were performed 5 hours (*left*) and 20 minutes (*right*) before the photograph was taken. The tests on the right show a typical end-point titration of a type I immediate wheal and flare reaction. The late-phase skin reaction (*left*) can be clearly seen at 5 hours, especially where a large immediate response has preceded it. Figures for allergen dilution are given. (b) An atopic eczema reaction on the back of a knee of a child allergic to rice and eggs.

Type III (c) Facial appearance in systemic lupus erythematosus (SLE). Lesions of recent onset are symmetrical, red and edematous. They are often most pronounced on the areas of the face which receive most light exposure, i.e. the upper cheeks and bridge of the nose, and

the prominences of the forehead. (d) Histology of acute inflammatory reaction in polyarteritis nodosa associated with immune complex formation with hepatitis B surface (HBs) antigen. A vessel showing thrombus (Thr) formation and fibrinoid necrosis (FN) is surrounded by a mixed inflammatory infiltrate, largely polymorphs.

Type IV (e) Mantoux test showing cell-mediated hypersensitivity reaction to tuberculin, characterized by induration and erythema. (f) Type IV contact hypersensitivity reaction to nickel caused by the clasp of a necklace. ((a), (b) and (e) kindly provided by Dr J. Brostoff; (c) by Dr G. Levene; (d) by Professor N. Woolf; (f) reproduced from British Society of Immunology teaching slides with permission of the Society and Dermatology Department, London Hospital.)

both these tests are negative, probably as a result of local synthesis of IgE antibodies.

Therapy

Allergen avoidance

If one considers the sequence of reactions from initial exposure to allergen right through to the production of atopic disease, it can be seen that several points in the chain provide legitimate targets for therapy (figure 14.3). Avoidance of contact with *potential* allergens is often impractical, although, to give one example, feeding infants cows' milk at too early an age is discouraged. After sensitization, avoidance where possible is obviously worthwhile but the reluctance of some parents to dispose of the family cat to stop little Algernon's wheezing is sometimes quite surprising.

Modulation of the immunologic response

Attempts to desensitize patients immunologically by repeated subcutaneous injections of allergen can lead to worthwhile improvement. This is thought to be due to the activation of TH1-type cells rather than TH2, resulting in production of increasing amounts of IgG rather than IgE. The IgG antibody will compete for antigen with IgE and will divert the allergen from contact with tissue-bound IgE. Other strategies attempt to inhibit the binding of IgE to its mast cell receptor using either a humanized anti-IgE which does not cross-link, or a small blocking peptide.

Mast cell stabilization

At the drug level, much relief has been obtained with agents such as inhalant isoprenaline and **sodium cromoglycate**, which render mast cells resistant to triggering. Sodium cromoglycate blocks chloride channel activity and maintains cells in a normal resting physiological state which probably accounts for its inhibitory effects on a wide range of cellular functions such as mast cell degranulation, eosinophil and neutrophil chemotaxis and mediator release, and reflex bronchoconstriction. Some or all of these effects are responsible for its anti-asthmatic actions.

Mediator antagonism

An important recent advance has been the introduction of long-acting inhaled β_2-**agonists** such as salmeterol and formoterol which are bronchodilators and protect against bronchoconstriction for over 12 hours. Potent **leukotriene**

antagonists such as zafirlukast also block constrictor challenges and clinical trials are encouraging.

Theophylline has been used in the treatment of asthma for more than 50 years and remains the single most prescribed drug for asthma worldwide. As a **phosphodiesterase (PDE) inhibitor** it increases intracellular cAMP, thereby causing bronchodilatation, inhibition of IL-5-induced prolongation of eosinophil survival and probably suppression of eosinophil migration into the bronchial mucosa.

Attacking chronic inflammation

Mild asthma involving mainly mast cell activation and eosinophil recruitment is treated with short-acting β_2-agonists and chromones but with increasing severity, activated T-cells dominate and **topical steroids** in increasing doses supplemented by long-acting β_2-agonists and theophylline are administered. More serious trials of inhaled cyclosporin A and other T-cell-specific drugs are overdue.

TYPE II: ANTIBODY-DEPENDENT CYTOTOXIC HYPERSENSITIVITY

This form of hypersensitivity is due to an abnormal antibody directed against a cell or a tissue. Such an antigen–antibody reaction will activate the complement cascade and the target will be destroyed by the full **complement** system up to C8 and C9 producing **direct membrane damage** (figure 14.6). Alternatively, combination with antibody will encourage the demise of that cell by promoting contact with phagocytes, either directly through the Fc receptor present on phagocytes, or by **immune adherence** where C3b on the antigen–antibody complex attaches to the CR1 receptor on the phagocytic cell. Target cells coated with low concentrations of IgG antibody can also be killed 'nonspecifically' through an extracellular nonphagocytic mechanism involving nonsensitized leukocytes which bind to the target by their specific receptors for the Cγ2 and Cγ3 domains of IgG Fc (figure 14.7). This so-called **antibody-dependent cell-mediated cytotoxicity (ADCC)** may be exhibited by both phagocytic and nonphagocytic myeloid cells (polymorphs and monocytes) and by large granular lymphocytes with Fc receptors, dubbed 'K-cells', which are almost certainly identical with the natural killer (NK) cells. Functionally, this extracellular cytotoxic mechanism would be expected to be of significance where the target is too large for ingestion by phagocytosis, for example large parasites and solid tumors.

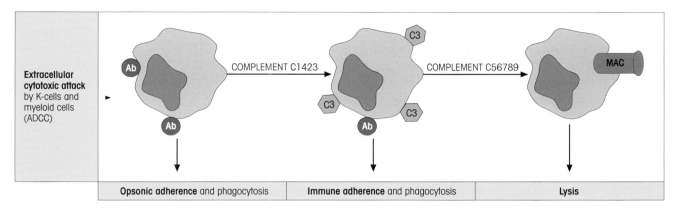

Figure 14.6 Type II: antibody-dependent cytotoxic hypersensitivity. Antibodies directed against cell surface antigens cause cell death not only by C-dependent lysis but also by adherence reactions leading to phagocytosis or through nonphagocytic extracellular killing by certain lymphoid and myeloid cells (antibody-dependent cell-mediated cytotoxicity).

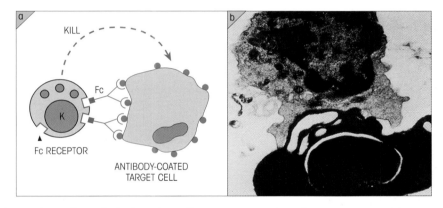

Figure 14.7 Killing of Ab-coated target by antibody-dependent cell-mediated cytotoxicity (ADCC). Fcγ receptors bind the effector to the target, which is killed by an extracellular mechanism. Human monocytes and IFNγ-activated neutrophils kill Ab-coated tumor cells using their FcγRI and FcγRII receptors; lymphocytes (NK cells) kill hybridoma targets through FcγRIII receptors. (a) Diagram of effector and target cells. (b) Electron micrograph of attack on Ab-coated chick red cell by a mouse large granular lymphocyte showing close apposition of effector and target and vacuolation in the cytoplasm of the latter. ((b) courtesy of P. Penfold.)

Type II reactions between members of the same species (alloimmune)

Transfusion reactions

Of the many different polymorphic constituents of the human red cell membrane, **ABO blood groups** form the dominant system. The antigenic groups A and B are derived from H substance by the action of glycosyl transferases encoded by A or B genes respectively. Individuals with both genes (group AB) have the two antigens on their red cells, while those lacking these genes (group O) synthesize H substance only. Antibodies to A or B occur when the antigen is absent from the red cell surface; thus a person of blood group A will possess anti-B and so on. These **isohemagglutinins** are usually IgM and probably belong to the class of 'natural antibodies'; they would be boosted through contact with antigens of the gut flora which are structurally similar to the blood group carbohydrates, so that the antibodies formed cross-react with the appropriate red cell type. If an individual is blood group A, they would be tolerant to antigens closely similar to A and would only form cross-reacting antibodies capable of agglutinating B red cells; similarly an O individual would make anti-A and anti-B (table 14.1). On transfusion, mismatched red cells will be coated by the isohemagglutinins and cause severe reactions.

129

Rhesus incompatibility

The **rhesus (Rh) blood groups** form the other major antigenic system, the RhD antigen being of the most consequence for isoimmune reactions. A mother with an RhD-negative blood group (i.e. *dd* genotype) can readily be sensitized by red cells from a baby carrying RhD antigens (*DD* or *Dd* genotype). This occurs most often at the birth of the first child when a placental bleed can release a large number of the baby's erythrocytes into the mother. The antibodies formed are predominantly of the IgG class and are able to cross the placenta in any subsequent pregnancy. Reaction with the D-antigen on the fetal red cells leads to the latter's destruction through opsonic adherence, giving hemolytic disease of the newborn (figure 14.8). For this reason **RhD-negative mothers are now treated prophylactically** with small amounts of avid IgG anti-D at the time of birth of the first child, and this greatly reduces the risk of sensitization. Another success for immunology!

Organ transplant rejection

Hyperacute graft rejection mediated by preformed anti-bodies in the graft recipient is a classic example of a cytotoxic reaction. Recipients may develop such antibodies as a result of previous blood transfusions or failed transplants. Following attachment of the blood supply to the new graft these antibodies attach to donor antigens resulting in very rapid hyperacute rejection.

Antibodies directed against surface transplantation antigens on the graft may also be important in longstanding allografts which have withstood the first onslaught of the cell-mediated reaction. These may be directly cytotoxic or cause adherence of phagocytic cells or 'nonspecific' attack by K-cells or they may lead to platelet adherence when combining with antigens on the surface of the vascular endothelium (see figure 15.3).

Autoimmune type II hypersensitivity reactions

A variety of organ-specific autoimmune diseases result from antibodies directed against various cell or tissue antigens. Autoantibodies to the patient's own red cells are produced in **autoimmune hemolytic anemia**. Red cells coated with these antibodies have a shortened half-life, largely through their adherence to phagocytic cells in the spleen. Antibodies to platelets result in autoimmune thrombocytopenia, and the serum of patients with Hashimoto's thyroiditis contains antibodies which, in the presence of complement, are directly cytotoxic to thyroid cells. In Goodpasture's syndrome (included here for convenience), antibodies to the basement membranes of kidney glomeruli and lung alveoli are present. Biopsies show these antibodies together with complement components bound to the basement membranes, where the action of the full complement system leads to serious damage (figure 14.9a).

Table 14.1 ABO blood groups and serum antibodies.

BLOOD GROUP (PHENOTYPE)	GENOTYPE	ANTIGEN	SERUM ANTIBODY
A	*AA, AO*	A	ANTI-B
B	*BB, BO*	B	ANTI-A
AB	*AB*	A and B	NONE
O	*OO*	H	ANTI-A ANTI-B

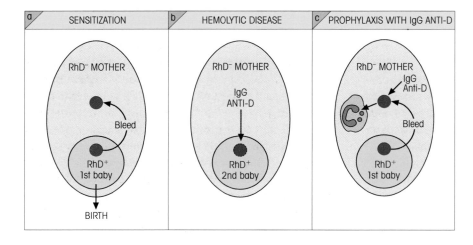

Figure 14.8 Hemolytic disease of the newborn due to rhesus incompatibility. (a) RhD+ve red cells from the first baby sensitize the RhD−ve mother. (b) The mother's IgG anti-D crosses the placenta and coats the erythrocytes of the second RhD+ve baby causing type II hypersensitivity hemolytic disease. (c) IgG anti-D given prophylactically at the first birth removes the baby's red cells through phagocytosis and prevents sensitization of the mother.

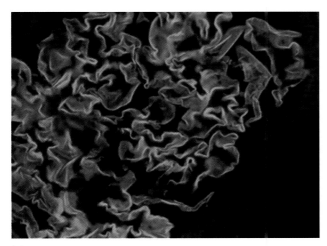

(a)

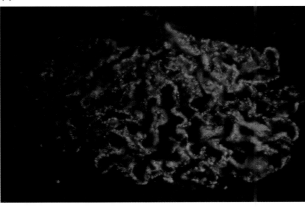

(b)

Figure 14.9 Glomerulonephritis: (a) due to linear deposition of antibody to glomerular basement membrane, here visualized by staining the human kidney biopsy with a fluorescent anti-IgG; and (b) due to deposition of antigen–antibody complexes, which can be seen as discrete masses lining the glomerular basement membrane following immunofluorescent staining with anti-IgG. Similar patterns to these are obtained with a fluorescent anti-C3. (Photographs kindly supplied by Dr S. Thiru.)

Type II drug reactions

Drugs may become coupled to body components and thereby undergo conversion from a hapten to a full antigen which will sensitize certain individuals. If IgE antibodies are produced, anaphylactic reactions can result. In some circumstances, particularly with topically applied ointments, cell-mediated hypersensitivity may be induced. In other cases where coupling to serum proteins occurs, the possibility of type III complex-mediated reactions may arise. In the present context we are concerned with those instances where the drug appears to form an antigenic complex with the surface of a formed element of the blood and evokes the production of antibodies which are cytotoxic for the cell–drug complex.

When the drug is withdrawn, the sensitivity is no longer evident. Examples of this mechanism have been seen in the **hemolytic anemia** sometimes associated with continued administration of chlorpromazine or phenacetin, in the **agranulocytosis** associated with the taking of aminopyrine or of quinidine, and the now classic situation of **thrombocytopenic purpura** which may be produced by Sedormid, a sedative of yesteryear. In the latter case, freshly drawn serum from the patient will lyse platelets in the presence, but not in the absence, of Sedormid; inactivation of complement by preheating the serum at 56°C for 30 minutes abrogates this effect.

Anti-receptor autoimmune diseases

Many cells are signaled by agents such as hormones through surface receptors to which they specifically bind. Autoantibodies directed against those receptors may give rise to disease by either blocking or depleting the receptor from the cell surface or by activating the receptor. As will be discussed more fully in Chapter 18, myasthenia gravis is a disorder due to an abnormal antibody directed against the acetylcholine receptors resulting in profound muscular weakness. In Graves' disease (thyrotoxicosis), however, the abnormal antibody stimulates the receptor for thyroid-stimulating hormone (TSH) resulting in uncontrolled production of thyroid hormones and in many cases, depending upon the time specificity of the antibodies, thyroid growth.

TYPE III: IMMUNE COMPLEX-MEDIATED HYPERSENSITIVITY

The body may be exposed to an excess of antigen over a protracted period in a number of circumstances. The union of such antigens with the subsequently formed antibodies forms insoluble complexes at fixed sites within the body where they may well give rise to acute inflammatory reactions (figure 14.10). When complement is fixed, the anaphylatoxins C3a and C5a will cause release of mast cell mediators resulting in increased vascular permeability. These same chemotactic factors and those released by mast cells, will lead to an influx of polymorphonuclear leukocytes, which attempt to phagocytose the immune complexes. This in turn results in the extracellular release of the polymorph granule contents, particularly when the complex is deposited on a basement membrane and cannot be phagocytosed (so-called 'frustrated phagocytosis'). The proteolytic enzymes (including neutral proteinases and collagenase), kinin-forming enzymes, polycationic proteins and reactive oxygen and nitrogen intermediates which are

131

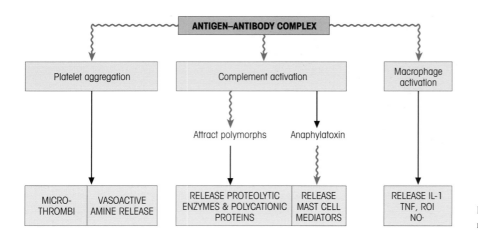

Figure 14.10 Type III immune complex-mediated hypersensitivity.

released from the polymorph will damage local tissues and intensify the inflammatory responses. Under appropriate conditions, platelets may be aggregated with two consequences: they provide yet a further source of vasoactive amines and may also form microthrombi, which can lead to local ischemia. Insoluble complexes taken up by macrophages cannot readily be digested and provide a persistent activating stimulus leading to release of the cytokines IL-1 and TNF, reactive oxygen intermediates and nitric oxide (figure 14.10) which further damage the tissue.

The outcome of the formation of immune complexes *in vivo* depends not only on the absolute amounts of antigen and antibody, but also on their *relative* proportions which govern the nature of the complexes and hence their distribution within the body. Between **antibody excess** and **mild antigen excess**, the complexes are rapidly precipitated and tend to be localized to the site of introduction of antigen, whereas in **moderate** to **gross antigen excess**, soluble complexes are formed. These small complexes containing C3b bind by immune adherence to CR1 complement receptors on the human erythrocyte and are transported to fixed macrophages in the liver where they are safely inactivated. If there are defects in this system, for example deficiencies in classical complement pathway components or perhaps if the system is overloaded, then the immune complexes are free in the plasma and widespread disease involving deposition in the kidneys, joints and skin may result.

Inflammatory lesions due to locally formed complexes

The Arthus reaction

Maurice Arthus found that injection of soluble antigen intradermally into hyperimmunized rabbits with high levels

of antibody, produced an erythematous and edematous reaction reaching a peak at 3–8 hours and then usually resolving. The lesion was characterized by an intense infiltration with polymorphonuclear leukocytes. The injected antigen precipitates with antibody and binds complement. Using fluorescent reagents, antigen, immunoglobulin and complement components can all be demonstrated in this lesion. Anaphylatoxin is soon generated and causes mast cell degranulation, the influx of polymorphs with release of polymorph granules, and local tissue injury. Local intravascular complexes will also cause platelet aggregation and vasoactive amine release resulting in erythema and edema.

Reactions to inhaled antigens

Intrapulmonary Arthus-type reactions to exogenous inhaled antigen appear to be responsible for the condition of hypersensitivity pneumonitis. The severe respiratory difficulties associated with **farmer's lung** occur within 6–8 hours of exposure to the dust from moldy hay. These patients are sensitized to thermophilic actinomycetes which grow in the moldy hay, and extracts of these organisms give precipitin reactions with the subject's serum and Arthus reactions on intradermal injection. Inhalation of bacterial spores present in dust from the hay introduces antigen into the lungs and a complex-mediated hypersensitivity reaction occurs. Similar situations arise in pigeon-fancier's disease, where the antigen is probably serum protein present in the dust from dried feces, in rat handlers sensitized to rat serum proteins excreted in the urine (figure 14.11), and in many other quaintly named cases of **extrinsic allergic alveolitis** resulting from continual inhalation of organic particles, for example cheese washer's disease (*Penicillium casei* spores), furrier's lung (fox fur proteins) and maple bark stripper's disease (spores of *Cryptostroma*). Although the initial

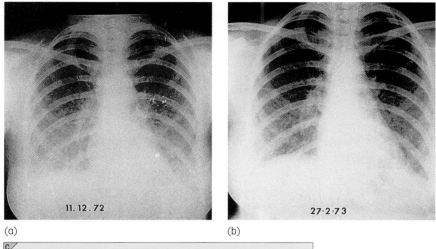

(a)　　　　　　　　　　(b)

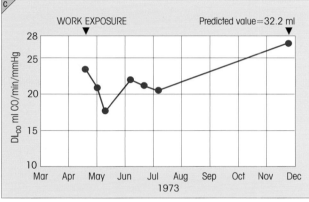

Figure 14.11 Extrinsic allergic alveolitis due to rat serum proteins in a research assistant handling rats (Type III hypersensitivity). Typical systemic and pulmonary reactions on inhalation and positive prick tests were elicited by rat serum proteins; precipitins against serum proteins in rat urine were present in the patient's serum. (a) Bilateral micronodular shadowing during acute episodes. (b) Marked clearing within 11 days after cessation of exposure to rats. (c) Temporary fall in pulmonary gas exchange measured by DL_{co} (gas transfer, single breath) following a 3-day exposure to rats at work (arrowed). (From Carroll K.B., Pepys J., Longbottom J.L., Hughes D.T.D. & Benson H.G. (1975) *Clinical Allergy* **5**, 443; figures kindly provided by Professor J. Pepys.)

damage in the lung is due to localized immune complexes, subsequent infiltration of macrophages and T-cells will result in the release of a variety of proinflammatory cytokines which produce further tissue damage.

Disease resulting from circulating complexes

Serum sickness

Injection of relatively large doses of foreign serum (e.g. horse antidiphtheria) used to be employed for various therapeutic purposes. Although horse serum containing specific antibodies is still used therapeutically (such as for the treatment of snake bite) injection of monoclonal antibodies originating in mice is not an uncommon procedure. Some individuals receiving foreign serum begin to synthesize antibodies against the foreign protein giving rise to a condition known as 'serum sickness', which appears about 8 days after the injection. This results from the deposition of soluble antigen–antibody complexes, formed in antigen excess, in small vessels throughout the body. The clinical manifesta-

tions include a rise in temperature, swollen lymph nodes, a generalized urticarial rash and painful swollen joints associated with a low serum complement and transient albuminuria. To be pathogenic, the complexes have to be of the right size—too big and they are snapped up smartly by the macrophages of the mononuclear phagocyte system, too small and they fail to induce an inflammatory reaction. Even when they are the right size, it seems that they will only localize in vessel walls if there is a change in vascular permeability. This may come about through release of 5-hydroxytryptamine (5HT; serotonin) from platelets reacting with larger complexes or through an IgE or complement-mediated degranulation of basophils and mast cells to produce histamine, leukotrienes and PAF. The effect on the capillaries is to cause separation of the endothelial cells and exposure of the basement membrane to which the appropriately sized complexes attach and attract polymorphs which give rise to the vasculitis so typical of immune complex-mediated disease. The skin, joints, kidneys and heart are particularly affected. As antibody synthesis increases, antigen is cleared and the patient normally recovers.

133

Immune complex glomerulonephritis

Following a number of chronic infections and autoimmune diseases **immune complexes are retained in or on the endothelial side of the glomerular basement membrane** (figure 14.12) where they build up as 'lumpy' granules staining for antigen, immunoglobulin and complement by immunofluorescence (figure 14.9b) and appear as large amorphous masses in the electron microscope. The inflammatory process damages the basement membrane, causing leakage of serum proteins and consequent proteinuria. Because serum albumin molecules are small they appear in the urine even with just minor degrees of glomerular damage.

Many cases of glomerulonephritis are associated with circulating complexes, and biopsies give a fluorescent staining pattern similar to that of figure 14.9b, which depicts DNA/anti-DNA/complement deposits in the kidney of a patient with SLE. Similar immune complex disease may follow various bacterial infections such as with certain strains of so-called 'nephritogenic' streptococci, in chronic parasitic infections such as quartan malaria, and in the course of chronic viral infections.

Deposition of immune complexes at other sites

The favored sites for immune complex deposition are the skin, joints and kidney. The vasculitic skin rashes which are a major feature of serum sickness are also characteristic of systemic and discoid lupus erythematosus (figure 14.5c), and biopsies of the lesions reveal amorphous deposits of Ig and C3 at the basement membrane of the dermal–epidermal junction. The necrotizing arteritis produced in rabbits by experimental serum sickness closely resembles the histology of polyarteritis nodosa, where immune complexes containing the HBs antigen of hepatitis B virus are present in the lesions (figure 14.5d). In some instances, drugs such as penicillin become antigenic after conjugation with body proteins and form complexes which mediate hypersensitivity reactions. The choroid plexus, being a major filtration site, is also favored for immune complex deposition and this could account for the frequency of central nervous disorders in SLE. Similarly, in subacute sclerosing panencephalitis, deposits containing Ig and measles Ag may be found in neural tissue.

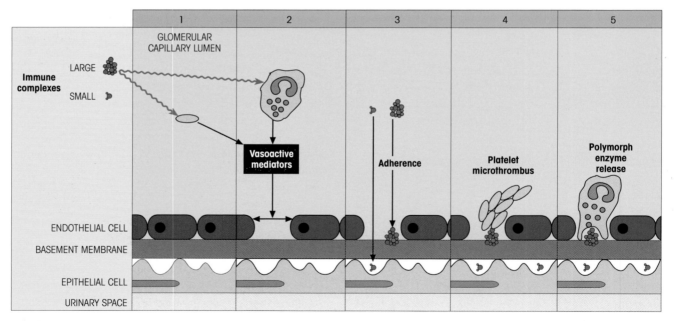

Figure 14.12 Deposition of immune complexes in the kidney glomerulus. (1) Complexes induce release of vasoactive mediators from basophils and platelets which cause (2) separation of endothelial cells, (3) attachment of larger complexes to exposed basement membrane, while smaller complexes pass through to epithelial side; (4) complexes induce platelet aggregation; (5) chemotactically attracted neutrophils release granule contents in 'frustrated phagocytosis' to damage basement membrane and cause leakage of serum proteins. Complex deposition is favored in the glomerular capillary because it is a major filtration site and has a high hydrodynamic pressure. Deposition is greatly reduced in animals depleted of platelets or treated with vasoactive amine antagonists.

TYPE IV: CELL-MEDIATED (DELAYED-TYPE) HYPERSENSITIVITY

This form of hypersensitivity is encountered as a reaction to numerous bacteria, viruses and fungi, in the contact dermatitis resulting from sensitization to certain simple chemicals, and in the rejection of transplanted tissues. Perhaps the best known example is the **Mantoux reaction** obtained by injection of tuberculin into the skin of an individual in whom previous infection with the mycobacterium has induced a state of cell-mediated immunity (CMI). The reaction is characterized by erythema and induration (figure 14.5e), which appears only after several hours (hence the term 'delayed') and reaches a maximum at 24–48 hours, thereafter subsiding. Histologically the earliest phase of the reaction is seen as a perivascular cuffing with mononuclear cells followed by a more extensive exudation of mono- and poly-morphonuclear cells. The latter soon migrate out of the lesion leaving behind a predominantly mononuclear cell infiltrate consisting of lymphocytes and cells of the monocyte-macrophage series. This contrasts with the essentially 'polymorph' character of the Arthus reaction.

The cellular basis of type IV hypersensitivity

Unlike the other forms of hypersensitivity which we have discussed, delayed-type reactivity cannot be transferred from a sensitized to a nonsensitized individual with serum antibody; lymphoid cells, in particular the T-lymphocytes, are required.

It cannot be stressed too often that the hypersensitivity lesion results from an exaggerated interaction between antigen and the *normal* cell-mediated immune mechanisms. Following earlier priming, memory T-cells recognize the antigen together with class II major histocompatibility complex (MHC) molecules on an antigen-presenting cell, and are stimulated into blast cell transformation and proliferation. The stimulated T-cells release a number of cytokines which function as mediators of the ensuing hypersensitivity response, particularly by attracting and activating macrophages if they belong to the T_H1 subset, or eosinophils if they are T_H2; they also help T_C precursors to become killer cells, which can cause tissue damage (figure 14.13).

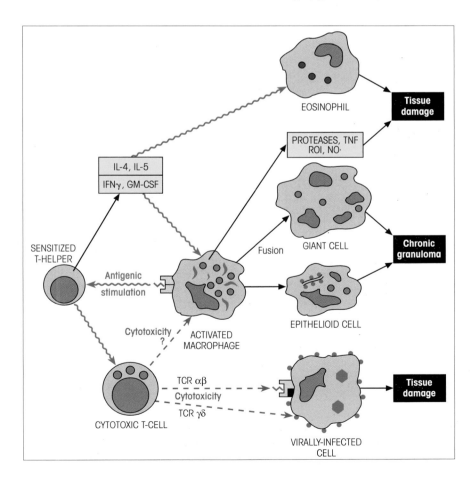

Figure 14.13 The cellular basis of Type IV hypersensitivity.

Tissue damage produced by type IV reactions

Infections

The development of a state of cell-mediated hypersensitivity to bacterial products is probably responsible for the lesions associated with bacterial allergy such as the cavitation, caseation and general toxemia seen in human tuberculosis, and the granulomatous skin lesions found in patients with the borderline form of leprosy. When the battle between the replicating bacteria and the body defenses fails to be resolved in favor of the host, persisting antigen provokes a chronic local delayed hypersensitivity reaction. Continual release of cytokines from sensitized T-lymphocytes leads to the accumulation of large numbers of macrophages, many of which give rise to arrays of epithelioid cells, while others fuse to form giant cells. Macrophages bearing bacterial antigen on their surface may become targets for killer T-cells and be destroyed. Further tissue damage will occur as a result of indiscriminate cytotoxicity by lymphokine-activated macrophages (and natural killer (NK) cells?). Morphologically, this combination of cell types with proliferating lymphocytes and fibroblasts associated with areas of fibrosis and necrosis is termed a **chronic granuloma** and represents an attempt by the body to wall off a site of persistent infection (figure 14.13).

The skin rashes in smallpox and measles and the lesions of herpes simplex may be largely attributed to delayed-type allergic reactions with extensive damage to virally infected cells by Tc cells. Cell-mediated hypersensitivity has also been demonstrated in the fungal diseases candidiasis, dermatomycosis, coccidioidomycosis and histoplasmosis, and in the parasitic disease leishmaniasis.

Contact dermatitis

The epidermal route of inoculation tends to favor the development of a T-cell response through processing by class II-rich dendritic Langerhans cells which migrate to the lymph nodes and present antigen to T-lymphocytes. Thus, delayed-type reactions in the skin are often produced by foreign materials capable of binding to body constituents, possibly surface molecules of the Langerhans cell, to form new antigens. The reaction is characterized by a mononuclear cell infiltrate peaking at 12–15 hours, accompanied by edema of the epidermis with microvesicle formation. Contact hypersensitivity can occur in people who become sensitized while working with chemicals such as picryl chloride and chromates, or who repeatedly come into contact with the substance urushiol from the poison ivy plant. p-Phenylene diamine in certain hair dyes, neomycin in topically applied ointments, and nickel salts formed from articles such as nickel jewellery clasps (figure 14.5f), can provoke similar reactions.

Other examples

Delayed hypersensitivity contributes significantly to the prolonged reactions which result from insect bites. In certain organ-specific autoimmune diseases, such as type I diabetes, cell-mediated hypersensitivity reactions undoubtedly provide the major engine for tissue destruction. Similarly in multiple sclerosis, T-cells sensitized to myelin basic protein play a major role in the production of demyelination.

REVISION

See the accompanying website (www.roitt.com) for multiple choice questions.

Excessive stimulation of the normal effector mechanisms of the immune system can lead to tissue damage, and we speak of hypersensitivity reactions, of which several types can be distinguished.

Type I: anaphylactic hypersensitivity
• Anaphylaxis involves contraction of smooth muscle and dilatation of capillaries.

• This depends upon the reaction of antigen with specific IgE antibody bound through its Fc to the mast cell.
• Cross-linking and clustering of the IgE receptors leads to release from the granules of mediators including histamine, leukotrienes and platelet activating factor, plus eosinophil and neutrophil chemotactic factors and the cytokines IL-3, -4, -5 and GM-CSF.
• IL-4 is involved in isotype switch to IgE.

Atopic allergy

• Atopy stems from an excessive IgE response to extrinsic antigens (allergens) which leads to local anaphylactic reactions at sites of contact with allergen.

• Hay fever and extrinsic asthma represent the most common atopic allergic disorders resulting from exposure to inhaled allergens.

• Serious prolongation of the response to allergen is caused by T-cells of TH2-type which recruit tissue-damaging eosinophils through release of IL-5. This TH2 bias is reinforced by NO produced by cytokine-stimulated airway epithelial cells.

• Many food allergies involve Type I hypersensitivity.

• Strong genetic factors include the propensity to make the IgE isotype.

• The offending antigen is identified by intradermal prick tests giving immediate wheal and erythema reactions, also by provocation testing and by RAST.

• Where possible, allergen avoidance is the best treatment.

• Symptomatic treatment involves the use of long-acting β_2-agonists and newly developed leukotriene antagonists. Chromones, such as sodium cromoglycate, block chloride channel activity thereby stabilizing mast cells and inhibiting bronchoconstriction. Theophylline, the single most prescribed drug for asthma, is a phosphodiesterase inhibitor which raises intracellular calcium; this causes bronchodilatation and inhibition of IL-5 effects on eosinophils. Chronic asthma is dominated by activated TH2 cells and is treated with topical steroids, supplemented where necessary by long-acting β_2-agonists and theophylline.

• Courses of antigen injection may desensitize by formation of blocking IgG or IgA antibodies or through T-cell regulation. T-cell epitope peptides may be manipulated to modulate the atopic state.

Type II: antibody-dependent cytotoxic hypersensitivity

• This involves the death of cells bearing antibody attached to a surface antigen.

• The cells may be taken up by phagocytic cells to which they adhere through their coating of IgG or C3b, or they may be lysed by the operation of the full complement system.

• Cells bearing IgG may also be killed by polymorphs and macrophages or by K-cells through an extracellular mechanism (antibody-dependent cell-mediated cytotoxicity).

• Examples are: transfusion reactions, hemolytic disease of the newborn through rhesus incompatibility, antibody-mediated graft destruction, autoimmune reactions directed against the formed elements of the blood and kidney glomerular basement membranes, and hypersensitivity resulting from the coating of erythrocytes or platelets by a drug.

Type III: complex-mediated hypersensitivity

• This results from the effects of antigen–antibody complexes through (i) activation of complement and attraction of polymorphonuclear leukocytes which release tissue-damaging mediators on contact with the complex, and (ii) aggregation of platelets to cause microthrombi and vasoactive amine release.

• Where circulating antibody levels are high, the antigen is precipitated near the site of entry into the body. The reaction in the skin is characterized by polymorph infiltration, edema and erythema maximal at 3–8 hours (Arthus reaction).

• Examples are: farmer's lung, pigeon-fancier's disease and pulmonary aspergillosis, where inhaled antigens provoke high antibody levels; reactions to an abrupt increase in antigen caused by microbial cell death during chemotherapy for leprosy or syphilis; and an element of the synovial lesion in rheumatoid arthritis.

• In relative *antigen excess*, soluble complexes are formed which are removed by binding to the CR1 C3b receptors on red cells. If this system is overloaded or if the classical complement components are deficient, the complexes circulate in the free state and are deposited under circumstances of increased vascular permeability at certain preferred sites—kidney glomerulus, joints, skin and choroid plexus.

• Examples are: serum sickness following injection of large quantities of foreign protein; glomerulonephritis associated with systemic lupus erythematosus (SLE) or infections with streptococci, malaria and other parasites; neurological disturbances in SLE and subacute sclerosing panencephalitis; polyarteritis nodosa linked to hepatitis B virus; and hemorrhagic shock in dengue viral infection.

Type IV: cell-mediated or delayed-type hypersensitivity

• This is based upon the interaction of antigen with primed T-cells and represents tissue damage resulting from inappropriate cell-mediated immunity reactions.

• A number of soluble cytokines including IFNγ are released which activate macrophages and account for the events which occur in a typical delayed hypersensitivity response such as the Mantoux reaction to tuberculin, i.e. the delayed appearance of an indurated and erythematous reaction which reaches a maximum at 24–48 hours and is characterized histologically by infiltration with mononuclear phagocytes and lymphocytes.

• Continuing provocation of delayed hypersensitivity by persisting antigen leads to formation of chronic granulomas.

• TH2-type cells producing IL-4 and IL-5 can also produce tissue damage through their ability to recruit eosinophils.

• CD8 T-cells are activated by class I major histocompatibil-ity antigens to become directly cytotoxic to target cells bearing the appropriate antigen.

• Examples are: tissue damage occurring in bacterial (tuberculosis, leprosy), viral (smallpox, measles, herpes), fungal (candidiasis, histoplasmosis) and parasitic (leishma-niasis, schistosomiasis) infections; contact dermatitis from exposure to chromates and poison ivy; insect bites; and psoriasis.

FURTHER READING

Chapel H. & Haeney M. (1993) *Essentials of Clinical Immunology*, 3rd edn. Blackwell Scientific Publications, Oxford. [Very broad account of the diseases involving the immune system. Good illustration by case histories and the laboratory tests available. Also MCQ. One reviewer questions the adequacy of the treatment of allergy.]

Erb K.J. (1999) Atopic disorders: a default pathway in the absence of infection? *Immunology Today* **20** (7), 317.

Kinet J.-P. (ed) (1999) Section on Atopic Allergy and other Hypersensi-tivities. *Current Opinion in Immunology* **11** (6).

CHAPTER 15

Transplantation

GRAFT REJECTION IS IMMUNOLOGIC

The replacement of diseased organs by a transplant of healthy tissue has long been an objective in medicine but has been frustrated to no mean degree by the uncooperative attempts by the body to reject grafts from other individuals. Before discussing the nature and implications of this rejection phenomenon, it would be helpful to define the terms used for transplants between individuals and species:

Autograft—tissue grafted back on to the original donor.

Isograft—graft between syngeneic individuals (i.e. of identical genetic constitution) such as identical twins or mice of the same pure line strain.

Allograft (old term, homograft)—graft between allogeneic individuals (i.e. members of the same species but different genetic constitution), e.g. man to man and one mouse strain to another.

Xenograft (heterograft)—graft between xenogeneic individuals (i.e. of different species), e.g. pig to man.

It is with the allograft reaction that we have been most concerned, and the most common allografting procedure is probably blood transfusion where the unfortunate consequences of mismatching are well known. Considerable attention has been paid to the rejection of solid grafts such as skin, and the sequence of events is worth describing. After suturing the allogeneic skin in place, the graft becomes vascularized within a few days, but between the 3rd and 9th day the circulation gradually diminishes and there is increasing infiltration of the graft bed with lymphocytes and monocytes but very few plasma cells. Necrosis begins to be visible macroscopically and within a day or so the graft is sloughed completely (figure M15.1.1).

First and second set rejection

It would be expected that if the reaction has an immunologic basis the second contact with antigen would represent a more explosive event than the first, and indeed the rejection

of a second graft from the same donor is much accelerated (Milestone 15.1). The initial vascularization is poor and may not occur at all. There is a very rapid invasion by polymorphonuclear leukocytes and lymphoid cells, including plasma cells, and thrombosis and acute cell destruction can be seen by 3–4 days. Second set rejection is not the fate of all subsequent allografts but only of those derived from the original donor or a related strain (figure M15.1.2). Grafts from new donors are rejected as first set reactions.

CONSEQUENCES OF MHC INCOMPATIBILITY

Class II MHC differences produce a mixed lymphocyte reaction (MLR)

When lymphocytes from individuals of different class II haplotype are cultured together *in vitro*, blast cell transformation and mitosis occurs, the T-cells of each population of lymphocytes reacting against MHC class II determinants on the surface of the other population. This constitutes the mixed lymphocyte reaction (MLR). The responding cells belong predominantly to a population of CD4$^+$ T-lymphocytes and are stimulated by the class II determinants present mostly on B-cells, macrophages and especially dendritic antigen-presenting cells. For many years the MLR was employed in transplantation laboratories to determine the degree of compatibility between individuals. With the introduction of very accurate molecular HLA testing the MLR is no longer routinely performed.

The graft-vs-host (g.v.h.) reaction

When competent T-cells are transferred from an HLA-incompatible donor to an immunosuppressed recipient who is incapable of rejecting them, the grafted cells survive and have time to recognize the host antigens and react immunologically against them. Instead of the normal transplantation reaction of host against graft, we have the reverse, the so-called graft-vs-host (g.v.h.) reaction. In the human, fever, anemia, weight loss, rash, diarrhea and splenomegaly are observed, with cytokines, especially tumor necrosis factor (TNF), being thought to be the major mediators of pathology. The 'stronger' the transplantation antigen difference, the more severe that reaction. G.v.h. may therefore be observed in immunologically anergic subjects receiving bone marrow grafts, for example for combined immunodeficiency (see p. 114) or for the re-establishment of bone marrow in subjects whose own marrow has been destroyed by massive doses of chemotherapy used to treat malignant disease (figure 15.1).

MECHANISMS OF GRAFT REJECTION

Lymphocytes mediate rejection

A primary role of lymphoid cells in first set rejection would be consistent with the histology of the early reaction showing infiltration by mononuclear cells with very few polymorphs or plasma cells (figure 15.2). The dramatic effect of experimental neonatal thymectomy on prolonging skin transplants, and the long survival of grafts on children with thymic deficiencies implicate the T-lymphocytes in these reactions. More direct evidence has come from *in vitro* studies showing that T-cells taken from mice rejecting an allograft could kill target cells bearing the graft antigens *in vitro*. Most of these T-cells are CD8+ cytotoxic cells which recognize class I alloantigens on the graft and mount a cytotoxic reaction against graft parenchymal and endothelial cells. Cytotoxicity results both from perforin/granzyme-based activities and from the apoptosis due to interactions between FasL on the activated cells and Fas on the target cells. CD4+ cells also play a major role in graft rejection by the secretion of the cytokines which mediate delayed hypersensitivity reactions. These include IFNγ, which activates

MILESTONE 15.1—THE IMMUNOLOGIC BASIS OF GRAFT REJECTION

The field of transplantation owes a tremendous debt to Sir Peter Medawar, the outstanding scientist who kick-started and inspired its development. Even at the turn of the century it was an accepted paradigm that grafts between unrelated members of a species would be unceremoniously rejected after a brief initial period of acceptance (figure M15.1.1). That there was an underlying genetic basis for rejection became apparent from Padgett's observations in Kansas City in 1932 that skin allografts between family members tended to survive for longer than those between unrelated individuals, and J.B. Brown's critical demonstration in St Louis in 1937 that monozygotic (i.e. genetically identical) twins accepted skin grafts from each other. However, it was not until Medawar's research in the early part of the Second World War, motivated by the need to treat aircrew with appalling burns, that rejection was laid at immunology's door. He showed that a second graft from a given donor was rejected more rapidly and more vigorously than the first, and further that an unrelated graft was rejected with the kinetics of a first set reaction (figure M15.1.2). This **second set rejection** is characterized by **memory** and **specificity** and thereby bears the hallmarks of an immunologic response. This of course was later confirmed by transferring the ability to express a second set reaction with lymphocytes.

The message was clear: to achieve successful transplantation of tissues and organs in the human, it would be necessary

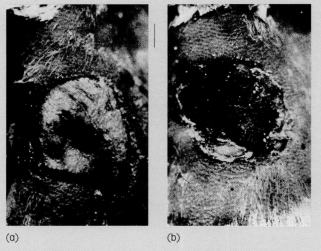

(a) (b)

Figure M15.1.1 Rejection of CBA skin graft by strain A mouse. (a) Ten days after transplantation; discolored areas caused by destruction of epithelium and drying of the exposed dermis. (b) Thirteen days after transplantation; the scabby surface indicates total destruction of the graft. (Photographs courtesy of Professor L. Brent.)

to overcome this immunogenetic barrier. Limited success was obtained by Murray, at the Peter Bent Brigham Hospital, and Hamburger in Paris, who grafted kidneys between dizygotic twins using sublethal X-irradiation. The key breakthrough came when Schwartz and Damashek's report on the immunosuppressive effects of the antimitotic drug 6-mercaptopurine

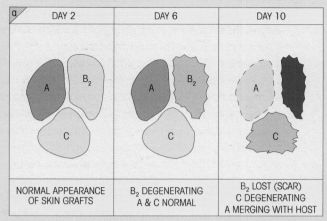

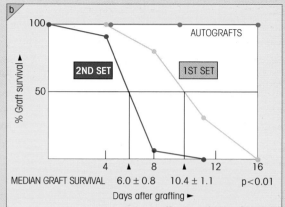

Figure M15.1.2 Memory and specificity in skin allograft rejection in rabbits. (a) Autografts and allografts from two unrelated donors, B and C, are applied to the thoracic wall skin of rabbit A which has already rejected a first graft from B (B_1). While the autograft A remains intact, graft C seen for the first time undergoes first set rejection, whereas a *second* graft from B (B_2) is sloughed off very rapidly. (b) Median survival times of first and second set skin allografts showing faster second set rejection. (From Medawar P.B. (1944) The behaviour and fate of skin autografts and skin homografts (allografts) in rabbits. *Journal of Anatomy* **78**, 176.)

was applied independently by Calne and Zukowski in 1960 to the prolongation of renal allografts in dogs. This was followed very rapidly by Murray's successful grafting in 1962 of an unrelated cadaveric kidney under the immunosuppressive umbrella of azathioprine, the more effective derivative of 6-mercaptopurine devised by Hutchings and Elion.

This story is studded with Nobel Prize winners and readers of a historical bent will gain further insight into the development of this field and the minds of the scientists who gave medicine this wonderful prize in *History of Transplantation; Thirty-five Recollections*, Terasaki P.I. (ed.) (1991) UCLA Tissue Typing Laboratory, Los Angeles, CA.

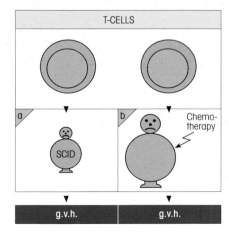

Figure 15.1 Graft-vs-host reaction. When competent T-cells are inoculated into a host incapable of reacting against them, the grafted cells are free to react against the antigens on the host's cells which they recognize as foreign. The ensuing reaction may be fatal. Two of many possible situations are illustrated. (a) A patient with severe combined immunodeficiency receives a graft from an HLA incompatible donor. (b) A leukemia patient post-chemotherapy receives a bone marrow transplant from an autologous donor.

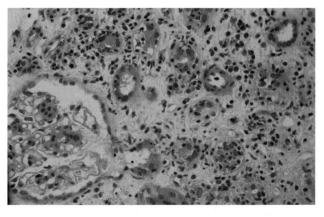

Figure 15.2 Acute rejection of human renal allograft showing dense cellular infiltration of interstitium by mononuclear cells. (Photograph courtesy of Drs M. Thompson and A. Dorling.)

and recruits macrophages and upregulates MHC antigen expression on the graft, IL-2, which promotes T-cell proliferation and CD8$^+$ cell activation, and lymphotoxin α, which is directly cytotoxic to allogeneic cells.

The allograft response is powerful

Remember, we defined the MHC by its ability to provoke the most powerful rejection of grafts between members of the same species. It transpires that **normal individuals have a very high frequency of alloreactive cells** (i.e. cells which react with allografts), which presumably accounts for the intensity of MHC-mismatched rejection. Whereas merely a fraction of one percent of the normal T-cell population is specific for a given single peptide, upwards of 10% of the T-cells react with alloantigens. The reason for this is that very large numbers of T-cells each specific for a foreign peptide presented in the groove of self MHC molecules, may cross-react with an allogeneic MHC molecule containing host peptides in its groove. Such a complex mimics self MHC with foreign peptide in its groove and because the T-cell repertoire is recognizing large numbers of previously unseen foreign antigens, large numbers of recipient T-cells are activated. This is the so-called 'direct pathway'. In addition it is clear that T-cells may recognize some allogeneic peptides presented on self MHC molecules, a process called the 'indirect pathway'. T-cells recognizing peptides derived from graft proteins are present in low frequency comparable to that observed with any foreign antigen. Nonetheless, a graft which has been in place for an extended period will have the time to expand this small population significantly so that later rejection will depend progressively on this pathway.

There are different forms of graft rejection

Hyperacute rejection is the most dramatic form of graft rejection, occurring within minutes of transplantation. It is due to the presence in the recipient of preformed antibodies directed against donor HLA or ABO antigens. Such antibodies will attach to the endothelial cells of the donor organ, fix complement and cause damage to these cells. This will produce aggregation of platelets which contributes to the vascular occlusion, seen in renal transplantation as glomerular microthrombi, which are so characteristic of this form of rejection. Fortunately, by ABO matching and by performing cross-matches in which patients are screened for pre-existing antibodies, hyperacute rejection is no longer a major problem in most transplant centers. It is worth pointing out that because humans have a variety of natural antibodies against animal tissue, hyperacute rejection is the major hurdle to xenogeneic transplants.

Acute early rejection occurring up to 10 days or so after transplantation is characterized by dense cellular infiltration (figure 15.2) and rupture of peritubular capillaries, and appears to be a cell-mediated hypersensitivity reaction mainly involving an attack by CD8$^+$ cells on graft cells whose MHC antigen expression has been upregulated by γ-interferon.

Acute late rejection, which occurs from 11 days onwards in patients suppressed with prednisone and azathioprine, is probably caused by the binding of immunoglobulin (presumably antibody) and complement to the arterioles and glomerular capillaries, where they can be visualized by immunofluorescent techniques. These immunoglobulin deposits on the vessel walls induce platelet aggregation in the glomerular capillaries leading to acute renal shutdown (figure 15.3). The possibility of damage to antibody-coated

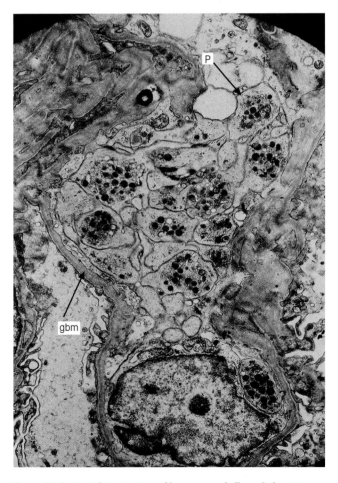

Figure 15.3 Acute late rejection of human renal allograft showing platelet (P) aggregation in a glomerular capillary (gbm) induced by deposition of antibody on the vessel wall (electron micrograph). (Photograph courtesy of Professor K. Porter.)

cells through antibody-dependent cell-mediated cytotoxicity must also be considered.

Chronic or late rejection may occur months or years after the initial transplant depending on the success of immunosuppressive therapy. The main pathologic feature is vascular injury and occlusion of the vessel due to proliferation of smooth muscle cells, and accumulation of T-cells and macrophages in the intima of the vessel wall. The cause of this graft arteriosclerosis is not clear but it may be due to delayed hypersensitivity which activates macrophages in the vessel wall with the release of various smooth muscle growth factors. There is also evidence of a humoral component in that deposits of antibodies against donor tissue, or antigen–antibody complexes have been detected in vascular endothelial cells and may give rise to occlusion of the vessels. It has been noticed that chronic rejection is more prominent in patients who initially showed even mild acute rejection and also in those who have chronic viral infections, especially with cytomegalovirus.

THE PREVENTION OF GRAFT REJECTION

Matching tissue types on graft donor and recipient

The value of matching tissue types

The greater the degree of identity between the various HLA antigens on donor and recipient tissues, i.e. the greater the degree of 'matching', the weaker the rejection of the graft.

Although improvements in operative techniques and the use of drugs such as cyclosporin A have greatly diminished the effects of mismatching HLA specificities on solid graft survival, nevertheless, most transplanters favor a high degree of matching, especially at the DR locus (see figure 15.4). The consensus is that matching at the DR loci is of greater benefit than the B loci, which in turn are of more relevance to graft survival than the A loci. Bone marrow grafts, however, require a high degree of compatibility, which is now afforded by the greater accuracy of the modern DNA typing methods.

Because of the many thousands of different HLA phenotypes (figure 15.4), it is usual to work with a large pool of potential recipients, so that when graft material becomes available the best possible match can be made. The position will be improved when the pool of available organs can be increased through the development of long-term tissue storage banks, but techniques are not good enough for this at present. Bone marrow cells fortunately, can be kept viable even after freezing and thawing. With a paired organ such as the kidney, living donors may be used; siblings provide the best chance of a good match (cf. figure 15.4). However, the use of living donors poses difficult ethical problems and there has been encouraging progress in the use of cadaver material.

Agents producing general immunosuppression

Graft rejection can be held at bay by the use of agents which nonspecifically interfere with the induction or expression of

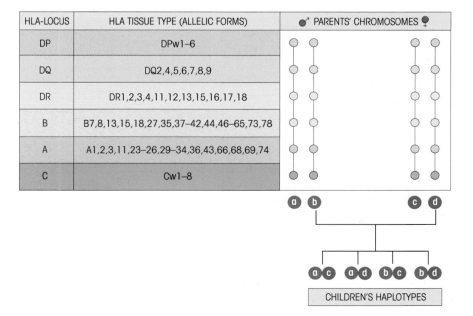

HLA-LOCUS	HLA TISSUE TYPE (ALLELIC FORMS)
DP	DPw1–6
DQ	DQ2,4,5,6,7,8,9
DR	DR1,2,3,4,11,12,13,15,16,17,18
B	B7,8,13,15,18,27,35,37–42,44,46–65,73,78
A	A1,2,3,11,23–26,29–34,36,43,66,68,69,74
C	Cw1–8

♂ PARENTS' CHROMOSOMES ♀

Ⓐ Ⓑ   Ⓒ Ⓓ

CHILDREN'S HAPLOTYPES

ⒶⒸ ⒶⒹ ⒷⒸ ⒷⒹ

Figure 15.4 Serologically defined HLA specificities and their inheritance. The complex lies on chromosome 6. Since there are several possible alleles at each locus, the probability of a random pair of subjects from the general population having identical HLA specificities is very low. However, there is a 1 : 4 chance that two siblings will be identical in this respect because each group of specificities on a single chromosome forms a haplotype which will be inherited en bloc, giving four possible combinations of paternal and maternal chromosomes. Parent and offspring can only be identical if the mother and father have one haplotype in common.

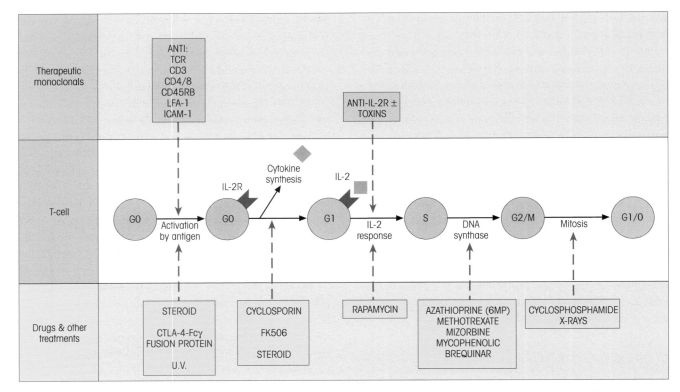

Figure 15.5 Immunosuppressive agents used to control graft rejection. These drugs act at many different points in the immune response. Simultaneous treatment with agents acting at sequential stages in development of the rejection response would be expected to synergize strongly and this is clearly seen with cyclosporin A and rapamycin.

the immune response (figure 15.5). Because these agents act on various parts of the cellular immune response, patients on immunosuppressive therapy tend to be susceptible to infections and more prone to the development of lymphoreticular cancers, particularly those with a known viral etiology.

Immunosuppressive drugs

Many of the immunosuppressive drugs now employed were first used in cancer chemotherapy because of their toxicity to dividing cells. Aside from the complications of blanket immunosuppression mentioned above, these antimitotic drugs are especially toxic for cells of the bone marrow and small intestine and must therefore be used with great care.

A very commonly used drug in this field is **azathioprine**, which has a preferential effect on T-cell-mediated reactions by inhibiting the synthesis of nucleic acid. The N-mustard derivative, **cyclophosphamide**, probably attacks DNA by alkylation and cross-linking, so preventing correct duplication during cell division. These agents appear to exert their damaging effects on cells during mitosis and for this reason

are most powerful when administered after presentation of antigen at a time when the antigen-sensitive cells are dividing.

Corticosteroids such as prednisone intervene at many points in the immune response, affecting lymphocyte recirculation and the generation of cytotoxic effector cells; in addition, their outstanding anti-inflammatory potency rests on features such as inhibition of neutrophil adherence to vascular endothelium in an inflammatory area and suppression of monocyte/macrophage functions such as microbicidal activity, release of proinflammatory cytokines and response to lymphokines. Corticosteroids form complexes with intracellular receptors, which then bind to regulatory genes and block transcription of TNF, IFNγ, IL-1, -2, -3 and -6 and MHC class II, i.e. they block expression of lymphokines and monokines whereas cyclosporin (see below) has its main action on lymphokines.

An exciting and entirely new group of fungal metabolites (figure 15.5) are having a dramatic effect in human transplantation and in the therapy of immunologic disorders, through their ability to target T-cells. **Cyclosporin A** (CsA), selectively blocks the transcription of IL-2 in activated T-cells and this will inhibit their proliferation and possibly the upregulation of the FasL on activated cytotoxic T-cells. Resting cells which carry the vital memory for immunity to microbial infections are spared and there is little toxicity for dividing cells in gut and bone marrow. Another T-cell-specific immunosuppressive drug, **FK506**, also blocks lymphokine production. The latest addition to the stable, **rapamycin**, is a macrolide like FK506, but in contrast acts to block signals induced by combination of IL-2 with its receptor.

Cyclosporin now has a proven place as first-line therapy in the prophylaxis and treatment of transplant rejection, and it has also been evaluated in a wide range of disorders where T-cell-mediated hypersensitivity reactions are suspected. Indeed, the benefits of cyclosporin in diseases such as idiopathic nephrotic syndrome, type 1 insulin-dependent diabetes, Behçet's syndrome, active Crohn's disease, aplastic anemia, severe corticosteroid-dependent asthma and psoriasis have been interpreted to suggest or confirm a pathogenic role for the immune system.

Targeting lymphoid populations

Anti-CD3 monoclonals are in widespread use as anti-T-cell reagents to successfully reverse acute graft rejection. They produce a complex 'flu-like' clinical syndrome which includes fever, chills, headache and gastrointestinal discomfort associated with an increase in serum γ-interferon (IFNγ), tumour necrosis factor α (TNFα) and often interleukin-2 (IL-2), presumably resulting from T-cell activation. Xenosensitization to the mouse monoclonal is a problem but this can be avoided by 'humanizing' the antibody (see p. 32).

The IL-2 receptor represents another potential target for blocking the immune response, and antibody to this receptor has, in association with other immunosuppressive drugs, been shown to reduce the frequency of acute kidney rejection. A somewhat similar strategy is to construct a fusion protein of IL-2 itself with PE-40, the truncated *Pseudomonas* exotoxin which should be taken up selectively by cells bearing IL-2 receptors.

IS XENOGRAFTING A PRACTICAL PROPOSITION?

Because the supply of donor human organs for transplantation lags seriously behind the demand, a widespread interest in the feasibility of using animal organs is emerging. Of even greater practical use is the possible transplantation of animal cells and tissues to treat disease. Transplants of animal pancreatic islet cells could cure diabetes, and implants of neuronal cells would be useful in Parkinson's disease and other brain disorders. Pigs are more favored than primates as donors, both on grounds of ethical acceptability and the hazards of zoonoses, although these animals have been shown to harbor endogenous retroviruses that can infect human cells *in vitro*. The first hurdle to be overcome is **hyperacute rejection** due to xenoreactive natural antibodies in the host. These activate complement in the absence of regulators of the human complement system such as decay accelerating factor, CD59 and MCP, which precipitates the hyperacute rejection phenomenon.

The next crisis is acute vascular rejection as antibodies are formed to the xenoantigens on donor epithelium.

Even as the immunologic problems are being overcome, the question of whether animal viruses might infect humans and cause man-made pandemics (xenozoonosis), still needs to be considered.

CLINICAL EXPERIENCE IN GRAFTING

Privileged sites

Corneal grafts survive without the need for immunosuppression. Because they are avascular they do not sensitize the recipient, although they become cloudy if the individual has been presensitized. Grafts of cartilage are successful in the same way but an additional factor is the protection afforded the chondrocytes by the matrix. With bone and artery it doesn't really matter if the grafts die because they can still provide a framework for host cells to colonize.

Kidney grafts

Thousands of kidneys have been transplanted and with improvement in patient management there is a high survival rate. Matching at the HLA-DR locus has a strong effect on graft survival (figure 15.6) but in the long term (5 years or more) the desirability of reasonable HLA-B, and to a lesser extent HLA-A, matching also becomes apparent.

Patients are partially immunosuppressed at the time of transplantation because uremia causes a degree of immunologic anergy. The combination of azathioprine and prednisone was commonly employed in the long-term management of kidney grafts but is now supplemented by cyclosporin A in the so-called **triple therapy**. One hopes that the synergy between cyclosporin and rapamycin will emerge as a powerful new therapeutic regimen. When transplantation is performed because of immune

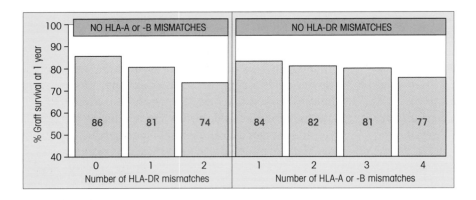

Figure 15.6 First cadaveric kidney graft survival in Europe on the basis of mismatches for HLA-A, B and DR. There is a significant influence of matching. (Data kindly supplied by Drs G. Opelz and Jacqueline Smits of the Eurotransplant International Foundation.)

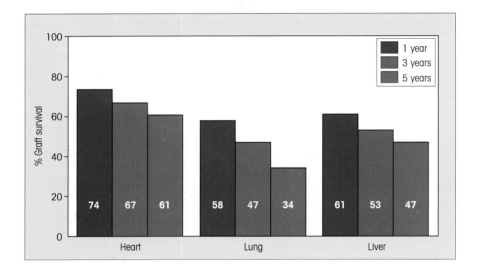

Figure 15.7 Graft survival rates for first heart, liver and lung transplantations in Eurotransplant. (Data kindly supplied by Dr Jacqueline Smits, Eurotransplant International Foundation.)

complex-induced glomerulonephritis, the immunosuppressive treatment used may help to prevent a similar lesion developing in the grafted kidney. Patients with glomerular basement membrane antibodies (e.g. Goodpasture's syndrome) are likely to destroy their renal transplants unless first treated with plasmapheresis and immunosuppressive drugs.

Heart transplants

The overall 1-year survival figure for heart transplants has moved up to over the 70% mark (figure 15.7), helped considerably by the introduction of cyclosporin A therapy. Full HLA matching is of course not practical but a single mismatch at the DR locus gave 90% survival at 3 years compared with a figure of 65% for two DR mismatches. Aside from the rejection problem it is likely that the number of patients who would benefit from cardiac replacement is

much greater than the number dying with adequately healthy hearts. More attention will have to be given to the possibility of xenogeneic grafts and mechanical substitutes.

Liver transplants

Survival rates for orthotopic liver grafts are not quite as high as those achieved with heart transplants (figure 15.7). The use of new preservatives now allows livers to be stored for 24 hours or more and has revolutionized the logistics of liver transplantation. To improve the prognosis of patients with primary hepatic or bile duct malignancies which were considered to be inoperable, transplantation of organ clusters with liver as the central organ has been designed, for example liver and pancreas, or liver, pancreas, stomach and small bowel or even colon.

Work is in progress on the transfer of isolated hepatocytes attached to collagen-coated microcarriers injected intraperitoneally for the correction of isolated deficiencies such as albumin synthesis. This attractive approach could have much wider applications, although in the distant future it will presumably run into competition from gene therapy.

Bone marrow grafting

Patients with certain immunodeficiency disorders and aplastic anemia are obvious candidates for treatment with bone marrow stem cells, as are leukemia patients treated radically with intensive chemotherapy and possibly whole-body irradiation in attempts to eradicate the neoplastic cells. Although bone marrow is the most often used source of stem cells, both umbilical cord blood and fetal liver are rich in stem cells and have been used for transplantation. For both these alternative sources, however, the major limitation is availability and the low absolute number of stem cells in a single sample. Another good source of stem cells is peripheral blood, which normally contains very small numbers of CD34+ stem cells, but these numbers rise dramatically following the administration of granulocyte colony-stimulating factor (G-CSF). Good results are being obtained with stem cell transplantation *in utero* for inherited blood disorders using CD34-enriched populations from paternal bone marrow.

Graft-vs-host disease is a major problem in bone marrow grafting

G.v.h. disease resulting from recognition of recipient antigens by allogeneic T-cells in the bone marrow inoculum represents a serious, sometimes fatal complication. The incidence of g.v.h. disease is reduced if T-cells in the grafted marrow are first purged with a cytotoxic cocktail of anti-T-cell monoclonals.

Successful results with bone marrow transfers require highly compatible donors if fatal g.v.h. reactions are to be avoided, and here siblings offer the best chance of finding a matched donor (figure 15.4). Undoubtedly non-HLA minor transplantation antigens are important and are more difficult to match. Acute g.v.h. disease occurring within the first 100 days following infusion of allogeneic marrow primarily affects the skin, liver and gastrointestinal tract. Current therapy uses cyclosporin with prednisone, but inclusion of methotrexate in this regimen is said to improve efficacy. Chronic g.v.h. disease (i.e. later than 100 days) has a relatively good prognosis if limited to skin and liver, but if multiple organs are involved, clinically resembling progressive systemic sclerosis, the outcome is poor.

Other organs

It is to be expected that improvement in techniques of control of the rejection process will encourage transplantation in several other areas — not cases of endocrine disorders where exogenous replacement therapy is convenient, but, for example, in diabetes where the number of transplants recorded is rising rapidly and the current success rate is around 40%. The 5-year survival rate of 34% for lung transplants is still less than satisfactory and one looks forward to the successful transplantation of skin for lethal burns.

Reports are coming in of experimental forays into the grafting of **neural tissues**. Mutant mice with degenerate cerebellar Purkinje cells which mimic the human condition, cerebellar ataxia, can be restored by engraftment of donor cerebellar cells at the appropriate sites. Clinical trials with transplantation of human embryonic dopamine neurons to reverse the neurological deficit in Parkinson's disease have been severely hampered by the excessive death of the grafted cells.

ASSOCIATION OF HLA TYPE WITH DISEASE

Association with immunologic diseases

An impressive body of data is accumulating which links specific HLA antigens with particular disease states in the human (table 15.1) and even more striking relationships may be uncovered as the complexity of the HLA-D region is unravelled. A significant association between a disease and a given HLA specificity does not imply that we have identified the disease susceptibility gene, because we might find an even better correlation with another HLA gene in linkage disequilibrium with the first. Linkage disequilibrium describes a state where closely linked genes on a chromosome tend to remain associated rather than being genetically randomized throughout the population.

With odd exceptions, HLA-linked diseases are intimately bound up with immunologic processes. By and large, the HLA-D-related disorders are autoimmune, with a tendency for DR3 or linked genes to be associated with organ-specific diseases. It has been suggested that HLA antigens might affect the susceptibility of a cell to viral attachment or infection, thereby influencing the development of autoimmunity to associated surface components. Inevitably though, because class II genes tend to dominate these relationships, the temptation is to think in terms of immune response genes controlling the nature of the reaction to the relevant autoantigen or to whatever might be a causative agent,

Table 15.1 Association of HLA with disease.

DISEASE	HLA ALLELE	RELATIVE RISK
a Class II associated		
Hashimoto's disease	*DR5	3.2
Primary myxedema	DR3	5.7
Thyrotoxicosis (Graves')	DR3	3.7
Insulin-dependent diabetes	DQ8	14
	DQ2/8	20
	DQ6	0.2
Addison's disease (adrenal)	DR3	6.3
Goodpasture's syndrome	DR2	13.1
Rheumatoid arthritis	DR4	5.8
Juvenile rheumatoid arthritis	DR8	8.1
Sjögren's syndrome	DR3	9.7
Chronic active hepatitis (autoimmune)	DR3	13.9
Multiple sclerosis	DR2,DR6	12
Narcolepsy	DQ6	38
Dermatitis herpetiformis	DR3	56.4
Celiac disease	DQ2	250
Tuberculoid leprosy	DR2	8.1
b Class I, HLA-B27 associated		
Ankylosing spondylitis	B27	87.4
Reiter's disease	B27	37.0
Post-salmonella arthritis	B27	29.7
Post-shigella arthritis	B27	20.7
Post-yersinia arthritis	B27	17.6
Post-gonococcal arthritis	B27	14.0
Uveitis	B27	14.6
Amyloidosis in rheumatoid arthritis	B27	8.2
c Other class I associations		
Subacute thyroiditis	B35	13.7
Psoriasis vulgaris	Cw6	13.3
Idiopathic hemochromatosis	A3	8.2
Myasthenia gravis	B8	4.4

(Data mainly from Ryder L.P., Andersen E. & Svejgaard A. (1979) HLA and disease Registry 1979. *Tissue Antigens*, supplement and Thorsby E. (1995) *The Immunologist* **3**, 51.) *DR specificities relate to 'old nomenclature'.

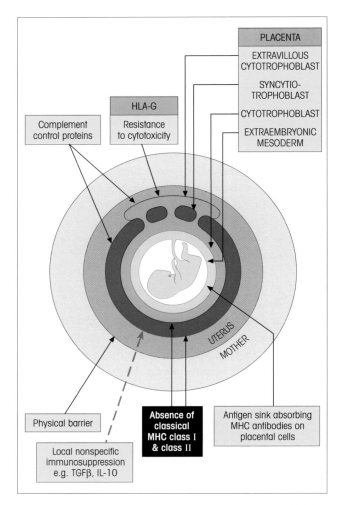

Figure 15.8 Mechanisms postulated to account for the survival of the fetus as an allograft in the mother.

perhaps through an ability to bind certain antigenic peptides. A given HLA-D allele may permit the binding of foreign peptides and cross-reacting self-epitopes; alternatively the complex with particular self-peptides could positively or negatively select either reactive or suppressive T-cells.

Insulin-dependent diabetes mellitus is associated with DQ8 and DQ2 but the strongest susceptibility is seen in the **DQ2/8 heterozygote**. The fact that two genes are necessary to determine the strongest susceptibility and the universality of this finding in all populations studied, implies that the DQ molecules themselves, not other molecules in linkage disequilibrium, are primarily involved in disease susceptibility. Possession of some subtypes of DQ6 gives a dominantly protective effect (table 15.1).

DR4 and, to a lesser extent, DR1 are risk factors for **rheumatoid arthritis** in white Caucasians. Analysis of DR4 subgroups, and of other ethnic populations where the influence of DR4 is minimal, has identified a particular linear sequence from residues 67–74 as the disease susceptibility element, and the variations observed are based on sharing of this sequence with other HLA-DR specificities. This stretch of amino acids is highly polymorphic and forms particular pockets in the peptide-binding cleft. As in diabetes, the DR2 allele is under-represented and DR2-positive patients have less severe disease, implying that a DR2-linked gene might be protective in some way.

The association with HLA in **ankylosing spondylitis** is quite remarkable; up to 95% of patients are of B27 phenotype as compared with around 5% in controls. The incidence of B27 is also markedly raised in other conditions when accompanied by sacroiliitis, for example Reiter's disease, acute anterior uveitis, psoriasis and other forms of infective sacroiliitis such as *Yersinia*, gonococcal and *Salmonella* arthritis. One suggestion is that a bacterial peptide may cross-react with a B27-derived sequence and provoke an autoreactive T-cell response.

Deficiencies in C4 and C2, which are MHC class III molecules, clearly predispose to the development of **immune complex disease** (see p. 112) and so it would be expected that the inheritance of null genes or alleles coding for the less active complement allotypes would increase the risk of rheumatological disorders and add yet further complexity to the correlations between HLA types and disease.

REPRODUCTIVE IMMUNOLOGY

The fetus is a potential allograft

In the human hemochorial placenta, maternal blood with immunocompetent lymphocytes does circulate in contact with the fetal trophoblast. We therefore have to explain how the fetus avoids allograft rejection, despite the development of an immunologic response in a proportion of mothers as evidenced by the appearance of antibodies and cytotoxic lymphocytes directed against paternal HLA antigens. In fact, prior sensitization with a skin graft fails to affect a pregnancy, showing that trophoblast cells are immunologically protected and indeed they are resistant to most cytotoxic mechanisms. Some of the many speculations which have been aired on this subject are summarized in figure 15.8.

Undoubtedly, the most important factor is the well-documented lack of both conventional class I and class II MHC antigens on the placental villous trophoblast, which protects the fetus from allogeneic attack. These fundamental changes in the regulation of MHC genes also lead to the unique expression of the nonclassical HLA-G protein on the extravillous cytotrophoblast. This may protect the trophoblast from killing by uterine endometrial large granular lymphocytes, which are an NK cell subset, since HLA-null lymphoblastoid cells transfected with HLA-G are resistant to NK lysis. This would be consistent with the 'missing self hypothesis', which postulates that MHC class I inhibits a positive signal from a potential target to the NK cell.

REVISION

See the accompanying website (www.roitt.com) for multiple choice questions.

Graft rejection is an immunologic reaction
• It shows specificity, the second set response is brisk, it is mediated by lymphocytes, and antibodies specific for the graft are formed.

Consequences of MHC incompatibility
• Class II MHC molecules provoke a mixed lymphocyte reaction of proliferation and blast transformation when genetically dissimilar lymphocytes interact.
• Class II differences are largely responsible for the reaction of tolerated grafted lymphocytes against host antigen (graft vs host (g.v.h.) reaction).

Mechanisms of graft rejection
• CD8 lymphocytes play a major role in the acute early rejection of first set responses.
• The strength of allograft rejection is due to the surprisingly large number of allospecific precursor cells. These derive mainly from the variety of T-cells which recognize allo-MHC plus self peptides plus a small number which directly recognize the allo-MHC molecule itself; later rejection increasingly involves allogeneic peptides presented by self MHC.

Different forms of graft rejection exist
• Preformed antibodies cause hyperacute rejection within minutes.
• Acute graft rejection is mediated mainly by cytotoxic T-cells.
• Acute late rejection of organ grafts from 11 days onwards is caused by Ig and C binding to graft vessels.
• Insidious and late rejection may be due to immune complex deposition.

Prevention of graft rejection
• Rejection can be minimized by cross-matching donor and graft for ABO and MHC tissue types.
• Rejection can be blocked by agents producing general

immunosuppression such as antimitotic drugs (e.g. azathioprine) or anti-inflammatory steroids. Cyclosporin A, FK506 and rapamycin represent exciting new groups of T-cell specific drugs. A number of T-cell specific monoclonal antibodies, such as anti CD3 and anti IL-2R, are useful in controlling graft rejection.

Xenografting

• The major hurdle to the use of animal organs is hyperacute rejection due to the presence of xenoreactive cross-reacting antibodies in the host.

Clinical experience in grafting

• Cornea and cartilage grafts are avascular and comparatively well tolerated.
• Kidney grafting gives excellent results and has been the most widespread, although immunosuppression must normally be continuous.
• High success rates are also being achieved with heart and liver transplants, particularly helped by the use of cyclosporin.
• Bone marrow grafts for immunodeficiency and aplastic anemia are accepted from matched siblings but it is difficult to avoid g.v.h. disease with allogeneic marrow. Stem cells may be obtained from umbilical cord blood or from peripheral blood especially after administration of G-CSF.

Association of HLA type with disease

• HLA specificities are often associated with particular diseases, e.g. HLA-B27 with ankylosing spondylitis, DR3 with Sjögren's syndrome, DR4 with rheumatoid arthritis, DQ2 and DQ8 with insulin-dependent diabetes mellitus and DR2,DQ6 with multiple sclerosis.
• The association may be related to an ability to bind particular antigenic peptides or to cross-react with certain infectious agents.

The fetus as an allograft

• Differences between MHC of mother and fetus may be beneficial to the fetus but as a potential graft it must be protected against transplantation attack by the mother.
• A major defense mechanism is the lack of classical class I and II MHC antigens on syncytiotrophoblast and cytotrophoblast which form the outer layers of the placenta.
• The extravillous cytotrophoblast expresses a nonclassical nonpolymorphic MHC class I protein, HLA-G, which may act to inhibit cytotoxicity by maternal NK cells.

FURTHER READING

Reisner Y. & Martelli M.J. (1999) Stem cell escalation enables HLA-disparate haematopoietic transplants in leukaemia patients. *Immunology Today* 20 (8), 343.

Rowe P. (1996) Xenotransplantation: from animal facility to the clinic. *Molecular Medicine* 2, 10.

Sykes M. (ed.) (1999) Section on Transplantation. *Current Opinion in Immunology* 11 (5).

Thorsby E. (1995) HLA-associated disease susceptibility. *The Immunologist* 3, 51.

Vince G.S. & Johnson P.M. (1996) Reproductive immunology: conception, contraception, and the consequences. *The Immunologist* 4 (5), 172.

CHAPTER 16

Tumor immunology

It has long been suggested that the allograft rejection mechanism represented a means by which the body's cells could be kept under **immunologic surveillance** so that altered cells with a neoplastic potential could be identified and summarily eliminated. For this to operate, cancer cells must display some new discriminating surface structure which can be recognized by the immune system. Two groups of tumor antigens have been described. Tumor-specific antigens (TSAs) are expressed on tumor cells but not normal cells and therefore might evoke an active immune response. Tumor-associated antigens (TAAs) are found on tumor cells but may also be present on normal tissue and therefore are unlikely to stimulate a significant response.

CHANGES ON THE SURFACE OF TUMOR CELLS (FIGURE 16.1)

Virally controlled antigens

A substantial minority of tumors arise through infection with **oncogenic viruses** including Epstein–Barr viruses (EBV) in lymphomas, human T-cell leukemia virus-1 (HTLV-1) in leukemia, and papilloma virus in cervical cancers. After infection, the viruses express genes homologous with cellular oncogenes which encode factors affecting growth, cell division and apoptosis. Failure to control these genes therefore leads to potentially malignant transformation. Virally derived peptides associated with surface MHC on the tumor cell behave as powerful transplantation antigens which generate specific cytotoxic T-cells (Tc).

Expression of normally silent genes

The dysregulated uncontrolled cell division of the cancer cell creates a milieu in which the products of normally silent genes may be expressed. Sometimes these encode differen-

tiation antigens normally associated with an earlier fetal stage. Thus tumors may express proteins normally expressed on fetal but not adult tissue. Such **oncofetal antigens** include α-fetoprotein (AFP), found on primary hepatocellular carcinoma cells, and carcino-embryonic antigen (CEA) expressed by gastrointestinal and breast carcinomas. Since these oncofetal antigens are released into the blood they may be used to diagnose these malignancies and to monitor progression of the disease.

The majority of tumor-specific antigens are either completely abnormal peptides or mutated forms of normal cellular proteins produced by tumor cells and complexed to class I MHC products. These peptides, which are not normally destined to be positioned in the surface plasma membrane, can still signal their presence to T-cells in the outer world by a processed peptide/MHC mechanism. One such group of tumor-specific antigens is encoded by families of genes that are normally silent in all normal tissues except human testis. They include the MAGE, BAGE or GAGE families of genes, which code for proteins found on the surface of a significant proportion of tumors, including melanomas and head and neck tumors. These patients often have circulating cytotoxic T-cells specific for these peptides, indicating that they can induce immune responses and therefore could be ideal targets for immunotherapy.

Mutant antigens

Other antigens are encoded by genes that are expressed in normal cells but are mutated in tumor cells. Such mutations may change as few as one amino acid. Single point mutations in oncogenes or tumor suppressor genes can account for the large diversity of antigens found on carcinogen-induced tumors. The gene encoding the p53 cell cycle inhibitor is a hotspot for mutation in cancer, while the oncogenic human *ras* genes differ from their normal counterpart by point mutations usually leading to single amino acid substitutions. Such mutations have been recorded in 40% of human colorectal cancers and their preneoplastic lesions, in

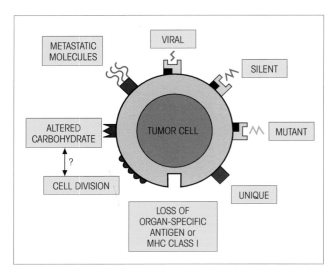

Figure 16.1 Tumor-associated surface changes. Surface carbohydrate changes may occur during cell division. An Ig idiotype on B-cell leukemia would be a unique antigen.

more than 90% of pancreatic carcinomas, in acute myelogenous leukemia and in preleukemic syndromes. The oncogene *HER-2/neu* encodes a membrane protein that is present on various human tumors, especially ovarian and breast carcinomas, where it could serve as a target for either monoclonal antibodies or cytotoxic T-cells.

Tissue-specific differentiation antigens

A tumor arising from a particular tissue may express normal differentiation antigens specific for that tissue. For example, prostatic tumors may carry prostate-specific antigen (PSA), which is also released into the serum and can be measured as a screening test for prostate cancer. Lymphoid cells at almost any stage in their differentiation or maturation may become malignant and proliferate to form a clone of cells which are virtually 'frozen' at a particular developmental stage because of defects in maturation. The malignant cells bear the markers one would expect of normal lymphocytes reaching the stage at which maturation had been arrested. Thus, chronic lymphocytic leukemia cells resemble mature B-cells in expressing surface class II and Ig, albeit of a single idiotype in a given patient. B-cell lymphomas will express on their surface CD19, CD20 and either kappa or lambda light chains depending on which light chain the original cell was carrying. Similarly, T-cell malignancies will carry the TCR with CD3 and other T-cell-specific cell surface antigens such as CD4, CD8, CD2, CD7 or the IL-2 receptor CD25. Using monoclonal antibodies directed against Ig and specific antigens on T- or B-cells, it has been possible to classify the

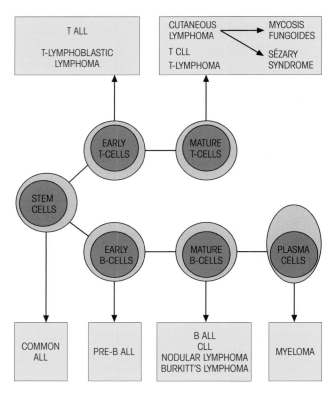

Figure 16.2 Cellular phenotype of human lymphoid malignancies. ALL = acute lymphoblastic leukemia; CLL = chronic lymphocytic leukemia. (After Greaves M.F. & Janossy G, personal communication.)

lymphoid malignancies in terms of the phenotype of the equivalent normal cell (figure 16.2).

Malignant tumors may lack class I MHC molecules

Malignant transformation of cells may be associated with loss or downregulation of class I MHC expression linked in most cases to increased metastatic potential. This presumably reflects their decreased vulnerability to T-cells but not NK cells. In breast cancer, for example, around 60% of metastatic tumors lack class I.

Changes in carbohydrate structure

The chaotic internal control of metabolism within neoplastic cells often leads to the presentation of abnormal surface carbohydrate structures. Abnormal mucin found in pancreatic and breast tissue can have immunologic consequences and can be recognized by cytotoxic T-cells or by antibody. Changes in surface carbohydrates can have a dramatic effect on malignancy. For example, lung cancer patients whose tumors showed deletion of blood group A had a much worse prognosis than those with continuous A expression.

IMMUNE RESPONSE TO TUMORS

Immune surveillance against strongly immunogenic tumors

The **immune surveillance theory** would predict that there should be more tumors in individuals whose immune systems are suppressed. This undoubtedly seems to be the case for **strongly immunogenic tumors**. There is a considerable increase in skin cancer in immunosuppressed patients living in high sunshine regions and, in general, transplant patients on immunosuppressive drugs are unduly susceptible to skin cancers, largely associated with papilloma virus, and EBV-positive lymphomas. Likewise, the lymphomas which arise in children with T-cell deficiency linked to Wiskott–Aldrich syndrome or ataxia telangiectasia, express EBV genes. On the other hand, there is no clear evidence that nonvirally induced, spontaneously developing tumors such as the common tumors in humans, have an increased incidence in immunodeficient individuals or athymic (nude) mice.

A role for acquired immune responses?

Various immunologic effector mechanisms against tumors have been described but it is unclear which of these mechanisms are important as protective antitumor responses. Cytotoxic CD8 cells (CTL) are thought to provide surveillance by recognizing and destroying tumor cells. They employ a variety of mechanisms to destroy tumor cells including exocytosis of granules containing the cytotoxic effector molecules perforin and granzyme and secretion of tumor necrosis factor which also has tumoricidal activities. Another and perhaps more important mechanism is based on direct effector–target interaction between Fas on target cells and FasL expressed on the cytotoxic T-cell. FasL activation of the membrane-bound Fas present on target cells leads to apoptosis of the tumor cell (figure 16.3). The role that cytotoxic T-cells (CTL) play in tumor immunity is unclear but patients with malignant disease have been shown to have both circulating and tumor-infiltrating lymphocytes which show cytotoxicity *in vitro* against the tumor cells. The mechanisms by which tumor cells resist this attack will be dealt with later.

A role for innate immunity?

Perhaps in speaking of immunity to tumors, one too readily thinks only in terms of acquired responses, whereas it is

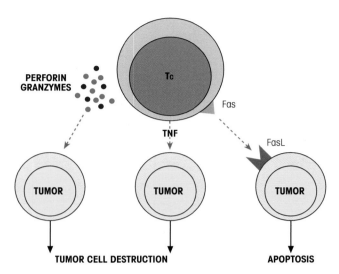

Figure 16.3 Mechanisms involved in cytotoxic T-lymphocyte destruction of tumors by cytotoxic T-cells.

now accepted that innate mechanisms are of significance. Macrophages, which often infiltrate a tumor mass, can destroy tumor cells in tissue culture through the copious production of reactive oxygen intermediates (ROI) and tumor necrosis factor (TNF). Similarly, natural killer (NK) cells subserve a function as the earliest cellular effector mechanism against dissemination of blood-borne metastases. Powerful evidence implicating these cells in protection against cancer is provided by beige mice, which congenitally lack NK cells. They die with spontaneous tumors earlier than their nondeficient littermates.

Resting NK cells are spontaneously cytolytic for certain, but by no means all, tumor targets; IL-2-activated cells (lymphokine-activated killer cells, or LAK cells) display a wider lethality. As was mentioned previously, recognition of class I imparts a **negative inactivating** signal to the NK cell implying conversely that downregulation of MHC class I, which tumors employ as a strategy to escape Tc cells, would make them **more susceptible to NK attack**.

Tumors develop mechanisms to evade the immune response

Most tumors occur in individuals who are not immunosuppressed, indicating that tumors themselves have mechanisms for escaping the innate or acquired immune systems. Several such mechanisms have been suggested (figure 16.4). Most important of these is that tumor cells have an inherent defect in antigen processing or presentation as they lack costimulatory molecules such as the B7 molecule. T-cell anergy occurs following antigen–MHC complex recognition

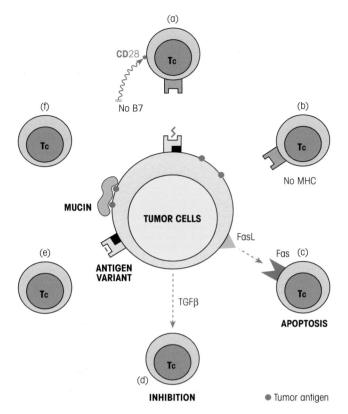

Figure 16.4 Mechanisms by which tumor cells escape destruction by the immune response. Tumor cells may (a) lack costimulatory molecules such as B7; (b) express reduced levels of class I MHC; (c) express FasL, which causes apoptosis of attacking Tc cells; (d) produce various cytokines which inhibit the immune response; (e) develop antigen-negative variants; (f) produce mucins which disguise their antigens. (Tc, cytotoxic T-cell.)

in the absence of costimulation. Tumor cells also lack other molecules which are important in activating T-cells especially MHC class II or adhesion molecules such as ICAM-1 or LFA-3. Furthermore, as has been previously indicated, many tumors express reduced or absent levels of class I MHC, which imparts resistance to cytotoxic T-cells although presumably increasing susceptibility to NK cells. Other tumors express functional FasL which confers resistance to these tumors by inducing apoptosis of autologous infiltrating lymphocytes which are known to express Fas. Tumors themselves may release various immunosuppressive factors such as transforming growth factor-β, which is a potent immunosuppressive cytokine having effects on many mediators of the immune response including a potent inhibitory effect on differentiation of cytotoxic T-cells. It is also likely that as tumors grow they tend to favor the selective outgrowth of antigen-negative variants, or they may produce

mucins which conceal or mask their antigens so that they are not recognized by the immune response.

APPROACHES TO CANCER IMMUNOTHERAPY

Nonspecific activation of the immune system

For many years the injection of adjuvants that nonspecifically stimulate the immune system has been used to augment other forms of chemotherapy. This treatment mainly activates macrophages and increases their production of IL-1 and costimulatory molecules, but this therapy is not generally adequate to eliminate tumors. The use of the tuberculosis vaccine, BCG, for the treatment of superficial bladder cancer is, however, a highly effective form of therapy which is used commonly in this disease.

Exploitation of acquired immune responses

Immunization with viral antigens

Based on the not unreasonable belief that certain forms of cancer (e.g. lymphoma) are caused by oncogenic viruses, attempts are being made to isolate the virus and prepare a suitable vaccine from it. In fact, large-scale protection of chickens against the development of Marek's disease lymphoma has been successfully achieved by vaccination with another herpes virus native to turkeys. In human Burkitt's lymphoma, work is in progress to develop a vaccine to exploit the ability of Tc cells to target **EBV-related antigens** on the cells of all Burkitt tumors. Similarly in patients with cervical cancer cytotoxic T-cells against the causative human papilloma virus (HPV) can be successfully induced using vaccinia virus expressing HPV genes.

Immunization with tumor-specific antigens

The identification of tumor-associated antigens has led to the commencement of clinical trials using the relevant peptides. The unique **idiotype** on monoclonal B-cell tumors with surface Ig offers a potentially feasible target for immunotherapy. This form of therapy, however, requires the preparation of a different vaccine for each patient. Other tumor-specific antigens and mutant peptide sequences are all possible candidates for immunotherapy such as the human melanoma-specific MAGE antigenic peptides. Various forms of immunization are possible including: the injection of peptide alone or with adjuvant; the use of recombinant defective viruses carrying the sequence encoding the protein; or the use of dendritic cells taken from the patient, treated with the antigen and reinfused back into the patient to be presented to T-helper cells.

Increasing the immunogenicity of tumors

Many tumors fail to stimulate an immune response because they lack the costimulatory molecule B7. Antigen–MHC interactions therefore, will result in T-cell anergy, which is a major limitation to the effective development of an immune response. The introduction of the costimulatory molecule B7 enhances the immunogenicity of the tumor so that the B7-transfected cells can activate resting T-cells to recognize and attack even nontransfected tumor cells (figure 16.5). Another approach is to transfect tumor cells with syngeneic MHC class II genes, to enable the transfected cells to present endogenously encoded tumor peptides to CD4 cells. This maneuver improves the antigen-presenting capability of tumor cells and significantly enhances their immunogenicity. A powerful method for inducing CTL responses against silent tumor antigens is to immunize with dendritic cells which have been previously loaded with the tumor peptides. This induces potent CTL responses against the established tumor.

Modification of tumors with cytokine genes

Tumor cells genetically modified with cytokine genes, such as those for IL-2, IL-12, IL-4 and GM-CSF, may serve as vaccines which enhance the systemic immune response but which in particular localize the cytokines to the environment of the tumor. Cells modified with IL-2 genes have been shown to enhance immunization by expanding and activating cytotoxic T-cells, while those modified by IL-12 genes move the focus of immunity from a TH2 response to a more protective TH1 response. Tumors producing IL-4 tend to attract macrophages and eosinophils, which accumulate in the vicinity of the tumor, and those producing GM-CSF stimulate specific T-cell immunity by enhancing development and activation of antigen-presenting cells.

Systemic cytokine therapy

As has been pointed out previously, the cytokine network is extremely complex and administration of a cytokine designed to stimulate one branch of the immune response may lead to inhibition of another portion of the response. In some cases administration of systemic cytokine has produced serious side-effects with life-threatening consequences.

IL-2 has been used in a number of experimental protocols with the idea of expanding cytotoxic T-cells and NK cells. A number of these patients had serious side-effects due to the production of other cytokines which produced fever, shock and a vascular leak syndrome. Another approach is to expand peripheral blood lymphocytes with IL-2 to generate large numbers of lymphokine-activated killer (LAK) cells which can be infused back into the patient to target the tumor cells. Administration of autologous LAK cells

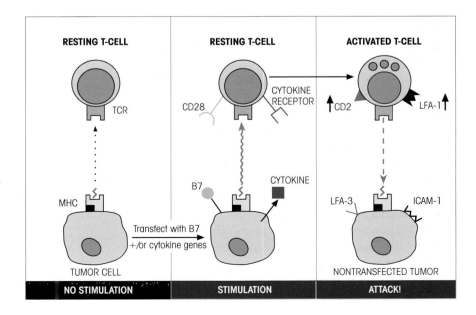

Figure 16.5 Immunotherapy by transfection with costimulatory molecules. The tumor can only stimulate the resting T-cell with the costimulatory help of B7 and/or cytokines such as GM-CSF, γ-interferon (IFNγ) and interleukins IL-2, -4 and -7. Once activated, the T-cell with upregulated accessory molecules can now attack the original tumor lacking costimulators.

together with high doses of IL-2 has led, in one study, to a considerable reduction in evaluable tumor in renal cancer patients.

TNF has powerful tumor-killing capability and can cause hemorrhagic necrosis and tumor regression. Unfortunately its systemic administration is associated with very severe toxicity due to its activation of the cytokine cascade.

In trials using the interferons IFNα and IFNβ, objective responses were seen in patients with various malignancies including a remarkable response rate of 80–90% among patients with hairy cell leukemia and mycosis fungoides.

With regard to the mechanisms of the antitumor effects, in certain tumors IFNs may serve primarily as antiproliferative agents. In others, activation of NK cells and macrophages may be important, while augmenting the expression of class I MHC molecules may make the tumors more susceptible to control by immune effector mechanisms. In some circumstances the antiviral effect could be contributory.

For diseases like renal cell cancer and hairy cell leukemia, IFNs have induced responses in a significantly higher proportion of patients than conventional therapies. However, in the wider setting, most investigators consider that the role of IFNs will be in combination therapy, for example with active immunotherapy or with various chemotherapeutic agents.

Monoclonal antibodies as magic bullets

Immunologists have for long been bemused by the idea of eliminating tumor cells by specific antibody or antibody linked to a killer molecule (immunotoxin). Not surprisingly, the 'magic bullet' devotees were greatly encouraged by experiments in which guinea-pig B-lymphoma cells were killed *in vitro* by anti-idiotype conjugated with ricin, a toxin of such devastating potency that one molecule entering the cell is lethal. The immunotoxins should have a reasonable half-life in the circulation, penetrate into tumors and not bind significantly to nontumor cells. Unfortunately in most human cancer patients, significant problems have arisen, including the development of an immune response against mouse proteins which in some cases limits therapy to one-time doses. Other practical problems include difficulties in moving the antibodies through the tortuous vessels found in tumors, and the development of mutant tumor cells that fail to express the target antigens.

Radioimmunoconjugates which carry a radiation source such as Tc-99 and In-111 to the tumor site for therapy or diagnosis are being intensively developed and have two advantages over toxins: they are nonimmunogenic and they can destroy adjacent tumor cells which have lost antigen. A

potent new antilymphoma drug employs a monoclonal antibody to the B-cell surface antigen CD20, to which is attached radioactive iodine. Another strategy is to target growth factor receptors present on the surface of tumor cells. Blocking of such receptors should deprive the cells of crucial growth signals. Herceptin is a monoclonal antibody that recognizes and binds to the HER/neu protein found on 30% of breast cancer cells. Because the protein is not present on normal cells the antibody selectively attacks the tumor causing its shrinkage in a substantial proportion of cases.

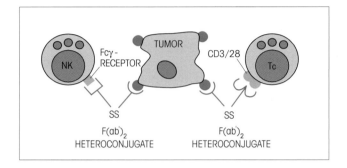

Figure 16.6 Focusing effector cells by heteroconjugates. Coupling F(ab') fragments of monoclonal antibodies specific for the tumor and an appropriate molecule on the surface of NK or Tc cells, provides the specificity to bring the effectors into intimate contact with the target cell.

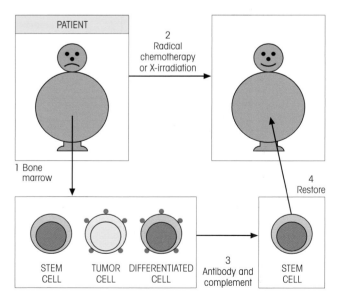

Figure 16.7 Treatment of leukemias by autologous bone marrow rescue. By using cytotoxic antibodies to a differentiation antigen present on leukemic cells and even on other normal differentiated cells, but absent from stem cells, it is possible to obtain a tumor-free population of the latter which can be used to restore hematopoietic function in patients subsequently treated radically to destroy the leukemic cells.

Genetic technology has now allowed the development of chimeric antibodies which have the variable antigen-binding region of a mouse monoclonal antibody, but with a human constant region. This molecule retains the specificity of the monoclonal but is much less immunogenic. Other options for immunologic attack using monoclonal antibodies are possible. For example, a mixture of **two bispecific heteroconjugates** of antitumor/anti-CD3 and antitumor/anti-CD28 should act synergistically to induce contact between a T-cell and the tumor to activate direct cytotoxicity (figure 16.6).

Another use of monoclonal antibodies is to **purge bone marrow grafts** of unwanted cells *in vitro* in the presence of complement from a foreign species. Thus, differentiation

antigens present on leukemic cells but absent from bone marrow stem cells, can be used to prepare tumor-free autologous stem cells to restore function in patients treated with chemotherapy or X-irradiation (figure 16.7).

Immunologic diagnosis of lymphoid neoplasias

With the availability of a range of monoclonal antibodies and improvements in immuno-enzymic and flow cytometric technology, great strides have been made in exploiting, for diagnostic purposes, the fact that malignant lymphoid cells, especially leukemias and lymphomas, display the markers of the normal lymphocytes which are their counterparts. Thus in the diagnosis of non-Hodgkin's lymphomas, the majority of which are of B-cell origin, the feature which is diagnostic is the synthesis of monotypic Ig, i.e. of one light chain only (figure 16.8a); in contrast, the population of cells at a site of reactive B-cell hyperplasia will stain for both kappa and lambda chains (figure 16.8b).

Plasma cell dyscrasias

Multiple myeloma

This is defined as a malignant proliferation of a clone of plasma cells secreting a monoclonal Ig. The myeloma or 'M' component in serum is recognized as a tight band on gel electrophoresis (figure 16.9) as all molecules in the clone are of course identical and have the same mobility. Since

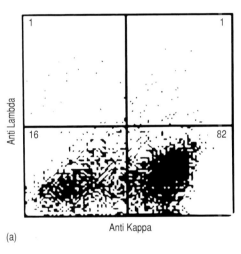

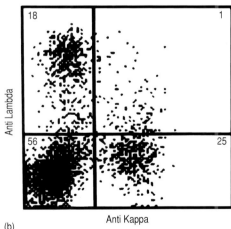

Figure 16.8 Use of flow cytometry to diagnose malignant lymphoma. Cells are dispersed and stained with fluorescein-labelled anti-kappa and anti-lambda. Lymphoma cells are monotypic and in this case stain with anti-kappa (a) while reactive lymphocytes are polytypic and stain with both anti-kappa and anti-lambda (b).

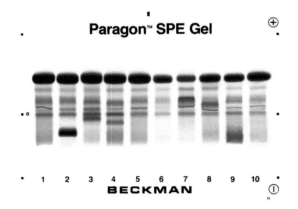

Figure 16.9 Myeloma paraprotein demonstrated by gel electrophoresis of serum. Lane 1, normal; lane 2, γ-paraprotein; lane 3, near β-paraprotein; lane 4, fibrinogen band in the γ-region of a *plasma* sample; lane 5, normal serum; lane 6, immunoglobulin deficiency (low γ); lane 7, nephrotic syndrome (raised α_2-macroglobulin, low albumin and Igs); lane 8, hemolysed sample (raised hemoglobin/haptoglobin in α_2 region); lane 9, polyclonal increase in Igs (e.g. infection, autoimmune disease); lane 10, normal serum. (Gel kindly provided by Mr A. Heys.)

Ig-secreting cells produce an excess of light chains, free light chains are present in the plasma of multiple myeloma patients, and can be recognized in the urine as Bence-Jones protein.

Immunodeficiency secondary to lymphoproliferative disorders

Immunodeficiency is a common feature in patients with lymphoid malignancies. The reasons for this are still obscure but it appears that the malignant cells interfere with the development of the corresponding normal cells. Thus in multiple myeloma the levels of normal B-cells and of non-myeloma Ig may be grossly depressed and the patients susceptible to infection with pyogenic bacteria.

REVISION

See the accompanying website (www.roitt.com) for multiple choice questions.

Changes on the surface of tumor cells
• Processed peptides derived from oncogenic viruses are powerful MHC-associated transplantation antigens.
• Some tumors express genes which are silent in normal tissues; sometimes they have been expressed previously in embryonic life (oncofetal antigens).
• Many tumors express weak antigens associated with point mutations in oncogenes such as *ras* and *HER-2/neu*.
• Many tumors express normal differentiation antigens specific for that tissue.
• Tumors may lack class I MHC molecules.
• Dysregulation of tumor cells frequently causes structural abnormalities in surface carbohydrate structures.

Immune response to tumors
• T-cells generally mount effective surveillance against tumors associated with oncogenic viruses or UV induction which are strongly immunogenic.
• More weakly immunogenic tumors are not controlled by T-cell surveillance, although sometimes low-grade responses are evoked.
• Cytotoxic T-cells may provide surveillance and cause tumor cell destruction or apoptosis.
• NK cells probably play a role in containing tumor growth and metastases. They can attack MHC class I negative tumor cells because the class I molecule imparts a negative inactivation signal to NK cells.

Tumor cells have a variety of mechanisms to evade the immune response

Approaches to cancer immunotherapy
• Nonspecific stimulation of the immune response may augment other forms of chemotherapy.

• Cancer vaccines based on oncogenic viral proteins can be expected.
• Immunization with tumor-specific peptides may be useful, but a different vaccine may be required for each patient. Effective melanoma-specific antigens have been identified. Immunogenic potency of a tumor antigen is greatly enhanced by dendritic cells pulsed with the antigen.
• Weakly immunogenic tumors provoke effective anti-cancer responses if transfected with costimulatory molecules such as B7 and cytokines IFNγ and IL-2, -4 and -7.
• Systemic cytokine therapy may be used to stimulate specific effector cells. IL-2-stimulated NK cells (LAK) are active against renal carcinoma. IFNγ and β are very effective in the T-cell disorders, hairy cell leukemia and mycosis fungoides.
• Monoclonal antibodies conjugated to toxins or radionuclides can target tumor cells or antigens associated with malignancy. Bifunctional antibodies can bring effectors such as NK and Tc close to the tumor target.
Monoclonal antibodies attached to an isotope may be used to image tumors.

Lymphoid malignancies
• The surface phenotype aids diagnosis.
• Multiple myeloma represents a malignant proliferation of a single clone of plasma cells producing a single 'M' band on electrophoresis.
• Bence-Jones protein consists of free light chains found in the urine of patients with multiple myeloma.
• Malignant lymphoid cells produce secondary immunodeficiency by suppressing differentiation of the corresponding normal lineage.

FURTHER READING

Begent R.H.J., Verhaar M.J., Chester K.A. *et al.* (1996) Clinical evidence of efficient tumor targeting based on single-chain Fv antibody selected from a combinatorial library. *Nature Medicine* **2** (9), 979.

Chattopadhyay U. (1999) Tumour immunotherapy: developments and strategies. *Immunology Today* **20** (11), 480.

Vitetta E. (ed.) (1999) Section on Cancer (Immunology). *Current Opinion in Immunology* **11** (5).

Witte O.N. & Boon T. (eds) (1995) Cancer. *Current Opinion in Immunology* **7**, 657. [Critical overviews of the whole field, which serious students are highly advised to read.]

CHAPTER 17

Autoimmune diseases
1 — Scope and etiology

THE SCOPE OF AUTOIMMUNE DISEASES

The monumental repertoire of the adaptive immune system has evolved to allow it to recognize and ensnare microbial molecules of virtually any shape, and in so doing has been unable to avoid the generation of lymphocytes which react with the body's own constituents. The term **'autoimmune disease'** applies to those cases where it can be shown that the **autoimmune process contributes to the pathogenesis of the disease** rather than situations where apparently harmless autoantibodies are formed following tissue damage, for example heart antibodies appearing after a myocardial infarction. These diseases count amongst the major medical problems of today's societies. There are, for example, over 6.5 million cases of rheumatoid arthritis in the USA, and Type 1 diabetes is the leading cause of end-stage renal disease.

The spectrum of autoimmune diseases

These disorders may be looked upon as forming a spectrum. At one end we have **'organ-specific diseases'** with organ-specific autoantibodies. **Hashimoto's disease** of the thyroid is an example: there is a specific lesion in the thyroid involving infiltration by mononuclear cells (lymphocytes, histiocytes and plasma cells), destruction of follicular cells and germinal center formation, accompanied by the production of circulating antibodies with absolute specificity for certain thyroid constituents (Milestone 17.1).

Moving towards the center of the spectrum are those disorders where the lesion tends to be localized to a single organ but the antibodies are nonorgan-specific. A typical example would be **primary biliary cirrhosis** where the small bile ductule is the main target of inflammatory cell infiltration but the serum antibodies present—mainly mitochondrial—are not liver-specific.

At the other end of the spectrum are the **'nonorgan-specific'** or **'systemic autoimmune diseases'** broadly belonging to the class of rheumatologic disorders, exemplified by **systemic lupus erythematosus (SLE)**, where neither lesions nor autoantibodies are confined to any one organ. Pathologic changes are widespread and are primarily lesions of connective tissue with fibrinoid necrosis. They are seen in the skin (the 'lupus' butterfly rash on the face is characteristic), kidney glomeruli, joints, serous membranes and blood vessels. In addition, the formed elements of the blood are often affected. A bizarre collection of autoantibodies is found, some of which react with the DNA and other nuclear constituents of all cells in the body.

An attempt to fit the major diseases considered to be associated with autoimmunity into this spectrum is shown in table 17.1.

Overlap of autoimmune disorders

There is a tendency for more than one autoimmune disorder to occur in the same individual; for example, patients with autoimmune thyroiditis (Hashimoto's disease or primary myxedema) have a much higher incidence of pernicious anemia than would be expected in a random population matched for age and sex (10% as against 0.2%). Conversely, both thyroiditis and thyrotoxicosis are diagnosed in pernicious anemia patients with an unexpectedly high frequency (table 17.2).

There is an even greater overlap in serological findings. Thirty percent of patients with autoimmune thyroid disease have concomitant parietal cell antibodies in their serum. Conversely, thyroid antibodies have been demonstrated in up to 50% of pernicious anemia patients. It should be stressed that these are not cross-reacting antibodies. The thyroid-specific antibodies will not react with stomach and vice versa. When a serum reacts with both organs it means that two populations of antibodies are present, one with specificity for thyroid and the other for stomach.

NATURE AND NURTURE

Autoimmune disorders are multifactorial

Undoubtedly, autoimmune diseases have a multifactorial etiology. Superimposed upon a genetically complex susceptibility, we might be dealing with some ageing process affecting the thymus or the lymphoid stem cells and their internal control of self-reactivity. Sex hormones and various environmental factors, particularly microbial agents, which could have a variety of effects on the target organs, the lymphoid system and the cytokine network may all contribute.

Genetic factors in autoimmune disease

Autoimmune phenomena tend to aggregate in certain families. For example, the first degree relatives (sibs, parents and children) of patients with Hashimoto's disease show a high incidence of thyroid autoantibodies (figure 17.1) and of overt and subclinical thyroiditis. Parallel studies have disclosed similar relationships in the families of pernicious anemia patients, in that gastric parietal cell antibodies are prevalent in relatives. There is now powerful evidence that multiple genetic components must be involved. The data on **twins** are unequivocal. When thyrotoxicosis or insulin-dependent diabetes mellitus (IDDM) occurs in twins there is

MILESTONE 17.1—THE DISCOVERY OF THYROID AUTOIMMUNITY

In an attempt to confirm Paul Ehrlich's concept of 'horror autotoxicus'—the body's dread of making anti-boxies to self—Rose and Witebsky immunized rabbits with rabbit thyroid extract in complete Freund's adjunvant. To what I would hazard was Witebsky's dismay and Rose's delight, this procedure resulted in the production of thyroid autoantibodies and chronic inflammatory destruction of the thyroid gland architecture (figure M17.1.1a and b).

Having noted the fall in serum γ-globulin which followed removal of the goiter in Hashimoto's thyroiditis and the simi-

larity of the histology (figure M17.1.1c) to that of Rose and Witebsky's rabbits, Roitt, Doniach and Campbell tested the hypothesis that the plasma cells in the gland might be making an autoantibody to a thyroid component, so causing the tissue damage and chronic inflammatory response. Sure enough, the sera of the first patients tested had precipitating antibodies to an autoantigen in normal thyroid extracts which was soon identified as thyroglobulin (figure M17.1.2).

In far off New Zealand (depending on your geographical location!), Adams and Purves, in seeking a circulating factor

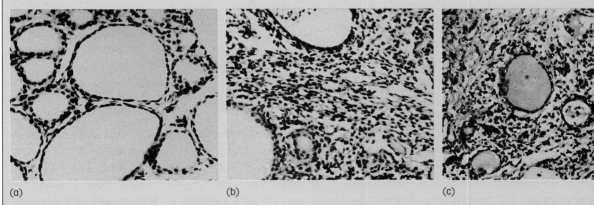

(a) (b) (c)

Figure M17.1.1 Experimental autoallergic thyroiditis.
(a) Control rat thyroid showing normal follicular architecture.
(b) Thyroiditis produced by immunization with rat thyroid extract in complete Freund's adjuvant; the invading chronic inflammatory cells have destroyed the follicular structure. (Based on the experiments of Rose N.R. & Witebsky E. (1956) Studies on organ specificity. V. Changes in the thyroid gland of rabbits following active immunization with rabbit thyroid extracts. *Journal of Immunology* 76, 417). (c) Similarity of lesions in spontaneous human autoimmune disease to those induced in the experimental model. Other features of Hashimoto's disease such as the eosinophilic metaplasia of acinar cells (Askenazy cells) and local lymphoid follicles are not seen in this experiment model, although the latter occur in the spontaneous thyroiditis of Obese strain chickens.

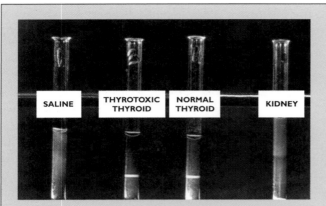

Figure M17.1.2 **Thyroid autoantibodies in the serum of a patient with Hashimoto's disease demonstrated by precipitation in agar.** Test serum is incorporated in agar in the bottom of the tube; the middle layer contains agar only while the autoantigen is present in the top layer. As serum antibody and thyroid autoantigen diffuse towards each other, they form a zone of opaque precipitate in the middle layer. Saline and kidney extract controls are negative (Based on Roitt I.M., Doniach D., Campbell P.N. & Hudson R.V. (1956) Autoantibodies in Hashimoto's disease. *Lancet* **ii**, 820.)

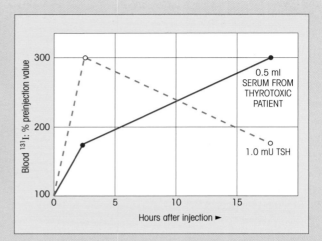

Figure M17.1.3 **The long-acting thyroid stimulator in Graves' disease.** Injection of TSH causes a rapid release of ^{131}I from the pre-labeled animal thyroid in contrast to the prolonged release which follows injection of serum from a thyrotoxic patient. (Based on Adams D.D. & Purves H.D. (1956) Abnormal responses in the assay of thyrotrophin. *Proceedings of the University of Otago Medical School* **34**, 11.)

which might be responsible for the hyperthyroidism of Graves' thyrotoxicosis, injected patient's serum into guinea-pigs whose thyroids had been prelabeled with ^{131}I, and followed the release of radiolabeled material from the gland with time. Whereas the natural pituitary thyroid-stimulating hormone (TSH) produced a peak in serum radioactivity some 4 hours or so after injection of the test animal, serum from thyrotoxic patients had a prolonged stimulatory effect (figure M17.1.3). The so-called *long-acting thyroid stimulator* (LATs) was ultimately shown to be an IgG mimicking TSH thorough its reaction with the TSH receptor but differing in its time-course of action, largely due to its longer half-life in the circulation.

a far greater concordance rate (i.e. both twins affected) in identical than in nonidentical twins. Furthermore, lines of animals have been bred which spontaneously develop autoimmune disease. In other words, **the autoimmunity is genetically programmed**.

These diseases are **genetically complex** and are **caused by an interplay of many different genes and environmental factors**. Dominant amongst the genetic associations with autoimmune diseases is linkage to the major histocompatibility complex (MHC). Numerous examples have been described, including the association between B27 and ankylosing spondylitis, the increased risk of IDDM for DQw8 individuals, the higher incidence of DR3 in Addison's disease and of DR4 in rheumatoid arthritis (see table 15.1). Some HLA molecules are associated with protection against autoimmune disease and in IDDM some molecules are associated with susceptibility, others with protection, whereas still others appear neutral. Figure 17.2 shows a multiplex family with IDDM in which the disease is closely linked to a particular HLA-haplotype.

It is not clear how particular structural variants of MHC molecules participate in autoimmunization and in fact the association may not be with the identified allele but with a closely related polymorphic gene. For example, the gene for familial hemochromatosis, a disorder that causes severe iron overload, is tightly linked to HLA-A3 and is said to be in linkage disequilibrium with it. Similarly the association of IDDM with DR3 and DR4 is almost certainly related to the linkage disequilibrium between these DR alleles and the susceptibility genes at the DQ locus. It is possible that the MHC glycoprotein may influence the outcome of positive and negative selection within the thymus and allow immature T-cells which are reactive with particular self antigens, to escape negative selection and mature. It is most likely, however, that a particular allelic form of the MHC molecule may have an exceptional capacity to present disease-inciting peptides to cytotoxic or helper T-cells.

Several other gene families may be important in susceptibility to autoimmune disease. We should remember that congenital deficiencies of the early classical complement components may predispose to vasculitis and an SLE-like syndrome. There may also be association with genes controlling the pattern of cytokine secretion or influencing the balance of TH1/TH2 subsets which could enhance susceptibility to IDDM or lead to resistance in otherwise predisposed subjects.

Hormonal influences in autoimmunity

There is a general trend for autoimmune disease to occur far more frequently in women than in men (figure 17.3), probably due to differences in hormonal patterns. Although the reason for the higher incidence of autoimmune disease in females is not clear, it is known that sex hormones can modify immune responses. Females generally produce more antibodies after an immune response than males, and excess amounts of estrogens have been observed in some patients with SLE. Similarly, administration of male hormones to mice with SLE reduces the severity of disease. Pregnancy is often associated with amelioration of disease severity, particularly in rheumatoid arthritis (RA), and there is sometimes a striking relapse after giving birth.

Table 17.1 Spectrum of autoimmune diseases.

ORGAN SPECIFIC	
↓	Hashimoto's thyroiditis
	Primary myxedema
	Thyrotoxicosis
	Pernicious anemia
	Autoimmune atrophic gastritis
	Addison's disease
	Premature menopause (few cases)
	Male infertility (few cases)
	Myasthenia gravis
	Insulin-dependent diabetes mellitus
	Goodpasture's syndrome
	Pemphigus vulgaris
	Pemphigoid
	Sympathetic ophthalmia
	Phacogenic uveitis
	(?? Multiple sclerosis ??)
	Autoimmune hemolytic anemia
	Idiopathic thrombocytopenic purpura
	Idiopathic leukopenia
	Primary biliary cirrhosis
	Active chronic hepatitis HB$_S$−ve
	Ulcerative colitis
	Sjögren's syndrome
	Rheumatoid arthritis
	Scleroderma
	Wegener's granulomatosis
	Poly/dermatomyositis
	Discoid lupus erythematosus
NONORGAN SPECIFIC	Systemic lupus erythematosus (SLE)

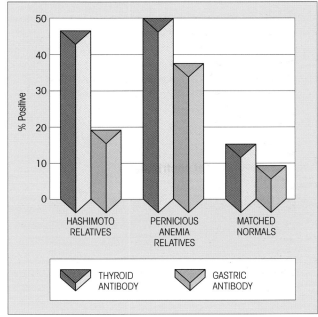

Figure 17.1 **The high incidence of thyroid and gastric autoantibodies in the first-degree relatives of patients with Hashimoto's disease or pernicious anemia.** Note the overlap of gastric and thyroid autoimmunity and the higher incidence of gastric autoantibodies in pernicious anemia relatives. In general, titers were much higher in patients than in controls. (Data from Doniach D. & Roitt I.M. (1964) *Seminars in Haematology* **1**, 313.)

Table 17.2 **Organ-specific and nonorgan-specific serological interrelationships in human disease.**

DISEASE	% POSITIVE REACTIONS FOR ANTIBODIES TO:			
	THYROID*	STOMACH*	NUCLEI*	IgG†
Hashimoto's thyroiditis	99.9	32	8	2
Pernicious anemia	55	89	11	
Sjögren's syndrome	45	14	56	75
Rheumatoid arthritis	11	16	50	75
SLE	2	2	99	35
Controls‡	0–15	0–16	0–19	2–5

*Immunofluorescence test
†Rheumatoid factor classical tests
‡Incidence increases with age and females > males

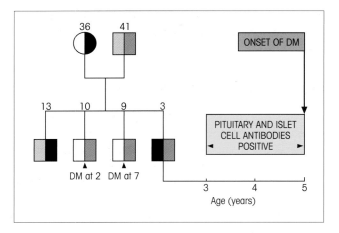

Figure 17.2 HLA-haplotype linkage and onset of insulin-dependent diabetes (DM). Haplotypes: (□) A3, B14, DR6; (■) A3, B7, DR4; (▨) A28, B51, DR4; and (▤) A2, B62, C3, DR4. Disease is linked to possession of the A2, B62, C3, DR4 haplotype. The 3-year-old brother had complement-fixing antibodies to the islet cell surface for 2 years before developing frank diabetes. (From Gorsuch A.N. *et al.* (1981) *Lancet* **ii**, 1363.)

Does the environment contribute?

Twin studies

Although the 50% concordance rate for the development of the autoimmune disease insulin-dependent diabetes mellitus (IDDM) in identical twins is considerably higher than that in dizygotic twins and suggests a strong genetic element, there is still 50% unaccounted for. In nonorgan-specific diseases such as SLE there is an even lower genetic contribution with a concordance rate of only 23% in same-sex monozygotic twins. This compares with 9% in same-sex dizygotic twins. There are also many examples where clinically unaffected relatives of patients with SLE have a higher incidence of nuclear autoantibodies if they are household contacts than if they live apart from the proband. Summing up, in some disorders the major factors are genetic, whereas in others, environmental influences seem to dominate.

Microbes

A number of autoimmune diseases following infectious episodes have been described, usually in genetically predisposed individuals: acute rheumatic fever follows group A streptococcal pharyngitis in patients with a hereditary susceptibility, and B3 coxsackievirus produces autoimmune myositis in certain mouse strains. In most cases of human chronic autoimmune disease, the problem is the long

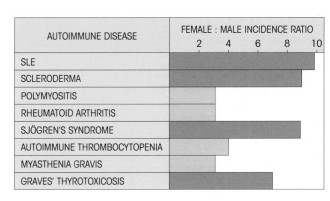

Figure 17.3 Increased incidence of autoimmune disease in females.

latency period, which makes it difficult to track down the initiating event and, secondly, viable organisms usually cannot be isolated from the affected tissues. The mechanism by which microbes may result in autoimmune disease is not clear but a number of mechanisms are possible.

1 Molecular mimicry in which immune responses directed against viruses or bacteria, may cross-react with self antigens (c.f. figure 17.6b(2)). Many organisms have been shown to possess antigenic determinants that are repeated in normal human tissue. For example, two envelope proteins of *Yersinia enterocolitica* share epitopes with the extracellular domain of the human thyroid-stimulating hormone (TSH) receptor. In rheumatic fever, antibodies produced to the *Streptococcus* also react with heart, and the sera of 50% of children with the disease who develop the neurological symptoms known as Sydenham's chorea have antibodies to neurones which can be absorbed out with streptococcal membranes. Colon antibodies present in ulcerative colitis have been found to cross-react with *Escherichia coli* 014. There is also some evidence for the view that antigens present on *Trypanosoma cruzi* may cross-react with cardiac muscle and peripheral nervous system antigens and provoke some of the immunopathologic lesions seen in Chagas' disease.

A large number of microbial peptide sequences with varying degrees of homology with human proteins have been identified (table 17.3) but the mere existence of a homology is no certainty that infection with that organism will necessarily lead to autoimmunity.

2 Microbes may act as adjuvants. Incorporation of many autologous proteins into adjuvants frequently endows them with the power to induce autoallergic disease in laboratory animals. This indicates that autoreactive T-cells are normally present and that they can be activated when presented with suitably altered autoantigens. Microbes often display adjuvant properties through their possession of polyclonal lymphocyte activators, such as bacterial endotoxins, which act by providing a nonspecific inductive signal for B-cell stimulation, so bypassing the need for specific T-cell help.

3 Microbes may activate lymphocytes polyclonally. The variety of autoantibodies detected in cases of infectious mononucleosis must surely be attributable to the polyclonal activation of B-cells by the Epstein–Barr (EB) virus. However, unlike the usual situation in human autoimmune disease, these autoantibodies tend to be IgM and, normally, do not persist when the microbial components are cleared from the body. In some instances microbes can act as superantigens that link CD4+ T-cells to antigen-presenting cells through the outer surfaces of the Vβ chain and the class II MHC glycoprotein. These may bring about the polyclonal stimulation of certain TCR Vβ families.

AUTOREACTIVITY COMES NATURALLY

It used to be thought that self–nonself discrimination was a simple matter of deleting autoreactive cells in the thymus, but it is now clear that this mechanism does not destroy all self-reactive lymphocytes. Processing of an autoantigen will lead to certain (dominant) peptides being preferentially expressed on antigen-presenting cells (APC) while others (cryptic) only appear in the MHC groove in very low concentrations which may fail to signal for negative selection of the corresponding T-cell in the thymus. Thus autoreactive T-cells specific for **cryptic epitopes** will survive in the repertoire but are not normally activated. There is also a subpopulation of B-cells which make low-affinity IgM autoantibodies. These antibodies, which do not normally cause tissue

damage, are demonstrable in comparatively low titer in the general population and their incidence increases steadily with age (figure 17.4).

Is autoantigen available to the lymphocytes?

Our earliest view, with respect to organ-specific antibodies at least, was that the antigens were sequestered within the organ, and through lack of contact with the lymphoreticular system failed to establish immunologic tolerance. Any mishap which caused a release of the antigen would then provide an opportunity for autoantibody formation. For a few body constituents this holds true, and in the case of sperm, lens and heart, for example, release of certain components directly into the circulation can provoke autoantibodies. But, in general, the experience has been that injection of *unmodified* extracts of those tissues concerned in the organ-specific autoimmune disorders does not readily elicit antibody formation.

CONTROL OF THE T-HELPER CELL IS PIVOTAL

The message then is that we are all sitting on a minefield of self-reactive cells, with potential access to their respective autoantigens, but since autoimmune disease is more the exception than the rule, the body has homeostatic mecha-

Table 17.3 Molecular mimicry: homologies between microbes and body components as potential cross-reacting T-cell epitopes.

Microbial molecule	Body component
Bacteria:	
Arthritogenic *Shigella flexneri*	HLA-B27
Klebsiella nitrogenase	HLA-B27
Proteus mirabilis urease	HLA-DR4
Mycobact. tuberculosis 65 kDa hsp	Joint (adjuvant arthritis)
Viruses:	
Coxsackie B	Myocardium
Coxsackie B	Glutamic acid decarboxylase
EBV gp110 ⎫	RA shared Dw4 T-cell epitope
E.coli DNAJ hsp ⎭	
HBV octamer	Myelin basic protein
HSV glycoprotein	Acetylcholine receptor
Measles hemagglutinin	T-cell subset
Retroviral gag p32	U-1 RNA

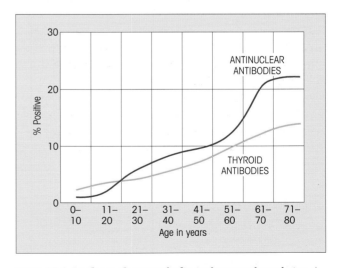

Figure 17.4 Incidence of autoantibodies in the general population. A serum was considered positive for thyroid antibodies if it reacted at a dilution of 1/10 in the tanned red cell test or neat in the immunofluorescent test and positive for antinuclear antibodies if it reacted at a dilution of 1/4 by immunofluorescence.

nisms to prevent them being triggered under normal circumstances. Accepting its limitations, figure 17.5 provides a framework for us to examine ways in which these mechanisms may be circumvented to allow autoimmunity to develop. It is assumed that the key to the system is control of the autoreactive T-helper cell since the evidence heavily favors the T-dependence of virtually all autoimmune responses; thus, interaction between the T-cell and MHC-associated peptide becomes the core consideration. We start with the assumption that these cells are unresponsive because of clonal deletion, clonal anergy, T-suppression or inadequate autoantigen presentation.

AUTOIMMUNITY CAN ARISE THROUGH BYPASS OF T-HELPERS

Provision of new carrier determinant

If autoreactive T-cells are tolerized and thereby unable to collaborate with B-cells to generate autoantibodies (figure 17.6a), provision of new carrier determinants to which no self-tolerance had been established would bypass this mechanism and lead to autoantibody production (figure 17.6b). Modification can be achieved through combination with a

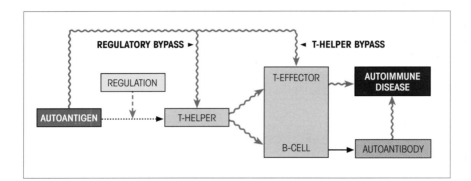

Figure 17.5 Autoimmunity arises through bypass of the control of autoreactivity. The constraints on the stimulation of self-reactive helper T-cells by autoantigen can be circumvented either through bypassing the helper cell or by disturbance of the regulatory mechanisms.

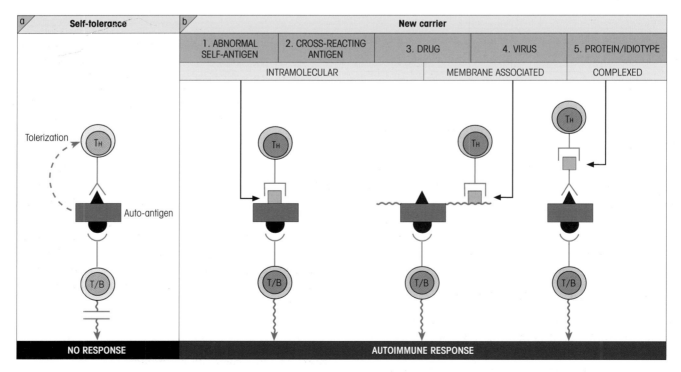

Figure 17.6 T-helper bypass through new carrier epitope (▨) generates autoimmunity. For simplicity, processing for MHC association has been omitted from the diagram. (a) The pivotal autoreactive T-helper is unresponsive either through tolerance or inability to see a cryptic epitope. (b) Different mechanisms providing a new carrier epitope.

drug (figure 17.6b.3); for example, the autoimmune hemolytic anemia associated with administration of α-methyldopa might be attributable to modification of the red-cell surface in such a way as to provide a carrier for stimulating B-cells which recognize the rhesus antigen. Similarly, a new helper determinant may arise through the insertion of viral antigen into the membrane of an infected cell (figure 17.6b.4).

Polyclonal activation

As indicated above, microbes such as the Epstein–Barr virus can activate B-cells in a polyclonal manner and this has been suggested as an important mechanism for the induction of autoimmunity. It is, however, difficult to see how a pan-specific polyclonal activation could give rise to the patterns of autoantibodies characteristic of the different auto-immune disorders without the operation of some antigen-directing factor.

AUTOIMMUNITY CAN ARISE THROUGH BYPASS OF REGULATORY MECHANISMS

Failure of Fas–FasL interaction

Failure of this interaction resulting from either absence of Fas or of FasL, has been demonstrated in various mouse strains susceptible to autoimmune disease. Either of these defects could result in persistence and survival of normally deleted helper T-cells specific for self antigens.

Defects in regulatory cells contribute to spontaneous autoimmunity

Normal animals have regulatory cells capable of damping down autoimmunity but they appear to be lost in certain models of autoimmune disease. For example, transfer of dia-betes by splenocytes from *diseased* non-obese diabetic (NOD) mice to appropriate recipients can be inhibited by a regula-tory subset still present in *young non-diabetic* animals.

Upregulation of T-cell interaction molecules

The majority of organ-specific autoantigens normally appear on the surface of the cells of the target organ in the context of class I but not class II MHC molecules. As such they cannot communicate with T-helpers and are therefore immunologi-cally silent. When class II genes are expressed, they endow the surface molecules with potential autoantigenicity

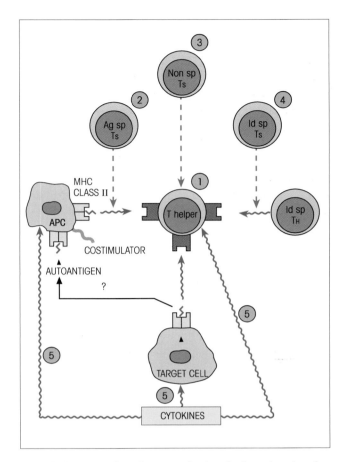

Figure 17.7 Bypass of regulatory mechanisms leads to triggering of autoreactive T-helper cells through defects in (1) tolerizability or ability to respond to or induce T-suppressors, or (2) expression of antigen-specific, (3) nonspecific or (4) idiotype-specific T-suppressors, or through (5) imbalance of the cytokine network producing derepres-sion of class II genes with inappropriate cellular expression of class II and presentation of antigen on target cell, stimulation of APC, and pos-sible activation of anergic T-helper.

(figure 17.7). For example, human thyroid cells in tissue culture express surface HLA-DR (class II) molecules after stimulation with IFNγ, and the glands of patients with Graves' disease (thyrotoxicosis) stain strongly with anti-HLA-DR reagents, indicating active synthesis of class II polypeptide chains. Inappropriate class II expression has also been reported on the bile ductules in primary biliary cirrho-sis and on endothelial cells and some β-cells in the diabetic pancreas.

TH1–TH2 imbalance with resulting overproduction of cytokines may induce autoimmunity

TH1 responses appear to be involved in the pathogenesis of a number of organ-specific autoimmune diseases by produc-

See the accompanying website (www.roitt.com) for multiple choice questions.

The immune system balances precariously between effective responses to environmental antigens and regulatory control of an array of potentially suicidal self molecules.

The scope of autoimmune diseases

• Autoimmunity is associated with certain diseases which form a spectrum. At one pole, exemplified by Hashimoto's thyroiditis, the autoantibodies and the lesions are **organ-specific** with the organ acting as the target for autoimmune attack; at the other pole are the **nonorgan-specific** or **systemic autoimmune diseases** such as SLE, where the autoantibodies have widespread reactivity and the lesions resemble those of serum sickness relating to deposition of circulating immune complexes.

• There is a tendency for organ-specific disorders such as thyroiditis and pernicious anemia to overlap in given individuals, while overlap of rheumatologic disorders is greater than expected by chance.

Genetic and environmental influences

• Multifactorial genetic factors increase predisposition to autoimmune disease: these include HLA tissue type, the predisposition to aggressive autoimmunity and the selection of potential autoantigens.

• Females have a far higher incidence of autoimmunity than males, perhaps due to hormonal influences.

• Twin studies indicate a strong environmental influence in many disorders; both microbial and nonmicrobial factors have been suspected.

• Microbes may initiate autoimmune disease by a number of mechanisms including molecular mimicry, or by acting as adjuvants or superantigens, or as polyclonal activators of the immune response.

Autoreactivity comes naturally

• Autoantigens are, for the most part, accessible to circulating lymphocytes which normally include autoreactive T- and B-cells. Dominant autoantigens will induce tol-erance but T-cells specific for peptides presented at low concentrations (cryptic epitopes) will be potentially autoreactive.

The T-helper is pivotal for control

• It is assumed that the key to the system is control of autoreactive T-helper cells which are normally unresponsive because of clonal deletion, clonal anergy, T-suppression or inadequate autoantigen processing.

Autoimmunity can arise through bypass of T-helpers

• Abnormal modification of the autoantigen through synthesis or breakdown, combination with a drug or cross-reaction with exogenous antigens, can provide new carrier determinants which can activate T-cells.

• B-cells and T-cells can be stimulated directly by polyclonal activators such as EB virus or superantigens.

• Failure of the Fas–FasL interaction can result in survival of normally deleted T-cells.

Autoimmunity can arise through bypass of regulatory mechanisms

• The derepression of class II genes could give rise to inappropriate cellular expression of class II so breaking the 'silence' between cellular autoantigen and autoreactive T-inducer.

• T_H1–T_H2 imbalance may result in overproduction of inflammatory cytokines.

• Defects in Fas–FasL interactions or in regulatory cells may permit the development of autoimmunity.

---

ing large quantities of inflammatory cytokines. Under normal circumstances this overproduction can be controlled by T_H2-derived cytokines, especially IL-10, which antagonizes IL-12, a cytokine crucial for the develoment of T_H1 cells. If an imbalance exists, unregulated IL-2 and IFNγ production can initiate autoimmunity. This may occur by increasing the concentration of processed intracellular autoantigens available to professional APCs and increasing their avidity for naive T-cells by upregulating adhesion mol-ecules, or even by making previously anergic cells responsive to antigen (figure 17.7).

FURTHER READING (SEE THE END OF CHAPTER 18)

Appelmelk B.J., Faller G., Claeys D., Kirchner T. & Vandenbroucke-Grauls C.M.J.E. (1998) Bugs on trial: the case of *Helicobacter pylori* and autoimmunity. *Immunology Today* **19** (7), 296.

Autoimmune diseases

2 — Pathogenesis, diagnosis and treatment

We have mentioned that despite certain exceptions as, for instance, myocardial infarction or damage to the testis, traumatic release of organ constituents does not in general elicit antibody formation. Destruction of thyroid tissue by therapeutic doses of radioiodine does not initiate thyroid autoimmunity, nor does damage to the liver in alcoholic cirrhosis result in the synthesis of mitochondrial antibodies, to give but two examples. We should now look at the evidence which bears directly on the issue of whether autoimmunity, however it arises, plays a **primary pathogenic role** in the production of tissue lesions in the group of diseases labeled as 'autoimmune'.

PATHOGENIC EFFECTS OF HUMORAL AUTOANTIBODY

Blood

Erythrocyte antibodies play a dominant role in the destruction of red cells in **autoimmune hemolytic anemia**. Normal red cells coated with autoantibody have a shortened half-life essentially as a result of their adherence to Fcγ receptors on phagocytic cells in the spleen. Lymphopenia occurring in patients with systemic lupus erythematosus (SLE) and rheumatoid arthritis (RA) may also be a direct result of antibody, since nonagglutinating antibodies coating these white cells have been reported in such cases.

In **Wegener's granulomatosis** antibodies to the usually intracellular proteinase III, the so-called antineutrophil cytoplasmic antibodies (ANCA) (figure 18.1) may react with the antigen on the surface of the cell causing activation and resulting degranulation and generation of reactive oxygen intermediates (ROI). Endothelial cell injury would then be a consequence of the release of superoxide anion and other ROI.

Platelet antibodies are responsible for **idiopathic thrombocytopenic purpura** (ITP) as IgG from a patient's serum when given to a normal individual causes a depres-

sion of platelet counts. The transient neonatal thrombocytopenia which may be seen in infants of mothers with ITP is explicable in terms of transplacental passage of IgG antibodies to the child.

The primary **antiphospholipid syndrome** is characterized by recurrent venous and arterial thromboembotic phenomena, recurrent fetal loss, thrombocytopenia and cardiolipin antibodies. Passive transfer of such antibodies into mice is fairly devastating, resulting in lower fecundity rates and recurrent fetal loss. The effect seems to be mediated through reaction of the autoantibodies with a complex of cardiolipin and β_2-glycoprotein 1, which inhibits triggering of the coagulation cascade, but may also activate the endothelial cells to increase prostacyclin metabolism, produce proinflammatory cytokines such as IL-6, and upregulate adhesion molecules.

Surface receptors

Thyroid

Under certain circumstances antibodies to the surface of a cell may stimulate rather than destroy. This is the case in **thyrotoxicosis** (Graves' disease), which is due to the presence of antibodies to TSH receptors (TSH-R) which seem to act in the same manner as TSH. Both operate through the adenyl cyclase system and both produce similar changes in ultrastructural morphology in the thyroid cell. When thyroid-stimulating antibodies (TSAb) from a thyrotoxic mother cross the placenta they cause the production of neonatal hyperthyroidism (figure 18.2), which resolves after a few weeks as the maternal IgG is catabolized.

There is a good correlation between the titer of TSAb and the severity of hyperthyroidism. Because TSAb act independently of the pituitary–thyroid axis, iodine uptake by the gland is unaffected by administration of thyroxine or triiodothyronine, whereas normally this would cause feedback inhibition and suppression of uptake; this forms the basis of an important diagnostic test for thyrotoxicosis. Graves' disease is often associated with exophthalmos, which might be due to a cross-reaction of antibodies to a 64 kDa membrane protein present on both thyroid and eye muscle.

Muscle

The transient muscle weakness seen in a proportion of babies born to mothers with **myasthenia gravis** is compatible with the transplacental passage of an IgG capable of inhibiting neuromuscular transmission. Strong support for this view is afforded by the consistent finding of antibodies to muscle acetylcholine receptors (ACh-R) in myasthenics and the depletion of these receptors within the motor endplates. In addition, myasthenic symptoms can be induced in animals by injection of monoclonal antibodies to ACh-R or by active immunization with the purified receptors themselves.

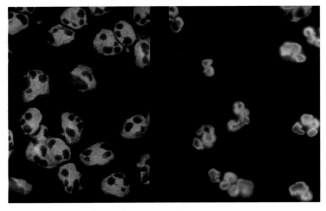

Figure 18.1 Antineutrophil cytoplasmic antibodies (ANCA). *Left:* cytoplasmic cANCA diffuse staining specific for proteinase III in Wegener's granulomatosis. *Right:* perinuclear p-ANCA staining by myeloperoxidase antibodies in periarteritis nodosa. Fixed neutrophils are treated first with patient's serum then fluorescein-conjugated anti-human Ig. (Kindly provided by Dr G. Cambridge.)

Glomerular basement membrane (g.b.m.)

In certain cases of glomerulonephritis, particularly those associated with lung hemorrhage (**Goodpasture's syndrome**), antibodies to g.b.m. can be picked up by immunofluorescent staining of kidney biopsies. These show *linear* deposition of IgG and C3 along the basement membrane of the glomerular capillaries (figure 14.9). Lerner and his colleagues eluted the g.b.m. antibody from a diseased kidney and injected it into a squirrel monkey. The antibody rapidly fixed to type IV collagen on the g.b.m. of the recipient animal and produced a fatal nephritis (figure 18.3). The lung changes in Goodpasture's syndrome are attributable to the antibody reacting with the same antigen in the basement membrane of pulmonary alveoli, and it is hard to escape the conclusion that the lesions in humans are the direct result of attack on these basement membranes by complement-fixing antibodies.

Heart

Neonatal lupus erythematosus is the most common cause of permanent **congenital complete heart block**. Almost all cases have been associated with high maternal titers of anti-Ro/SS-A antibodies. The mother's heart is unaffected. The key observation is that anti-Ro binds to neonatal rather than adult cardiac tissue and alters the transmembrane action potential by inhibiting repolarization. IgG anti-Ro reaches the fetal circulation by transplacental passage but although maternal and fetal hearts are exposed to the autoantibody, only the latter is affected.

The ability of β-hemolytic streptococci to elicit cross-reactive autoantibodies which damage heart muscle underlies the pathogenesis of acute rheumatic fever. Although antibodies to the streptolysin O exotoxin (ASO) are found in low titer in many patients following streptococcal infection, high and increasing titers are strongly

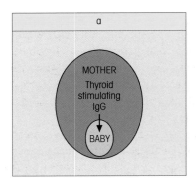

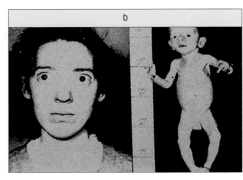

Figure 18.2 Neonatal thyrotoxicosis. (a) The autoantibodies which stimulate the thyroid through the TSH receptors are IgG and cross the placenta. (b) The thyrotoxic mother therefore gives birth to a baby with thyroid hyperactivity which spontaneously resolves as the mother's IgG is catabolized. (Photograph courtesy of Dr A. MacGregor.)

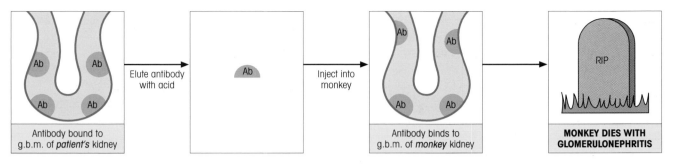

Figure 18.3 **Passive transfer of glomerulonephritis** to a squirrel monkey by injection of antiglomerular basement membrane (anti-g.b.m.) antibodies isolated by acid elution from the kidney of a patient with Goodpasture's syndrome. (After Lerner R.A., Glascock R.J. & Dixon F.J. (1967) *Journal of Experimental Medicine* **126**, 989.)

suggestive of acute rheumatic fever or post-streptococcal glomerulonephritis.

Other tissues

Many other organ-specific autoimmune diseases are associated with specific antibodies directed to those organs. An antibody pathogenesis for **pemphigus vulgaris** is favored by the recognition of an autoantigen on stratified squamous epithelial cells which is localized to the intercellular junctions of the epidermal cells. In some **infertile males**, agglutinating antibodies cause aggregation of the spermatozoa and interfere with their penetration into the cervical mucus. Pernicious anemia, which manifests as a deficiency of vitamin B_{12}, is due to immunologic attack on parietal cells with neutralization of residual intrinsic factor by the corresponding autoantibodies.

PATHOGENIC EFFECTS OF COMPLEXES WITH AUTOANTIGENS

Systemic lupus erythematosus (SLE)

Where autoantibodies are formed against soluble components to which they have continual access, complexes may be generated which can give rise to lesions similar to those occurring in serum sickness. A variety of different autoantigens are present in lupus, many of them within the nucleus, with the most pathognomonic being **double-stranded DNA** (**dsDNA**). Anti-dsDNA is enriched in eluates of renal tissue from patients with lupus nephritis where it can be identified, in complexes containing complement, by immunofluorescent staining of kidney biopsies from patients with evidence of renal dysfunction. The staining pattern with a

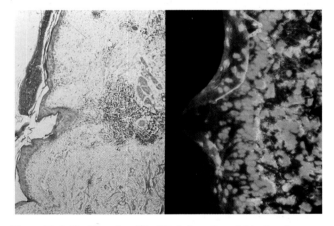

Figure 18.4 **The 'lupus band' in SLE.** *Left:* section of skin showing slight thickening of the dermo-epidermal junction with underlying scattered inflammatory cells and a major inflammatory focus in the deeper layers. Low power H & E. *Right:* green fluorescent staining of a skin biopsy at higher power showing deposition of complexes containing IgG (anti-C3 gives the same picture) on the basement membrane at the dermo-epidermal junction. (Kindly provided by Professor D. Isenberg.)

fluorescent anti-IgG or anti-C3 is punctate or 'lumpy-bumpy' (figure 14.9b), in marked contrast with the linear pattern caused by the g.b.m. antibodies in Goodpasture's syndrome (figure 14.9a; p. 131). Deposition of complexes is widespread, as the name implies, and although 40% of patients eventually develop kidney involvement, lesions are often present in the skin, joints, muscle, lung and brain (figure 18.4). During the active phase of the disease, serum complement levels fall as components are binding to immune aggregates in the kidney and circulation.

It is worth recalling that normal clearance of immune complexes requires an intact classical complement cascade and that absence of an early complement protein predisposes to immune complex disease. Thus, although homozygous complement deficiency is a rare cause of SLE—the archetypal immune complex disorder—it represents the most powerful disease susceptibility genotype so far identified as more than 80% of cases with homozygous C1q and C4 deficiency develop an SLE-like disease.

Rheumatoid arthritis

Morphological evidence for immunologic activity

The joint changes in rheumatoid arthritis (RA) are in essence produced by the **malign growth of the synovial cells** as a pannus overlaying and destroying cartilage and bone (figure 18.5). The synovial membrane, which surrounds and maintains the joint space, becomes intensely cellular as a result of considerable immunologic hyper-reactivity. There is infiltration of large numbers of T-cells, mostly CD4, in various stages of activation, usually associated with dendritic cells and macrophages; clumps of plasma cells are frequently observed and sometimes even secondary follicles with germinal centers are present as though the synovium had become an active lymph node. There is widespread expression of surface HLA-DR (class II) on T- and B-cells, dendritic and synovial lining cells and macrophages, indicative of activation by inflammatory cytokines. Indeed numerous cytokines, including IL-1, TNF and a variety of chemokines, are produced which provide an intense stimulus to the synovial lining cells. These undergo transformation into the invasive pannus with release of hydrolytic enzymes that, together with products of degranulated neutrophils, bring about cartilage destruction and joint erosion. Significant improvement in rheumatoid arthritis has been shown in patients treated with anti-TNF agents.

IgG autosensitization and immune complex formation

Autoantibodies to the IgG Fc region, known as **antiglobulins** or **rheumatoid factors**, are the hallmark of the disease, being demonstrable in virtually all patients with RA. The majority are IgM antiglobulins, the detection of which provides a very useful clinical test for rheumatoid arthritis.

IgG aggregates, presumably products of the infiltrating plasma cells, can be regularly detected in the synovial tissues and in the joint fluid where they give rise to typical acute inflammatory reactions with fluid exudates.

The production of tissue damage

The activated synovial cells grow out as a malign pannus (cover) over the cartilage and at the margin of this advancing granulation tissue breakdown can be seen (figure 18.5c), almost certainly as a result of the release of enzymes, ROIs and especially of IL-1, IL-6 and TNFα. The secreted products of the stimulated macrophage can activate chondrocytes to exacerbate **cartilage breakdown**, and osteoclasts to bring about **bone resorption** which is a further complication of severe disease. Immune complexes of rheumatoid factor and IgG when present in the joint space may initiate an Arthus reaction leading to an influx of polymorphs which release ROIs and lysosomal enzymes. These include neutral proteinases and collagenase which can **damage the articular cartilage** by breaking down proteoglycans and collagen fibrils. The contribution of these immune complexes to the pathogenesis of RA is built into the overview presented in figure 18.6, where it will be seen that a role for the T-cells must not be overlooked and will be discussed in the following section.

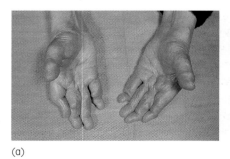
(a)

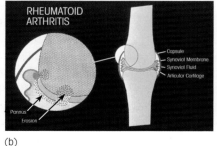
(b)

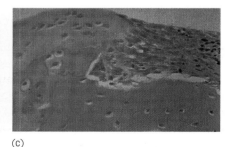
(c)

Figure 18.5 Rheumatoid arthritis (RA). (a) Hands of a patient with chronic RA showing classical swan-neck deformities. (b) Diagrammatic representation of a diarthrodial joint showing bone and cartilaginous erosions beneath the synovial membrane-derived pannus.

(c) Histology of pannus showing clear erosion of bone and cartilage at the cellular margin. ((a) Kindly given by Dr D. Isenberg; (c) by Dr L.E. Glynn.)

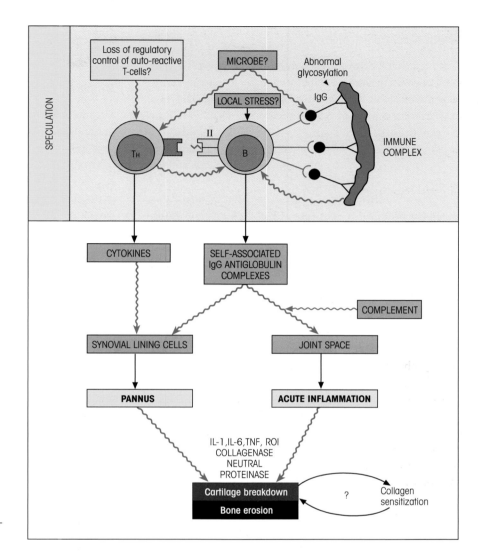

Figure 18.6 Immune pathogenesis of rheumatoid arthritis and speculation on the induction of autoimmunity. The identity of the peptide(s) associated with the class II molecule is unknown.

T-CELL-MEDIATED HYPERSENSITIVITY AS A PATHOGENIC FACTOR IN AUTOIMMUNE DISEASE

Rheumatoid arthritis again

The chronically inflamed synovium is densely crowded with activated T-cells and their critical role in the disease process is emphasized by the beneficial effects of cyclosporin and anti-CD4 treatments, and by the increased risk of disease associated with DR1 and certain DR4 alleles. The ability of T-cells to secrete a variety of proinflammatory cytokines and to induce macrophage synthesis of TNFα will drive pannus development with consequent erosion of cartilage and bone (figure 18.6).

Insulin-dependent diabetes mellitus (IDDM)

IDDM is a multifactorial autoimmune disease the major feature of which is a T-cell infiltration of the islets of Langerhans and progressive T-cell-mediated destruction of insulin-producing β-cells. Delay in onset of disease can be achieved by early treatment with cyclosporin A, since this drug targets T-cell cytokine synthesis so specifically. Autoantibodies against insulin and islet cells are present in the circulation but it is not clear if these are the result of T-cell-mediated injury or if they play some role in the causation of the disease. The disease is strongly linked to certain HLA genes and the majority of Caucasian patients are HLA-DQw8.

173

Multiple sclerosis (MS)

The idea that MS could be an autoimmune disease has for long been predicated on the morphological resemblance to experimental allergic encephalomyelitis (EAE). This is a demyelinating disease leading to motor paralysis which can be produced by immunizing experimental animals with myelin basic protein (MBP) in complete Freund's adjuvant or by transferring TH1-cells from an affected to a naive animal.

There is a large body of evidence suggesting that MS is mediated by T-helper cells directed at CNS myelin components occurring in individuals with certain class II MHC alleles. The demyelination is accompanied by infiltration of T-cells and macrophages and a variety of cytokines and adhesion molecules are overexpressed in the brain. Furthermore, the CNS of patients shows a clear expansion of activated CD4-cells specific for MBP. Another feature of MS is the presence of oligoclonal immunoglobulins in the CSF of patients. Their specificity and significance in the pathogenesis of the disease remains unknown.

Psoriasis

Given the evidence for T-cell-mediated pathogenesis, the isolation of clones specific for group A β-hemolytic streptococci from guttate skin lesions has fostered the thought that pathology is initiated by exotoxin (i.e. superantigen) recruited T-cells and is maintained by specific cells reacting both with streptococcal M protein and a cryptic skin epitope, possibly a keratin variant presented by cytokine-activated keratinocytes.

DIAGNOSTIC VALUE OF AUTOANTIBODY TESTS

Serum autoantibodies frequently provide valuable diagnostic markers, and the salient information is summarized in table 18.1. These tests may prove of value in screening for people at risk, for example relatives of patients with autoimmune diseases such as diabetes, thyroiditis patients for gastric autoimmunity and vice versa, and ultimately the general population if the sociological consequences are fully understood and acceptable.

TREATMENT OF AUTOIMMUNE DISORDERS

Metabolic control

The major approach to treatment, not unnaturally, involves manipulation of immunologic responses (figure 18.7). However, in many organ-specific diseases, metabolic control is usually sufficient, for example thyroxine replacement in primary myxedema, insulin in juvenile diabetes, vitamin B_{12} in pernicious anemia, antithyroid drugs for Graves' disease, and so forth.

Anti-inflammatory drugs

Corticosteroids have long been used to treat autoimmune diseases as they not only suppress various aspects of the immune response but also control the inflammatory lesions and particularly the influx of neutrophils and other phagocytic cells. Patients with severe myasthenic symptoms respond well to high doses of steroids, and the same is true for serious cases of other autoimmune disorders such as SLE and immune complex nephritis. In RA, steroids are very effective and accelerate the induction of remission. Selectins and adhesion molecules on endothelial cells and leukocyte integrins appear to be downregulated and this seriously impedes the influx of inflammatory cells into the joint. Another approach is to neutralize TNFα with a humanized monoclonal antibody which provides lasting benefit especially if combined with methotrexate.

Immunosuppressive drugs

Because it blocks lymphokine secretion by T-cells, cyclosporin A is an anti-inflammatory drug and, since lymphokines like IL-2 are also obligatory for lymphocyte proliferation, cyclosporin is also an antimitotic drug. It is of proven efficacy in a variety of autoimmune diseases, as are the conventional nonspecific antimitotic agents such as azathioprine, cyclophosphamide and methotrexate, usually given in combination with steroids. The general immunosuppressive effect of these agents, however, places the patients at much greater risk from infections.

Plasmapheresis

Plasma exchange to remove the abnormal antibodies and lower the rate of immune complex deposition in SLE provides only temporary benefit. Successful results have been obtained in a number of autoimmune diseases, especially

Table 18.1 Autoimmunity tests and diagnosis.

DISEASE	ANTIBODY	COMMENT
Hashimoto's thyroiditis	Thyroid	Distinction from colloid goiter, thyroid cancer and subacute thyroiditis Thyroidectomy usually unnecessary in Hashimoto goiter
Primary myxedema	Thyroid	Tests +ve in 99% of cases. If suspected hypothyroidism assess 'thyroid reserve' by TRH stimulation test
Thyrotoxicosis	Thyroid	High titers of cytoplasmic Ab indicate active thyroiditis and tendency to post-operative myxedema: anti-thyroid drugs are the treatment of choice although HLA-B8 patients have high chance of relapse
Pernicious anemia	Stomach	Help in diagnosis of latent PA, in differential diagnosis of non-autoimmune megaloblastic anemia and in suspected subacute combined degeneration of the cord
Insulin-dependent diabetes mellitus (IDDM)	Pancreas	Insulin Ab early in disease. GAD Ab standard test for IDDM. Two or more autoAb seen in 80% of new onset children or prediabetic relatives but no controls
Idiopathic adrenal atrophy	Adrenal	Distinction from tuberculous form
Myasthenia gravis	Muscle ACh receptor	When positive suggests associated thymoma (more likely if HLA-B12) positive in >80%
Pemphigus vulgaris and pemphigoid	Skin	Different fluorescent patterns in the two diseases
Autoimmune hemolytic anemia	Erythrocyte (Coombs' test)	Distinction from other forms of anemia
Sjögren's syndrome	Salivary duct cells, SS-A, SS-B	
Primary biliary cirrhosis	Mitochondrial	Distinction from other forms of obstructive jaundice where test rarely +ve Recognize subgroup within cryptogenic cirrhosis related to PBC with +ve mitochondrial Ab
Active chronic hepatitis	Smooth muscle anti-nuclear and 20% mitochondrial	Smooth muscle Ab distinguish from SLE Type 1 classical in women with Ab to nuclei, smooth muscle, actin and asialoglycoprotein receptor. Type 2 in girls and young women with anti-LKM-1 (cyt P450)
Rheumatoid arthritis	Antiglobulin, e.g. SCAT and latex fixation Antiglobulin + raised agalacto-Ig	High titer indicative of bad prognosis Prognosis of rheumatoid arthritis
SLE	High titer antinuclear, DNA Phospholipid	DNA antibodies present in active phase Ab to double-stranded DNA characteristic; high affinity complement-fixing Ab give kidney damage, low affinity CNS lesions Thrombosis, recurrent fetal loss and thrombocytopenia
Scleroderma	Nucleolar	
Wegener's granulomatosis	Neutrophil cytoplasm	Antiserine protease closely associated with disease; treatment urgent

when the treatment has been applied in combination with antimitotic drugs.

Immunologic control strategies

T-cell vaccination

If we regard autoreactive T-cells as tissue-destroying pathogens, it becomes clear that these T-cells if rendered inactive may be employed as vaccines to prevent and perhaps treat the disease. Administration of such autologous T-cells may induce the regulatory network to specifi-

cally control destructive T-cells, and such an approach has successfully been employed to control EAE in experimental animals. Trials in multiple sclerosis using a TCR peptide vaccine embodying the Vβ5.2 sequence expressed on T-cells specific for MBP show promise (figure 18.8.5).

Manipulation of regulatory mediators

In most solid organ-specific autoimmune diseases it is the TH1 cells which are pathogenic, and attempts to switch the phenotype to TH2 should be beneficial. Administration of

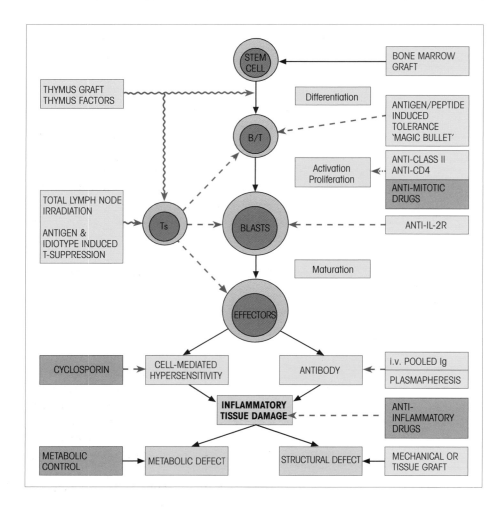

Figure 18.7 **The treatment of autoimmune disease.** Current conventional treatments are in dark orange; some feasible approaches are given in lighter orange boxes. (In the case of a live graft, bottom right, the immunosuppressive therapy used may protect the tissue from the autoimmune damage which affected the organ being replaced.)

interleukin-4 (IL-4), which deviates the immune response from TH1 to TH2, has been shown in EAE to downregulate or inhibit the destructive T-cell process. β-Interferon (IFNβ) inhibits the synthesis of IFNγ and has a number of suppressive effects on T-cell-mediated inflammation. These regulatory activities provide the basis for the therapeutic use of IFNβ in MS, where it significantly reduces both the frequency and the severity of the clinical exacerbations and is considered the first drug proven to improve the natural course of the disease.

Idiotype control with antibody

The powerful immunosuppressive action of anti-idiotype antibodies suggests that it may be useful in controlling autoantibody production. Curiously, **intravenous injection of Ig pooled from many normal donors** is of benefit in a number of autoimmune blood diseases. The inhibitory effects suggest that we are dealing with anti-idiotypic reactions; it is as though the normal pool was re-establishing a properly controlled network.

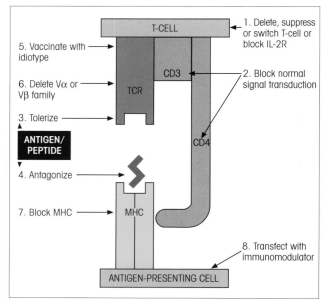

Figure 18.8 **Strategic options for therapy based on T-cell targeting.**

Manipulation by antigen

The object is to present the offending antigen in sufficient concentration and in a form which will occupy the antigen-binding cleft on MHC molecules to prevent binding by the autoantigen. One strategy is to design high-affinity peptide analogs differing by only one amino acid which bind obstinately to the appropriate MHC molecule and antagonize the response to autoantigen (figure 18.8.4). Since we express several different MHC molecules, this should not impair microbial defenses unduly. Clinical improvement has been achieved in patients with exacerbating-remitting MS given Cop1, a random copolymer of alanine, glutamic acid, lysine and tyrosine meant to simulate MBP.

We have already noted that because the mucosal surface of the gut is exposed to a horde of powerfully immunogenic microorganisms, it has been important for the immune defenses of the gut to evolve mechanisms which deter TH1-type responses. This objective is attained by the stimulation of cells which release immunosuppressive cytokines. Thus feeding antigens should tolerize TH1 cells and this has proved to be a successful strategy for blocking EAE and other experimental autoimmune diseases. MS patients fed bovine myelin daily for 1 year showed reduced numbers of MBP-specific T-cells as compared to patients given placebo, and there was some suggestion that MS symptoms were reduced in a proportion of patients.

The tolerogen can also be delivered by inhalation of peptide aerosols and this could be a very attractive way of generating antigen-specific T-cell suppression. Intranasal peptides have been used successfully to block various experimental autoimmune diseases and treatment can be effective even *after* induction of disease.

Monoclonal antibody treatment

Several groups are trying to evolve a strategy based upon the 'magic bullet', the essence of which is to fashion different types of cytotoxic weaponry which selectively home onto the lymphocytes bearing specific surface receptors. One approach is to specifically target the TCR expressed in a particular autoimmune disease. Another is to employ antibodies specific for CD4 as a general immunosuppressive. Antibodies to the IL-2 receptor give even better results as they target only activated T-cells and do not affect the overall immune responsiveness of the recipient.

Gene therapy

The antigen specificity of memory T-cells in autoimmune disease makes them ideal candidates for delivering transgene products to autoimmune lesions. For example, autoreactive T-cells removed from an animal and then genetically modified to express an immunosuppressive IL-10 transgene, inhibited the onset of EAE in experimental animals. Similarly, autoreactive T-cells may be genetically modified to produce therapeutic transgene growth factors for repairing tissue damaged during the autoimmune process or to deliver anti-inflammatory cytokines to autoimmune lesions.

REVISION

See the accompanying website (www.roitt.com) for multiple choice questions.

Pathogenic effects of humoral autoantibody
• Direct pathogenic effects of human autoantibodies to blood, surface receptors and several other tissues are listed in table 18.2.
• Passive transfer of disease is seen in 'experiments of nature' in which transplacental passage of maternal IgG autoantibody produces a comparable but transient disorder in the fetus.

Pathogenic effects of complexes with autoantigens
• Immune complexes, usually with bound complement, appear in the kidneys, skin and joints of patients with SLE, associated with lesions in the corresponding organs.
• Most patients with RA produce autoantibodies to IgG (rheumatoid factors) as a result of immunologic hyperreactivity in the deeper layers of the synovium. The IgG rheumatoid factors self-associate to form complexes.
• These give rise to acute inflammation in the joint space and stimulate the synovial lining cells to grow as a malign pannus which produces erosions in the underlying cartilage and bone through the release of IL-1, IL-6, TNFα,

Table 18.2 Direct pathogenic effects of humoral antibodies.

DISEASE	AUTOANTIGEN	LESION
Autoimmune hemolytic anemia	Red cell	Erythrocyte destruction
Lymphopenia (some cases)	Lymphocyte	Lymphocyte destruction
Idiopathic thrombocytopenic purpura	Platelet	Platelet destruction
Wegener's granulomatosis	PMN proteinase III	PMN-induced endothelial injury
Anti-phospholipid syndrome	Cardiolipin/$\beta 2$–glycoprotein1 complex	Recurrent thromboembotic phenomena
Male infertility (some cases)	Sperm	Agglutination of spermatozoa
Pernicious anemia	H^+/K^+-ATPase, gastrin receptor	Block acid production
Hashimoto's disease	Thyroid peroxidase surface antigen	Cytotoxic effect on thyroid cells in culture
Primary myxedema	TSH receptor	Blocking of thyroid cell
Thyrotoxicosis	TSH receptor	Stimulation of thyroid cell
Goodpasture's syndrome	Glomerular basement membrane	Complement-mediated damage to basement membrane
Myasthenia gravis	Acetylcholine receptor	Blocking and destruction of receptors
Lambert–Eton syndrome	Presynaptic Ca channel	Neuromuscular defect
Acanthosis nigricans (type B) and ataxia telangiectasia with insulin resistance	Insulin receptor	Blocking of receptors
Atopic allergy (some cases)	β-Adrenergic receptors	Blocking of receptors
Congenital heart block	Ro/SS-A	Distort fetal cardiac membrane action potential
Celiac disease	Endomysium	Small intestinal inflammation

prostaglandin E_2, collagenase, neutral proteinase and reactive oxygen intermediates.

T-cell-mediated hypersensitivity as a pathogenic factor
• Suppression of disease by cyclosporin or anti-CD4 treatment is strong evidence for T-cell involvement. So is an HLA-linked risk factor.
• There is a prevailing view that organ-specific inflammatory lesions are caused by autoreactive pathogenic T_H1 cells.
• Activated T-cells are abundant in the rheumatoid synovium and their production of TNFα and GM-CSF complements the immune complex stimulus for pannus formation.
• The onset of IDDM is delayed by cyclosporin, HLA-DQ risk factors are prominent, and T-cell proliferative responses to β-islet cell antigens reflect prognosis of disease.
• Similarity to experimental allergic encephalomyelitis, a demyelinating disease induced by immunization with myelin in complete Freund's adjuvant, has made autoimmunity the front-running hypothesis in MS. Approximately one-third of the IL-2 or IL-4 activatable T-cells in the CSF of MS patients are specific for myelin and there is a strong association with certain class II alleles.

Diagnostic value of autoantibody tests
• A wide range of serum autoantibodies now provides valuable diagnostic markers.

Treatment of autoimmune disorders
• Therapy conventionally involves metabolic control and the use of anti-inflammatory and immunosuppressive drugs.
• Plasma exchange may be of value especially in combination with antimitotic drugs.
• A whole variety of potential immunologic control therapies are under intensive investigation. These include T-cell vaccinations, switching the immune response from T_H1 to T_H2, idiotype manipulations and attempts to induce antigen-specific unresponsiveness particularly to T-cells using peptides.
• Other approaches are to induce oral tolerance or to attack

Table 18.3 Comparison of organ-specific and nonorgan-specific diseases.

ORGAN-SPECIFIC (e.g. THYROIDITIS, GASTRITIS, ADRENALITIS)	NONORGAN-SPECIFIC (e.g. SYSTEMIC LUPUS ERYTHEMATOSUS)
DIFFERENCES	
Antigens only available to lymphoid system in low concentration	Antigens accessible at higher concentrations
Antibodies and lesions organ-specific	Antibodies and lesions nonorgan-specific
Clinical and serologic overlap – thyroiditis, gastritis and adrenalitis	Overlap SLE, rheumatoid arthritis, and other connective tissue disorders
Familial tendency to organ-specific autoimmunity	Familial connective tissue disease
Lymphoid invasion, parenchymal destruction by cell-mediated hypersensitivity and/or antibodies	Lesions due to deposition of antigen–antibody complexes
Therapy aimed at controlling metabolic deficit or tolerizing T-cells	Therapy aimed at inhibiting inflammation and antibody synthesis
Tendency to cancer in organ	Tendency to lymphoreticular neoplasia
Antigens evoke organ-specific antibodies in normal animals with complete Freund's adjuvant	No antibodies produced in animals with comparable stimulation
Experimental lesions produced with antigen in Freund's adjuvant	Diseases and autoantibodies arise spontaneously in certain animals (e.g. NZB mice and hybrids)
SIMILARITIES	
Circulating autoantibodies react with normal body constituents Patients often have increased immunoglobulins in serum Antibodies may appear in each of the main immunoglobulin classes particularly IgG and are usually high affinity and mutated Greater incidence in women Disease process not always progressive; exacerbations and remissions Association with HLA Spontaneous diseases in animals genetically programmed Autoantibody tests of diagnostic value	

sensitized T-cells with monoclonal antibodies. The antigen specificity of autosensitized T-cells make them ideal carriers of transgene products which may be beneficial in autoimmune diseases

• The accompanying comparison of organ-specific and nonorgan-specific autoimmune disorders (table 18.3) gives an overall view of many of the points raised in these last two chapters.

FURTHER READING

Albania S., Keystone E.C., Nelson J.L. *et al.* (1995) Positive selection in autoimmunity: abnormal immune responses to bacterial dnaJ antigenic determinant in patients with early rheumatoid arthritis. *Nature Medicine* 1, 448–452.

Appelmelk B.J., Faller G., Claeys D., Kirchner T. & Vandenbroucke-Grauls C.M.J.E. (1998) Bugs on trial: the case of *Helicobacter pylori* and autoimmunity. *Immunology Today* 19 (7), 296.

Austen K.F., Burakoff S.J., Rosen F.S. & Strom T.B. (eds) (1996) *Therapeutic Immunology*. Blackwell Science, Oxford.

Chapel M. & Haeney M. (1993) *Essentials of Clinical Immunology*, 3rd edn. Blackwell Scientific Publications, Oxford.

Flavell R.A. & Hafler D.A. (eds) (1999) Section on Autoimmunity. *Current Opinion in Immunology* 11 (6).

Gelfand E.W. (ed.) (1996) Intravenous immune globulin: mechanisms of action and model disease states. *Clinical and Experimental Immunology* 104 (Suppl. 1), 1–97.

Kingsley G., Lanchbury J. & Panayi G. (1996) Immunotherapy in rheumatic disease. *Immunology Today* 17, 9–12.

Lanzavacchia A. (1993) Identifying strategies for immune intervention. *Science* 260, 937–944.

Lokki M-J. & Colten H.R. (1995) Genetic deficiencies of complement. *Annals of Medicine* 27, 451–459.

McInnes I.B., Leung B.P., Sturrock R.D., Field M. & Liew F.Y. (1997) Interleukin-15 mediates T cell-dependent regulation of tumor necrosis factor-α production in rheumatoid arthritis. *Nature Medicine* 3, 189–195.

Selimena M. *et al.* (1990) Autoantibodies to GABA-ergic neurones and pancreatic β-cells in stiff man syndrome. *New England Journal of Medicine* 322, 1555. [Fun to read just for the title!]

Shoenfeld Y. & Isenberg D. (1989) *The Mosaic of Autoimmunity (The Factors associated with Autoimmune Disease)*. Elsevier, Amsterdam. [An excellent account.]

Shoenfeld Y. & Isenberg D.A. (eds) (1993) *Natural Autoantibodies. Their Physiological Role and Regulatory Significance*. CRC Press, Boca Raton, FL.

Sieper J. & Kingsley G. (1996) Recent advances in the pathogenesis of reactive arthritis. *Immunology Today* **17**, 160–163.

Song Y-H., Li Y. & Maclaren N.K. (1996) The nature of autoantigens targeted in autoimmune endocrine diseases. *Immunology Today* **17**, 232–238.

Stites D.P., Stobo J.D. & Wells I.V. (eds) (1994) *Basic and Clinical Immunology*, 7th edn. Appleton & Lange, Norwalk, USA.

Thomas J. & Lipsky P.E. (1996) Could endogenous self-peptides presented by dendritic cells initiate rheumatoid arthritis? *Immunology Today* **17**, 559–564.

Thompson R.A. (ed.) (1985) Laboratory investigation of immunological disorders. *Clinics in Immunology and Allergy*, Vol. 5. W.B. Saunders, London.

Thompson R.A. (series ed.) *Recent Advances in Clinical Immunology*. Churchill Livingstone, Edinburgh.

Tian J., Olcott A., Hanssen L., Zekzer D. & Kaufman D.L. (1999) Antigen-based immunotherapy for autoimmune disease: from animal models to humans? *Immunology Today* **20** (4), 190.

Todd J.A. (1996) Human genetics: transcribing diabetes. *Nature* **384** (6608), 407–408.

Vandenbark A.A. *et al.* (1996) Treatment of multiple sclerosis with T-cell receptor peptides. *Nature Medicine* **2**, 1109–1115.

Weetman A.P. (ed.) (1991) *Autoimmune Endocrine Disease*. Cambridge University Press, Cambridge, UK.

Weiner H.L. & Mayer L.F. (1996) Oral tolerance: mechanisms and applications. *Annals of the New York Academy of Science* **778**, 1–453.

Wicker L. & Wekerle H. (eds) (1995) Autoimmunity. *Current Opinion in Immunology* **6**, 783–852. [Several critical essays in each annual volume.]

Index